Practitioner's Guide to
Clinical Neuropsychology

CRITICAL ISSUES IN NEUROPSYCHOLOGY

Series Editors

Antonio E. Puente
University of North Carolina, Wilmington

Cecil R. Reynolds
Texas A & M University

Current Volumes in this Series

Practitioner's Guide to Clinical Neuropsychology

Robert M. Anderson, Jr.
Honolulu, Hawaii

Plenum Press • New York and London

Library of Congress Cataloging in Publication Data

Anderson, Robert M., 1943–
    Practitioner's guide to clinical neuropsychology / Robert M. Anderson, Jr.
        p.   cm.— (Critical issues in neuropsychology).
    Includes bibliographical references and index.
    ISBN 0-306-44616-2
    1. Clinical neuropsychology. 2. Neuropsychiatry. 3. Neuropsychological tests. I. Title.
II. Series.
    [DNLM: 1. Nervous System Diseases—diagnosis. 2. Neuropsychological Tests. 3.
Mental Disorders—diagnosis. WL 141 A549p   1994]
    RC341.A53   1994
    616.89—dc20
    DNLM/DLC   94-2057
    for Library of Congress   CIP

10 9 8 7 6 5 4 3 2

ISBN 0-306-44616-2

© 1994 Plenum Press, New York
A Division of Plenum Publishing Corporation
233 Spring Street, New York, N.Y. 10013

Printed in the United States of America

To
Robert M. Anderson and Jean Perz Anderson
and to the memory of
Yum Joe Leong and Gladys Chock Leong

Foreword

It is customary to note in a foreword that the book being introduced fills a need that is not satisfied by what is available in the literature. In this case, however, there seems to be no question. Despite the proliferation of books and journals in clinical neuropsychology, no single reference work for professionals provides a comprehensive guide to practice. If we divide clinical practice into assessment, treatment, and planning, we find that it is all here. Other sections focus on factors other than impairment of brain function that could influence test results—such as age and education—and a brief section reviews characteristics of the various disorders that commonly come to the attention of neuropsychologists.

Particularly notable in this book is that these terms are not narrowly defined. Dr. Anderson does not limit assessment to clinical neuropsychological testing, nor does he limit consideration of treatment to cognitive rehabilitation. Numerous outcomes are considered, such as independent self-care, driving, and occupational status. The book takes the stance that the practicing clinician ideally provides comprehensive services to his or her patients, and need not be limited to providing testing services, limited interventions, or treatment planning. This approach reflects a developing maturity in the field, with professional neuropsychologists no longer being restricted, or restricting themselves, to activities associated solely with testing. This growth parallels developments in psychology as a whole, in which practicing psychologists are increasingly functioning as health care providers rather than narrowly focused specialists.

In pursuing this path, while Anderson reviews the commonly used neuropsychological assessment methods and batteries; other sections cover record review, behavioral observation, and interviewing. While these sections are brief, they remind us that assessment is a comprehensive process involving not only tests, but talking to patients and their relatives and other associates, observing patients in their everyday activities, integrating assessment findings generated by other disciplines, and placing current findings into a historical context. The latter two are generally achieved through an informed reading and evaluation of clinical records.

Regarding treatment, the book's broad focus goes beyond the traditional role of neuropsychologists in cognitive rehabilitation, and perhaps coma stimulation. There are also chapters on psychotherapy and behavior modification. Issues such as treatment and management of agitation, aggression, loss of motivation, impairment of daily living skills, and the impact of brain injury on family members are discussed. Pertinent issues related to pain management and treatment of post-traumatic stress disorder are also briefly mentioned.

An entire section of the book is devoted to functional outcomes. This material is particularly relevant to recent discussions of the ecological validity of neuropsychological tests. If these tests can predict not only medical neurological status but also functional deficits experienced when interacting with a normal environment, then they might be particularly useful in the assessment of permanent disability and in the necessary rehabilitation planning. Clinicians are often asked to use their assessments to predict whether a patient can return to the community. In many cases, a return to work or school has to be considered and the appropriate accommodations and rehabilitation programs have to be designed, implemented, and monitored.

Practicing neuropsychologists frequently participate in disability evaluations, and have to make judgments about the client's capacity to return to driving, work, or school. Anderson provides descriptions of important distinctions among deficits, disabilities, and competencies, not only as these terms are used by psychologists, but also as they are used in vocational and forensic settings. Sound advice is provided to neuropsychologists concerning communication in this area, including avoiding referring to specific tests without description, avoiding the technical vocabulary of the neurosciences without adequate definition, and becoming knowledgable about the legal and technical terminology used in disability determination and vocational rehabilitation.

The section describing the various neurobehavioral disorders is notable for adherence to a standard outline that considers descriptive, epidemiologic, neuropathological, assessment, treatment, and prognostic components. The review of neuropsychological findings through expected levels and patterns of performance will be particularly useful to clinicians, but the related material can provide either a good brief review or a summarized introduction to disorders with which the clinician may not be familiar. This section also reflects contemporary trends in the field, with sections on neuropsychological aspects of human immunodeficiency virus infection and on schizophrenia and depression—two psychiatric disorders that are of increasing interest to neuropsychologists.

This book should readily find itself on the desks of practicing clinicians who may make daily use of it to "look things up," to gain brief orientations to unfamiliar areas, and to correlate individual patient findings with what appears in the literature. While it is not a "handbook" in the way the term is used in science, it fully meets the dictionary definition of a handbook as a small reference book providing specific information or instruction about a subject. This book is notably contemporary and deals with areas that are relatively new to neuropsychology and not touched upon in more traditional texts. There is a broadening of the concept of assessment beyond neuropsychological testing, a broadening of how treatment is conceptualized ranging beyond neuropsychologically based cognitive rehabilitation, and extensive consideration of functional outcome. In essence, it is a practical book for practitioners, something clinical neuropsychology has been lacking.

Gerald Goldstein

Veterans Administration Medical Center, Highland Drive
Pittsburgh, Pennsylvania

Preface

I became aware of the need for a concise clinical neuropsychology reference book while I was a postdoctoral fellow in a large, acute-care hospital (University of Rochester Medical Center). Patients needed to be evaluated rapidly but accurately, and often little time was available for extensive research on their varied conditions. An easily accessible reference source would have been very helpful, but none existed.

Practitioner's Guide to Clinical Neuropsychology is intended to fill this need. It is intended to provide practicing neuropsychologists and neuropsychologists-in-training with an easily accessible summary of neuropsychological tests, neuropsychiatric disorders, and the relationships of test performance to the disorders and treatment recommendations. Chapter 1 describes the purpose and limitations of this book in detail.

I am indebted to my mentors: Grover Maxwell, Karl Pribram, and Anthony Marsella. My editors, Antonio Puente and Eliot Werner, helped me to plan and complete the book and saw it through to publication. They continued to encourage me even when the project proved to be more complex and to take more time than was originally anticipated. Timothy Orrell read the entire manuscript and provided many helpful suggestions. David Bremer, Demetria Leong, and William Tsushima read and critiqued large portions of the book. Their efforts resulted in substantial improvements in the work. Peter Como, James Craine, Warren Rice, and Abraham Spevack contributed significantly to my understanding of and enthusiasm for clinical neuropsychology. The support of my friends and colleagues Amanda Armstrong, Bob Brown, Michael Compton, Joe Gonsalves, Brian Goodyear, Gary Gunderson, Harold Hall, Karuna Joshi-Peters, Morris Kaneshiro, Valerie McClain, Dennis McLaughlin, Dan Reed, John Schumacher, Marilyn Strauss, Douglas Umetsu, Tony Wong, and Neil Young has been invaluable. Terri Needels, Provost of Forest Institute of Professional Psychology at Hawaii, has been very encouraging and supportive of this project.

The resources and staff members of the Hawaii Medical Library and the Hamilton Library of the University of Hawaii were quite helpful.

Many others have contributed in a variety of ways to this book. Among them are my patients, from whom I have learned about the brain and behavior, about courage in the face of extreme personal adversity, and to whom I would like to extend my gratitude.

Robert M. Anderson, Jr.

Honolulu

ix

Notice

This book is not intended as a substitute for appropriate education and training in clinical neuropsychology, as outlined in the International Neuropsychological Society/Division 40 (Clinical Neuropsychology) of the American Psychological Association's (APA) education and training guidelines. To determine the definition of a clinical neuropsychologist, consult Division 40 of APA and the National Academy of Neuropsychology. Furthermore, readers should be thoroughly familiar with and adhere to the American Psychological Association Ethical Principles.

This book provides the reader with an accessible summary of neuropsychological assessment techniques, neuropsychiatric disorders, and relevant psychosocial therapies and supports. Its purpose is to orient and provide some guidelines for the practicing clinical neuropsychologist or neuropsychology fellow. It is *not* a comprehensive handbook and is *not* intended to be used as a ''cookbook.'' Readers should consult the references cited throughout the book to obtain a full understanding of the subject areas covered. Neuropsychological evaluations should be administered and interpreted only by individuals with requisite training and experience (Hess & Hart, 1990).

The information on medical assessment and treatment provided in this book is *not* intended to be used as guidelines by practicing physicians. This information has been included to provide neuropsychologists and other readers with an understanding of the medical context within which neuropsychological evaluation and psychosocial therapy often take place.

REFERENCE

Hess, A. L., & Hart, R. (1990). The specialty of neuropsychology. *Neuropsychology, 4,* 49–52.

Contents

I

Introduction

Overview

This book provides the practitioner with an easily accessible summary of neuropsychological tests, neuropsychiatric disorders, and the relationships of test performance to the disorders and to treatment recommendations. It is not intended as a comprehensive handbook of clinical neuropsychology. Instead, it provides the practitioner with a concise outline of information relevant to clinical neuropsychology. The practitioner is encouraged to consult the references cited in the text for a more detailed treatment of topics.

The book is divided into six parts:

   I. Introduction
   II. Factors That Influence Test Performance
   III. Assessment Strategies and Instruments
   IV. Deficits, Competencies, and Disabilities
   V. Psychosocial Therapies
   VI. Disorders

They are ordered according to the way in which they might be used in conducting a neuropsychological evaluation: (1) An evaluation may begin by a thorough clinical history of the patient; (2) interview and formal testing are completed, as well as an accounting of possible confounding variables; (3) strengths and weaknesses are determined; (4) a diagnosis may be made; (5) inferences are made about everyday activities; (6) recommendations are made for therapy.

Part I, the Introduction, contains an overview of the book and summaries of three methods of neuropsychological assessment. The use of the book in neuropsychological evaluation and report writing is described.

Part II describes the effects of sensorimotor impairments, handedness, demographic variables (age, education, gender, ethnicity), anxiety, amotivation, and fatigue on neuropsychological test performance. Although improved norms may assist the practitioner in taking the effects of demographic variables into account, knowledge of the effects of these variables on performance and the ability to structure a battery to minimize these effects or to take them into account in interpretation is critical to accurate evaluation. In a sense, a good clinical neuropsychological assessment is not unlike any psychological experiment that is designed to control—or at least minimize—the influence of extraneous factors. This part is placed before the others because assessment and control of these variables is a precondition for conducting and accurately interpreting a neuropsychological evaluation.

Part III describes the data-gathering techniques used in clinical neuropsychology. These techniques include review of records, interview, behavioral observation, and formal testing.

Part IV addresses the translation of interview and test information into judgments about strengths and weaknesses, everyday abilities, and occupational and academic functioning. Issues relevant to special evaluations such as Social Security disability and Workers' Compensation evaluations are also addressed.

If deficits are demonstrated, referral may be made to appropriate professionals and agencies and recommendations may be made for psychosocial therapies. Part V briefly reviews some of the therapies commonly provided for patients with neuropsychiatric disorders.

Part VI synthesizes all the foregoing information in the context of specific neuropsychiatric disorders. Their medical and neuropsychological profiles are outlined. The disorders include closed head injury, stroke, epilepsy, degenerative neurological disorders, brain tumors, human immunodeficiency virus, alcoholism, neurotoxic disorders, schizophrenia, and depression.

Clinical neuropsychology has become a vast and rapidly growing area of knowledge and an expanding clinical profession. It is impossible for a single book to contain all the relevant information. Of necessity, some limitations had to be observed in presenting information in a condensed format.

First of all, the subject matter of this book is restricted to adult clinical neuropsychology. An attempt has been made to include current information. Due to the rate of growth and change in the field, some of the information contained in this book may be out of date by the time of publication. The reader is encouraged to corroborate the information contained in this book with other sources.

The descriptions of tests provided in part III do not include summaries of the psychometric features of the tests. Although this information is essential to deciding whether a test can be used appropriately, it was excluded due to space limitations. The reader is referred to the test manuals and to *Reliability and Validity in Neuropsychological Assessment* (Franzen, 1989).

This book does not contain case examples. The reason for excluding them is not that case studies lack importance; experience in evaluating and treating specific cases under supervision is essential to education and to the development of understanding in clinical neuropsychology. Case examples using a WAIS-centered, hypothesis-testing approach may be found in *The Neuropsychology Casebook* (Orsini *et al.*, 1988). Walsh (1987) has also provided a representative set of case studies. Case examples using the Halstead–Reitan Neuropsychological Battery are available in *The Halstead–Reitan Neuropsychological Test Battery* (Reitan & Wolfson, 1993). Case examples using the Luria–Nebraska Neuropsychological Battery may be found in *Interpretation of the Luria–Nebraska Neuropsychological Battery,* Volume 1 (Moses *et al.*, 1983a) and *Interpretation of the Luria–Nebraska Neuropsychological Battery,* Volume 2 (Moses *et al.*, 1983b).

This book does not provide a detailed description of the relationships between cognitive functions and brain function. The reader is referred to *Neuropsychology, Neuropsychiatry, and Behavioral Neurology* (Joseph, 1990), *Neuropsychology: A Clinical Approach* (Walsh, 1987), and *Fundamentals of Human Neuropsychology* (Kolb & Whishaw, 1985).

REFERENCES

Franzen, M. D. (1989). *Reliability and validity in neuropsychological assessment.* New York: Plenum Press.
Joseph, R. (1990). *Neuropsychology, neuropsychiatry, and behavioral neurology.* New York: Plenum Press.
Kolb, B., & Whishaw, I. Q. (1985). *Fundamentals of human neuropsychology* (2nd ed.). New York: W. H. Freeman.
Moses, J. A., Golden, C. J., Ariel, R., & Gustavson, J. L. (1983a). *Interpretation of the Luria–Nebraska neuropsychological battery* (Vol. 1). New York: Grune & Stratton.

Moses, J. A., Golden, C. J., Wilkening, G. N., McKay, S. E., & Ariel, R. (1983b). *Interpretation of the Luria–Nebraska neuropsychological battery* (Vol. 2). New York: Grune & Stratton.

Orsini, D. L., Van Gorp, W. G., & Boone, K. B. (1988). *The neuropsychology casebook*. New York: Springer-Verlag.

Reitan, R. M., & Wolfson, D. (1993). *The Halstead–Reitan Neuropsychological Test Battery* (2nd ed.). Tucson, AZ: Neuropsychology Press.

Walsh, K. (1987). *Neuropsychology: A clinical approach*. Edinburgh: Churchill Livingston.

Flexible Approaches

The Boston Process Approach originated in the efforts of Dr. Edith Kaplan to apply the distinction made by Werner (1937) between "process" and "achievement" in development to understanding impaired function in patients with brain damage (Milberg *et al.*, 1986). The method emphasizes the modification of test items and analysis of test performance with the goal of understanding the patient's individual cognitive strategies. It uses a core set of tests that may be supplemented by satellite tests. The core often contains a modified version of the Wechsler Adult Intelligence Scale—Revised (WAIS-R) along with other tests that assess intellectual and conceptual functions, memory functions, language functions, visuoperceptual functions, academic skills, self-control, and motor functions. A listing of tests commonly used may be found in Milberg *et al.* (1986). The modified version of the WAIS-R (Wechsler, 1981), termed the WAIS-R-NI, is available from the Psychological Corporation (Kaplan *et al.*, 1991). The modified version provides for a more detailed recording of the patient's cognitive strategy and supplementary items for some of the subtests. The modifications for each subtest are summarized in the corresponding subtest's review in Part III of this book. For example, Circle and Cow puzzles have been added to the Object Assembly subtest. The Circle can be solved by using contour information, while the Cow cannot be solved by contour information and demands a piece-by-piece analysis (Kaplan, 1988). Qualitative analysis of the patient's performance along such dimensions as featural or contextual can assist in making inferences about lateralizing and localizing lesions (Milberg *et al.*, 1986).

Norms have not been provided for the revised administrations of the WAIS-R subtests. However, norms have been provided for *scatter scores* for the WAIS-R subtests. *Scatter points* are scored if there is an absolute difference between two consecutive item scores. The scatter score on a subtest is the total scatter points.

The WAIS and WAIS-R are often used as the core of a flexible neuropsychological battery. Kaufman (1990) has reviewed the literature on the use of the WAIS and WAIS-R in the assessment of brain damage. He has concluded that "patients with damage to the *right* hemisphere, whether damage is unilateral or accompanied by damage to the left hemisphere as well, are very likely to manifest a V [verbal] > P [performance] profile" (Kaufman, 1990, p. 280). Patients with unilateral damage to the *left* hemisphere may show a slight P > V, but it is almost as likely that they will show V > P or no V–P discrepancy. There can be numerous causes of P > V discrepancies other than brain damage (Kaufman, 1990).

Norms for the WAIS-R are provided for ages 16–17, 18–19, 20–24, 25–34, 35–44, 45–54, 55–64, 65–69, and 70–74 (Wechsler, 1981). Ivnik *et al.* (1992) have provided norms for adults aged 56–97.

Exemplars of the hypothesis-testing approach may be found in the work of A. R. Luria (1966, 1973). In this approach, "the neuropsychological examination can be viewed as a series of experiments that generate explanatory hypotheses in the course of testing them'' (Lezak, 1983, pp. 100–101). Diagnosis proceeds by the successive elimination of alternative diagnostic hypotheses. Hypotheses are generated on the basis of medical records, interviews, and information from the referring source (Orsini *et al.,* 1988). Tests are then selected on the basis of the hypotheses and administered to determine the degree of impairment or preservation of cognitive functions. Tests are also selected to survey the functional areas (Orsini *et al.,* 1988). After deficits are identified on screening, additional tasks may be administered to more carefully delineate the nature of the dysfunction.

Advocates of the hypothesis-testing approach generally select tests to be administered from a set of commonly used tests. Orsini *et al.* (1988) have provided a list of tests organized by functional area. Lezak (1983) also provides a list of tests for a core battery: WAIS-R, Symbol Digit Modalities Test (SDMT), Rey Auditory–Verbal Learning Test (RAVLT), paragraph learning, Subtracting Serial 7's (SSS), draw a house or bicycle, Rey–Osferrieth Complex Figure Test: Copy (ROCFT), motor test, Wisconsin Card Sorting Test (WCST), and Trail Making Tests A & B (TMTA&B). This battery is supplemented by numerous tests that Lezak (1983) has described in her classic, encyclopedic *Neuropsychological Assessment.*

Hamsher (1990) has described a flexible battery approach that uses (among others) the tests developed by Benton and his colleagues. Kane (1991) has described the flexible battery approach and compared it to fixed batteries.

Cohen and Mapou (1988) have advocated the use of the hypothesis-testing approach in rehabilitation and treatment planning. Assessment focuses on relevant areas of cognitive functioning. In each evaluation, assessment is made of the following areas: (1) Arousal and Attentional Functioning, (2) Executive Functioning, (3) Language Functioning, (4) Visuospatial Functioning, (5) Reasoning and Problem-Solving Abilities, and (6) Learning and Memory Functioning.

REFERENCES

Cohen, R. F., & Mapou, R. L. (1988). Neuropsychological assessment for treatment planning: A hypothesis-testing approach. *Journal of Head Trauma Rehabilitation. 3,* 12–23.

Hamsher, K. deS. (1990). Specialized neuropsychological assessment methods. In G. Goldstein & M. Hersen (Eds.), *Handbook of psychological assessment* (2nd ed.) (pp. 256–279). New York: Pergamon Press.

Ivnik, R. J., Malec, J. F., Smith, G. E., Tangalos, E. G., Petersen, R. C., Kokmen, E., & Kurland, L. T. (1992). Mayo's older Americans normative studies: WAIS-R norms for ages 56 to 97. *The Clinical Neuropsychologist, 6,* 1–30.

Kane, R. L. (1991). Standardized and flexible batteries in neuropsychology: An assessment update. *Neuropsychology Review, 2,* 281–339.

Kaplan, E. (1988). A process approach to neuropsychological assessment. In T. Boll & B. K. Bryant (Eds.), *Clinical neuropsychology and brain function: Research, measurement, and practice* (pp. 129–167). Washington, DC: American Psychological Association.

Kaplan, E., Fein, D., Morris, R., & Delis, D. (1991). *WAIS-R-NI Manual: WAIS-R as a neuropsychological instrument.* San Antonio: Psychological Corporation.

Kaufman, A. S. (1990). *Assessing adolescent and adult intelligence.* Boston: Allyn & Bacon.

Lezak, M. (1983). *Neuropsychological assessment* (2nd ed.). New York: Oxford University Press.

Luria, A. R. (1966). *Higher cortical functions in man.* New York: Basic Books.

Luria, A. R. (1973). *The working brain.* New York: Basic Books.

Milberg, W. P., Hebben, N., & Kaplan, E. (1986). The Boston process approach to neuropsychological assessment. In I. Grant & K. M. Adams (Eds.), *Neuropsychological assessment of neuropsychiatric disorders* (pp. 65–86). New York: Oxford University Press.

Orsini, D. L., Van Gorp, W. G., & Boone, K. B. (1988). *The neuropsychology casebook.* New York: Springer-Verlag.

Wechsler, D. (1981). *Wechsler Adult Intelligence Scale—Revised.* New York: Psychological Corporation.

Werner, H. (1937). Process and achievement: A basic problem of education and developmental psychology. *Harvard Educational Review, 7,* 353–368.

Halstead–Reitan Neuropsychological Battery

The Halstead–Reitan Neuropsychological Battery (HRNB) was designed to assess reliably, validly, and completely the behavioral correlates of brain function (Reitan, 1986). The HRNB consists of measures in six categories: (1) input; (2) attention, concentration, and memory; (3) verbal abilities; (4) spatial, sequential, and manipulative abilities; (5) abstraction, reasoning, logical analysis, and concept formation; and (6) output (Reitan & Wolfson, 1993). It consists of the Halstead Category Test (CT), Speech Sounds Perception Test (SSPT), Seashore Rhythm Test (SR), Tactual Performance Test (TPT), TMTA&B, Reitan–Klove Sensory–Perceptual Examination (RKSPE), Reitan–Indiana Aphasia Examination (RIAE), Lateral Dominance Examination (LDE), and Halstead Finger Tapping Test (FTT) (Reitan & Wolfson, 1993). The WAIS is usually included in the battery. With the exception of the LDE, all of these tests are described in the Part III of this book.

Input or sensory functions are evaluated by the RKSPE and the Tactile Form Recognition Test (TFRT). These tests assess central processing in addition to basic sensory functioning. Although attention and concentration are involved in all tasks, the SSPT and SR are not too complicated or difficult but require close attention. Verbal functioning is assessed on the Reitan–Indiana Aphasia Screening Test (AST), SSPT, and the Verbal subtests of the WAIS. Visual–spatial abilities are assessed by the WAIS Performance subtests, the drawings of the Aphasia Screening Test (AST), and TMTA&B. Abstraction is assessed by the Halstead CT and TMTB. Output or motor functions are evaluated by the Halstead Finger Oscillation or FTT and Grip Strength (GS) Test, generally uncomplicated or "pure" tests of motor functioning. The TPT involves more central processing and both motor and sensory processing (Reitan, 1986).

Reitan and Wolfson (1993) have described the following procedure for interpreting the HRNB:

1. Reference is made to the WAIS to determine the patient's previous intellectual abilities. Reitan and Wolfson (1990) have stated that there is insufficient evidence available to justify substitution of the WAIS-R for the WAIS. If the Information, Comprehension, Similarities, and Vocabulary scores are good, they may be used as a comparison standard for neuropsychological tests.
2. Interpretation proceeds by reviewing scores on the measures most sensitive to brain damage: Halstead Impairment Index, CT, TMTB, and the Localization component of the TPT. Significant depression of these scores relative to Wechsler scores suggests

the possibility that the patient has suffered a neuropsychological deficit resulting from brain damage.

3. The third interpretive step involves inferences from patterns and relationships among test results to lateralization and localization of cerebral damage. This may involve: (a) WAIS—VIQ vs PIQ and subtest scatter, (b) bilateral disparity on the TPT, (c) bilateral disparity on the FTT, (d) dysphasia, (e) constructional dyspraxia, and (f) lateralized deficits on the Sensory Perceptual Examination.

4. The next step in interpretation is discernment of the course of the lesion.

5. The final step in diagnostic neuropsychological interpretation involves synthesizing all the data and drawing inferences about the neurological disorder (Reitan & Wolfson, 1993).

Several indices have been proposed to diagnose brain dysfunction from the HRNB. The Halstead Impairment Index is calculated on the basis of seven measures: (1) CT, (2) TPT-Time, (3) TPT-Memory, (4) TPT-Localization, (5) SR, (6) SSPT, and (7) FTT. The number of measures impaired relative to cutoff points recommended by Halstead is divided by the total number of tests. Brain damage is suggested by a ratio of 0.5 or greater (Reitan & Wolfson, 1993).

The Average Impairment Rating was developed by Russell *et al.* (1970) and is a commonly used summary score for the HRNB.

The Neuropsychological Deficit Scale is composed of 42 variables that are organized according to the four methodological approaches in the battery: (1) level of performance, (2) pathognomonic signs, (3) patterns and relationships, and (4) right/left comparisons. Variables in each of these categories are assigned values from 0 to 3, where 3 represents the greatest level of impairment or discrepancy. Summary scores can serve as an indicator of severity of neuropsychological deficit. A computer program that calculates these scores is available from the Reitan Neuropsychology Laboratory.

An excellent set of norms is available for age (20–34, 35–39, 40–44, 45–49, 50–54, 55–59, 60–64, 65–69, 70–74, and 75–80) crossed by education (6–8, 9–11, 12, 13–15, 16–17, 18+) and gender (Heaton *et al.,* 1991). T scores are obtained by first finding the scaled score corresponding to the raw score. The scaled scores may have interpretive value in their own right because they provide a comparison to a performance standard. T scores are then located. T scores may be useful in answering questions such as "(a) How adequate is this test result for a person with this subject's age, education, and sex? and (b) What is the likelihood that a neurologically normal person would obtain this T score?" (Heaton *et al.,* 1991, p. 35). A computer program based on these norms has received a mixed review (Fuerst, 1993).

The HRNB has been demonstrated to possess adequate reliability (Boll, 1981; Franzen, 1989). Although studies have generally demonstrated adequate validity, controversy regarding the HRNB's diagnostic efficiency persists (Franzen, 1989; Goldstein, 1990).

Reitan (1986) has delineated several limitations of the battery. Although memory functioning is assessed on several of the tests of the HRNB (CT, Localization and Memory of TPT), he has suggested that "in individual cases it might be of value to include supplementary tests of memory for clinical evaluation" (Reitan, 1986, p. 10). He also suggested that tests assessing motor functioning might be supplemented in some cases. Although verbal functioning is assessed by the WAIS Verbal subtests, the SSPT, and the AST, there is not an adequate assessment of verbal problem-solving (Reitan, 1986). Reitan has suggested the possible addition of the Word Finding Test (Reitan, 1972).

REFERENCES

Boll, T. J. (1981). The Halstead–Reitan Neuropsychology Battery. In S. B. Filskov & T. J. Boll (Eds.), *Handbook of clinical neuropsychology* (pp. 577–607). New York: Wiley-Interscience.

Franzen, M. D. (1989). *Reliability and validity in neuropsychological assessment.* New York: Plenum Press.

Fuerst, D. R. (1993). A review of the Halstead–Reitan Neuropsychological Battery norms program. *The Clinical Neuropsychologist, 7,* 96–103.

Goldstein, G. (1990). Comprehensive neuropsychological assessment batteries. In G. Goldstein & M. Hersen (Eds.), *Handbook of psychological assessment* (2nd ed.) (pp. 197–227). New York: Pergamon Press.

Heaton, R. K., Grant, I., & Matthews, C. G. (1991). *Comprehensive norms for an expanded Halstead–Reitan Battery: Demographic corrections, research findings, and clinical applications.* Odessa, FL: Psychological Assessment Resources.

Reitan, R. M. (1972). Verbal problem solving as related to cerebral damage. *Perceptual and Motor Skills, 34,* 515–524.

Reitan, R. M. (1986). Theoretical and methodological bases of the Halstead–Reitan Neuropsychological Test Battery. In I. Grant & K. M. Adams (Eds.), *Neuropsychological assessment of neuropsychiatric disorders* (pp. 3–30). New York: Oxford University Press.

Reitan, R. M., & Wolfson, D. (1990). A consideration of the comparability of the WAIS and WAIS-R. *The Clinical Neuropsychologist, 4,* 80–85.

Reitan, R. M., & Wolfson, D. (1993). *The Halstead–Reitan Neuropsychological Test Battery* (2nd ed.). Tucson: Neuropsychology Press.

Russell, E. W., Neuringer, C., & Goldstein, G. (1970). *Assessment of brain damage: A neuropsychological key approach.* New York: Wiley-Interscience.

4

Luria–Nebraska
Neuropsychological Battery

The Luria–Nebraska Neuropsychological Battery (LNNB) is a standardized battery of neuropsychological tasks designed to assess a broad range of neuropsychological functions. It consists of 269 items (Form I) or 279 items (Form II) comprised of over 700 discrete tasks. The battery is based on A. R. Luria's theories and neuropsychological evaluation (Luria, 1966), especially as reported in *Luria's Neuropsychological Investigation* (Christensen, 1975). The LNNB consists of 11 (Form I) or 12 (Form II) scales: C1 (Motor Functions), C2 (Rhythm), C3 (Tactile Functions), C4 (Visual Functions), C5 (Receptive Speech), C6 (Expressive Speech), C7 (Writing), C8 (Reading), C9 (Arithmetic), C10 (Memory), C11 (Intellectual Processes), and C12 (Intermediate Memory—Form II). Each of these scales is described in Part III of this book. They are composed of sets of heterogeneous items. The scales are further broken down into factor scales. Localization scales have been developed to assist the examiner in making inferences about the locus of brain damage. Impaired performance is determined on any of these scales by comparison with the *critical level*. The critical level is corrected for age and education and is calculated for each patient using the following equation: Critical level = 68.8 + (0.214 × Age) − (1.47 × Education). If a scale exceeds the critical level, the possibility of impairment on that scale is suggested. Elevations on two or more scales are suggestive of brain damage. Revised norms have been published for the LNNB— Form II (Moses *et al.*, 1992).

Since the clinical scales are composed of sets of heterogeneous items, caution must be exercised in interpreting elevations on these scales. For example, an elevation on the C1-Motor Functions scale does not necessarily imply impaired motor functioning per se, but could result from an inability to visually perceive upper-extremity positions modeled by the examiner. An analysis of the specific items failed and qualitative aspects of performance is essential to proper and complete interpretation of the battery.

None of the items in the scales is presumed to measure only a single function. According to Luria's theory of brain function, observable behaviors are the result of molecular skills and invariably involve a coordination of several functionally linked brain areas (Golden *et al.*, 1992). "Failure to perform a given task successfully can be the result of an impairment in any of the component molecular (nonobservable) skills that comprise the functional chain" (Franzen, 1989, pp. 109–110). By comparing performance across similar items that differ in their single-task requirements, the dysfunctional unit may be isolated.

Four levels of interpretation are described in the manual (Golden *et al.*, 1985). The first level concerns the determination of whether significant brain injury exists. What the patient can or cannot do is described at the second level. Probable causes of the patient's behavior (brain–behavior relationships) are described at the third level. The fourth level involves the integration of all findings into a description of how the patient's brain is functioning. Franzen (1989) has suggested a five-step interpretation of the LNNB: (1) clinical scales above the critical level are noted, (2) scatter among scales is examined, (3) localization and factor scales are compared to the critical level, (4) performance on items is examined, and (5) qualitative aspects of performance are examined.

Adequate reliability and validity have been demonstrated for the LNNB (Franzen, 1989; Golden, 1989; Golden & Maruish, 1986). Several studies have found similar rates of diagnostic accuracy for the HRNB and the LNNB (Goldstein & Shelly, 1984; Kane *et al.*, 1985).

As is true for any battery of neuropsychological tests, the LNNB cannot be expected to answer every neuropsychological assessment question. Franzen (1989) has noted that the LNNB does not assess reading comprehension and cannot distinguish between average and superior performance. It relies heavily on the verbal mediation of behavior and is deficient in complex visuomotor tasks. The LNNB may not be well suited for aphasia syndrome classification (Crosson & Warren, 1982; Moses & Maruish, 1990). It lacks complex items and may therefore be insensitive to existing deficits in high-level functioning (Purisch & Sbordone, 1986). This book provides LNNB users with descriptions of additional tests or alternative sets of tests that may supplement the LNNB in areas that are either not assessed or underassessed by the LNNB.

REFERENCES

Christensen, A. L. (1975). *Luria's neuropsychological investigation.* New York: Spectrum.
Crosson, B., & Warren, R. L. (1982). Use of the Luria–Nebraska Neuropsychological Battery in aphasia: A conceptual critique. *Journal of Consulting and Clinical Psychology, 50,* 22–31.
Franzen, M. D. (1989). *Reliability and validity in neuropsychological assessment.* New York: Plenum Press.
Golden, C. J. (1989). The Luria–Nebraska Neuropsychological Battery. In C. S. Newmark (Ed.), *Major psychological assessment methods,* Volume II (pp. 165–198). Boston: Allyn & Bacon.
Golden, C. J., & Maruish, M. (1986). The Luria–Nebraska Neuropsychological Battery. In D. Wedding, A. M. Horton, & J. Webster (Eds.), *The neuropsychology handbook: Behavioral and clinical perspectives* (pp. 161–193). New York: Springer.
Golden, C. J., Purisch, A. D., & Hammeke, T. A. (1985). *Luria–Nebraska Neuropsychological Battery: Forms I and II: Manual.* Los Angeles: Western Psychological Services.
Golden, C. J., Zillmer, E., & Spiers, M. (1992). *Neuropsychological assessment and intervention.* Springfield, IL: Charles C. Thomas.
Goldstein, G., & Shelly, C. (1984). Discriminative validity of various intelligence and neuropsychological tests. *Journal of Consulting and Clinical Psychology, 52,* 383–389.
Kane, R. L., Parsons, O. A., & Goldstein, G. (1985). Statistical relationships and discrimination accuracy of the Halstead–Reitan, Luria–Nebraska, and Wechsler IQ scores in the identification of brain damage. *Journal of Clinical and Experimental Neuropsychology, 7,* 211–223.
Luria, A. R. (1966). *Higher cortical functions in man.* New York: Basic Books.
Moses, J. A., & Maruish, M. E. (1990). A critical review of the Luria–Nebraska Neuropsychological Battery. XI. Critiques and rebuttals: Part two. *International Journal of Clinical Neuropsychology, 12,* 37–45.
Moses, J. A., Schefft, B. K., Wong, J. L., & Berg, R. A. (1992). Revised norms and decision rules for the Luria–Nebraska Neuropsychological Battery, Form II. *Archives of Clinical Neuropsychology, 7,* 251–269.
Purisch, A. D., & Sbordone, R. J. (1986). The Luria–Nebraska Neuropsychological Battery. In G. Goldstein & R. E. Tarter (Eds.), *Advances in clinical neuropsychology,* Volume 3 (pp. 291–316). New York: Plenum Press.

Neuropsychological Evaluations and Reports

REFERRAL QUESTIONS

Neuropsychological evaluations are often initiated through referral from a professional person or an agency. A wide variety of referral questions of varying relevance and specificity may be encountered. The referral may describe complaints and behavioral observations that prompted the referral. It may contain a brief history and an explicit statement of the purpose of the referral. Referrals are commonly made to: (1) clarify diagnostic issues; (2) assess cognitive and/or emotional strengths and weaknesses for placement in a rehabilitation program (Alfano & Finlayson, 1987); (3) determine limitations on and supports needed for community living, school, and work; and (4) determine the existence, extent, and etiology of brain injury as evidence in forensic cases (Walsh, 1991). Referral questions may be as cryptic and obscure as "evaluate for organicity" or "neuropsychological consultation." Consulting the referral source often helps to clarify the referral question.

Inappropriate referrals are sometimes received. Again, consultation with the referral source is recommended. As the field of clinical neuropsychology matures, indications for referral for neuropsychological evaluation will be made more specific. For example, Franklin *et al.* (1990) have suggested specific criteria for referral of patients with multiple sclerosis.

NEUROPSYCHOLOGICAL EVALUATION

According to Hamsher (1990, p. 266), it is essential "to keep one's eye keenly fixed on the referral question." The same test result may have to be interpreted differently in different circumstances. Neuropsychologists work in a wide variety of clinical settings with great variability in referral questions and situational parameters. The practitioner should have a variety of assessment strategies and instruments in his or her repertoire. For example, the HRNB is not likely to be appropriate for an agitated head-injury patient. A brief mental status examination would generally not provide a sufficient evaluation of a testable patient for return to work. No one strategy or set of tests is appropriate in all circumstances.

If the practitioner is using a flexible battery approach and if circumstances allow, the battery should assess all basic areas of cognitive functioning—areas of functioning dependent on the brain. These areas include orientation, attention, memory, intelligence, communication, visual–spatial ability, sensory functioning, motor functioning, executive functioning, and personality. The battery should include tests that relate to the brain generally as well as tests that relate to specific cortical areas (Reitan, 1988). Berent (1991) has suggested that tests be selected on the basis of: (1) their capacity to generate data that will answer the referral question, (2) their psychometric merits, (3) their conventional acceptance and use, and (4) the training of the individual administering the tests. The tests discussed in Part III of this book are organized according to cognitive or functional area to assist in flexible battery development.

If a diagnosis is unknown or testing is being done solely to evaluate cognitive functioning, Part III may be consulted for a listing of tests that assess specific areas of cognitive functioning. The test description includes information about modalities in which the test may be administered and in which the patient's responses are to be made. This information can assist the examiner in tailoring the examination for patients with impairments in sensory, motor, or cognitive functioning. Information on localization in Part III and comparison with expected results of testing in Part VI may assist in diagnosis.

If a neurological disorder is suspected, the practitioner can consult Part VI for background information, expected neuropsychological test results, and probable areas of cognitive impairment. This information can assist the examiner in selecting a collection of tests that can best assess the disorder. Part III may be consulted for information on any of the selected tests. If the diagnosis is supported, Part VI may again be consulted for suggestions for treatment recommendations for inclusion in a neuropsychological report.

If the practitioner is using a standard battery and a deficit is noted, it may be useful to further define the deficit by adding tests that assess that area of functioning in more detail. Part III may provide suggestions for these additional tests. As noted above, the profile of cognitive functioning can be compared to that expected for a given disorder as outlined in Part VI.

Part IV may be of assistance in making inferences from test results to activities of daily living, driving, academics, and work.

The practitioner may refer to Part V for a listing of possible therapeutic modalities.

NEUROPSYCHOLOGICAL REPORT

Report-writing styles vary greatly with practitioner, referral question, and setting. In some settings, a brief one- or two-page report summarizing findings and recommendations may be preferred to allow for expeditious communication. At the other extreme, a forensic evaluation may necessitate a lengthy, detailed description of all interview and test results. Experience and feedback from referral sources can assist the practitioner in tailoring his or her reports to be accurate and useful.

Identifying Information

Name, birth date, address, and other identifying information is recorded.

Reason for Referral

The referral source and question are briefly stated. It is important to clarify the referral question as much as possible, since this question will suggest the form the evaluation will take (e.g., comprehensiveness and relevancy of specific tests, issues to be explored in interview).

Pertinent Social and Medical History

Relevant history is presented as obtained from records review and interview.

Behavioral Observations

Observations of the patient's behavior and ways of relating to significant others are recorded.

Tests Administered

A list of tests administered and sources of information is provided.

Test Results

Test results are often organized by test or by area of functioning. The latter approach is used in this book because it gives the test results a meaningful organization. One problem with this approach results from the multifactorial nature of neuropsychological tests. Tests rarely assess only one area of cognitive functioning and are therefore difficult to classify. In this Test Results section, the test data are presented. Inferences about brain function and everyday abilities are minimal. Inferences are reserved for the Summary and Interpretation section of the report.

Test results are presented under the following headings:

Orientation

Attention/Concentration

Memory

Intelligence, General Knowledge, and Social Understanding

Speech/Language

Arithmetic

Visual–Spatial Functioning

Tactile Functioning

Motor Functioning

Executive Functioning

Personality

Summary and Interpretation

Strengths and weaknesses are summarized and inferences regarding brain impairment, diagnosis, and prognosis are made.

Diagnostic Impression

ICD-9 or DSM-III-R diagnosis is made.

Recommendations

Recommendations relevant to the referral (e.g., independent living, return to work or school, or appropriateness for rehabilitation or psychotherapy) are made. Referrals to appropriate agencies or professionals may be suggested. The necessity for further or repeat evaluation is assessed.

It should be noted that this is only one of many valid formats for writing neuropsychological reports and that there are numerous circumstances that require deviance from this format.

Providing feedback to clients is an essential part of the assessment process. When providing feedback, it is important to discuss common sources of bias and error in the assessment (Pope, 1992). Gass and Brown (1992) have listed steps in providing feedback to brain-injured patients as follows: (1) review the purpose of the testing, (2) define the tests, (3) explain test results and behavior, (4) describe strengths and weaknesses, and (5) address diagnostic and prognostic issues. Great care should be exercised in projecting the course of recovery or decline and in making diagnostic statements. Feedback must be tailored to fit the patient's behavior and capabilities.

REFERENCES

Alfano, D. P., & Finlayson, M. A. J. (1987). Clinical psychology in rehabilitation. *The Clinical Neuropsychologist, 1,* 105–123.

Berent, S. (1991). Modern approaches to neuropsychological testing. In D. Smith, D. Treiman, & M. Trimble (Eds.), *Advances in neurology,* Volume 55 (pp. 423–437). New York: Raven Press.

Franklin, G. M., Nelson, L. M., Heaton, R. K., & Filley, C. M. (1990). Clinical perspectives on the identification of cognitive impairment. In S. M. Rao (Ed.), *Neurobehavioral aspects of multiple sclerosis* (pp. 161–179). New York: Oxford University Press.

Gass, C. S., & Brown, M. C. (1992). Neuropsychological test feedback to patients with brain dysfunction. *Psychological Assessment, 4,* 272–277.

Hamsher, K. deS. (1990). Specialized neuropsychological assessment methods. In G. Goldstein & M. Hersen (Eds.), *Handbook of psychological assessment* (2nd ed.) (pp. 256–279). New York: Pergamon Press.

Pope, K. S. (1992). Responsibilities in providing psychological test feedback to clients. *Psychological Assessment, 4,* 268–271.

Reitan, R. M. (1988). Integration of neuropsychological theory, assessment, and application. *The Clinical Neuropsychologist, 2,* 331–349.

Walsh, K. W. (1991). *Understanding brain damage: A primer of neuropsychological evaluation* (2nd ed.). Edinburgh: Churchill Livingston.

Factors That Influence Test Performance

A number of variables that affect test performance may confound the interpretation of a neuropsychological evaluation. These variables must be properly assessed and their effects controlled or taken into account through the use of appropriate norms or correction factors. If this assessment is not made, impairment may be wrongly diagnosed when the patient's performance is actually in the normal range relative to appropriately matched peers. Or an impaired performance might be attributed to brain dysfunction when it actually resulted from peripheral injury.

A number of these variables are reviewed in the following chapters: peripheral motor and sensory functioning, handedness, age, education, gender, ethnicity, anxiety, amotivation, and fatigue. Methods for minimizing the confounding effects of peripheral sensorimotor impairments are suggested. Methods for assessing handedness and for using this information in interpreting test results are reviewed. The effects of demographic variables (e.g., age, education, gender, and ethnicity) on test performance and the use of appropriate norms to take these effects into account is discussed. Finally, the assessment of and significance for performance of states such as anxiety, amotivation, and fatigue are discussed.

Peripheral Motor and Sensory Impairments

MOTOR IMPAIRMENTS

In a neuropsychological evaluation, inferences are made from behavior to brain function and to cognitive processes dependent on brain function. To infer from impaired behavior to brain dysfunction, it is essential that impairment due to peripheral nervous system (PNS) dysfunction (including the spinal cord), muscular atrophy, arthritis, and other physical problems be ruled out. For example, an inference might be made from severely impaired finger-tapping speed of the right hand to dysfunction in the contralateral (left) hemisphere. However, if the *extensor digitorum* or *extensor indicis* tendons of the right hand were severed, this alone could result in severely impaired finger-tapping speed and an inference to brain dysfunction would not be warranted.

Often, a neurological or physical examination of the patient with information on more peripheral neurological and motoric abilities and physical disabilities is available in the patient's medical history. If this history is not available, a neurological evaluation is recommended.

If there are no PNS, orthopedic, or other physical problems, then inferences about brain function can be made more cleanly. Such absence of physical problems is often not the case. Many patients referred for neuropsychological evaluation have multiple injuries and medical problems, often involving the PNS, musculature, and bones. For these patients, the neuropsychological evaluation must be designed and interpreted in such a way that the influence of peripheral impairment is minimized and does not confound inferences to brain function and cognition.

Inferences from tests that involve lateral comparisons of motoric function such as the FTT, the Grooved Pegboard (GP) test, the GS test, and the TPT to cortical functioning are especially subject to contamination from peripheral motor impairment. Inferences from tests that involve motor performance, such as the Visual Reproduction subtest of the Wechsler Memory Scale—Revised (VR-WMS-R), the ROCFT:C&M, and the Block Design subtest of the WAIS-R (BD-WAIS-R), to visual–spatial functioning and cortical functioning are also subject to contamination. The norms for these tests are inappropriate if there is either unilateral or bilateral motor dysfunction (Swiercinsky, 1987). Allowances must be made for motor impairment or slowing due to peripheral causes or for use of tests that assess the area of functioning yet are not dependent on peripheral functioning. Time limits may need to be extended or eliminated on some tests even though this variation invalidates available norms (Kaplan *et al.,* 1991).

Patients who are dysarthric may need to respond by writing. If the patient is unable to respond by writing, he or she may be able to respond by pointing. Items may have to be presented in a multiple-choice format as in the Peabody Picture Vocabulary Test—Revised (PPVT-R) and the alternate multiple-choice tests for the WAIS-R (Kaplan *et al.,* 1991).

This *Practitioner's Guide* can assist the neuropsychologist in assessing patients with motor impairment. For each test or subtest reviewed in Part III of this book, there is a subsection headed *Response Modalities.* This subsection describes the general motoric require-ments for the test and indicates whether the test is *timed* (i.e., a higher score is obtained for a faster time or greater production in a specific period of time), *time-limited* (i.e., a set time period is allowed for the completion of the task), *paced* (i.e., the responses must keep up with a set pace), or *untimed* (i.e., no time limit is placed on completion of the task). These Response Modalities subsections can be of assistance to the neuropsychologist in constructing a battery of tests appropriate to patients with peripheral motoric impairments. The procedure would be as follows: (1) Peripheral motor impairments and strengths are noted. (2) Candidates for the battery are selected from the tests in Part III to answer the referral question and to assess the major areas of cognitive functioning. (3) The Response Modalities subsections of the test discussions are examined to determine which tests do not require the patient's peripherally impaired motor ability or response speed. (4) Tests are then selected that both address the pertinent issues of the neuropsychological evaluation and avoid dependence on peripherally impaired areas of motor functioning. If tests dependent on the impaired area of functioning must be used, this dependence can be clearly recognized, and the neuropsycholo-gist can take it into account when interpreting the test results.

For example, suppose that a patient who had suffered a very severe traumatic brain injury 10 years ago is referred for neuropsychological evaluation. The referral source requests a general evaluation of cognitive functioning to assess the patient's readiness for vocational training. According to the patient's medical history, brainstem and spinal cord injury resulted in severely impaired upper and lower extremity motor functioning with left extremities slightly more impaired than right. The patient is able to control an electric wheelchair by manipulating a joystick with the right hand. The patient is right-handed and can barely write, but can point. Speech, visual acuity, and hearing are grossly intact. With the listing of peripheral strengths and weaknesses completed, tests appropriate for assessment of each major area of cognitive functioning would be selected. By reference to the Response Modalities subsections of tests in Chapter 16 in Part III of this book, tests that require rapid, dextrous upper extremity motor responses would be eliminated and a selection made from the remaining tests. The Digit Symbol subtest of the WAIS-R (DSym-WAIS-R) and the Visual Search and Attention Test (VSAT) would be eliminated and a choice made from the Digit Span subtest of the WAIS-R (DS-WAIS-R) or WMS-R (DS-WMS-R), the Visual Memory Span subtest of the WMS-R (VMS-WMS-R), the Mental Control subtest of the WMS-R (MC-WMS-R), the Paced Auditory Serial Addition Test (PASAT), SSS, and the SDMT (Oral). Since the Continuous Performance Test (CPT) requires a *rapid* simple motor response, performance might be impaired by the patient's peripheral injury. Nevertheless, the information obtained from this test would be useful. This same procedure would be followed for other assessment areas and a battery appropriate for this patient constructed. It should be noted that not *all* tests involving dextrous motor functioning would be eliminated. The FTT and GS might be administered to assess the extent of the patient's motor impairment. However, a hazardous inference about cortical functioning on the basis of finger-tapping and grip strength would be avoided. One possible selection of tests for this patient would be as follows: clinical interview, the WAIS-R Verbal subtests and Picture Completion (PC-WAIS-R), WMS-R with the exception of VR,

Hooper Visual Organization Test (HVOT), Raven's Performance Matrices (RPM), WCST, the Reading subtest of the Wide Range Achievement Test—Revised (R-WRAT-R), and selected subtests of the Boston Diagnostic Aphasia Examination (BDAE), RKSPE, and Minnesota Multiphasic Personality Inventory—2 (MMPI-2).

SENSORY IMPAIRMENTS

Inferences to cognitive and cortical functioning from the behavior observed during a neuropsychological evaluation are often made under the assumption that sensory information is being received by the cortex and peripheral impairment has been ruled out. Gross evaluation of visual, auditory, and tactile acuity is usually included in the neuropsychological evaluation. The medical history may contain information on peripheral sensory functioning. In the interview, the patient is asked about visual impairments, glasses, hearing problems, hearing aids, and tactile abilities. If glasses or hearing aids are required, they should be used during the testing. Visual acuity can be assessed using a simple eye chart. Visual fields should be at least grossly assessed for each eye alone and for both eyes together as in the RKSPE by wiggling a finger in the periphery of the fields. The ability or inability of the patient to hear speech is usually apparent in the interview. If the patient is severely impaired, audition can be grossly assessed by asking simple questions or stating simple commands to determine whether the patient can respond appropriately. Audition is also grossly evaluated in the RKSPE by the examiner's rubbing his or her index finger and thumb near each of the patient's ears. Tactile functioning may be evaluated with an aesthesiometer to determine the patient's threshold for two-point discrimination at various places on the hand. A gross evaluation is also performed as part of the RKSPE by touching the patient on the back of the hand. Consistent unilateral errors on double simultaneous stimulation may suggest contralateral cortical impairment, if errors are not noted on single, unilateral stimulation (Reitan & Wolfson, 1993). Consistent errors on single, unilateral stimulation may be due to peripheral impairment or cortical impairment such as a scotoma or visual field cut.

If a patient has visual acuity problems not correctable by glasses, a sheet magnifier may used in administering tests such as the PC-WAIS-R (Kaplan et al., 1991). More severe uncorrectable visual problems and blindness will dictate emphasis or total reliance on tests that do not depend on the visual modality. For example, the TPT may be used to assess spatial skills, learning, and memory. The patient may finger-trace the shapes and their relative locations on a large surface while the examiner imitates and records the finger-tracing in pencil. The TPT Memory and Location norms will be of limited usefulness (Swiercinsky, 1987). Orally presented verbal tests requiring oral responses will need to be used to assess most areas of cognitive functioning.

Accommodations may need to be made for cortically mediated visual impairment in some instances. For example, if a patient has severe visual neglect, performance may be impaired on Picture Arrangement (PA-WAIS-R) solely due to cortically mediated visual neglect or inattention. Since there are numerous tests designed to assess visual neglect, the finding of impaired performance on PA-WAIS-R need not be used to assess neglect, yet such a finding would be contaminated by the possibility that the impairment was due to neglect. To avoid this problem, Kaplan et al. (1991) suggest that the cards be placed vertically in the intact visual field and the patient be asked to sequence the cards from top to bottom. A similar procedure may be used for a variety of test materials (Heaton & Heaton, 1981).

If a patient is unable to hear or understand spoken language, the information may be presented in written or printed form in the visual modality. Again, it should be noted that norms may be compromised.

Patients who are congenitally hearing-impaired will generally communicate primarily with American Sign Language (ASL). English syntax is different from that of ASL (Swiercinsky, 1987). Signs are broader in meaning and vocabulary is significantly reduced. The typical congenitally hearing-impaired individual reads English at the sixth-grade level, the reason being that the preferred form of communication is ASL. An ASL interpreter may communicate instructions and interpret for the interview, but interpretation may be invalid for individual test items. For example, if an interpreter signs, "How are a ball and a wheel alike?," the interpreter must gesture a specific ball and a specific wheel. The specific gestures destroy the intent of eliciting a general characteristic of all balls and all wheels.

General mathematical ability may be a better indicator of general intellectual functioning than English vocabulary. Concept formation and learning may be better assessed with relatively language-free tests such as the Halstead CT, BD-WAIS-R, and WCST. Language-free tests are preferred for memory assessment (Swiercinsky, 1987).

This *Practitioner's Guide* can be of assistance in designing batteries to assess patients with sensory impairment. For each test or subtest reviewed in Part III, there is a subsection headed *Presentation Modalities*. This subsection describes the general sensory (visual, auditory, or tactile) and information-processing (verbal or nonverbal) requirements for the test. These Presentation Modalities subsections can be of assistance to the neuropsychologist in constructing a battery of tests appropriate to patients with peripheral sensory impairments or information-processing deficits. The procedure would be as follows: (1) Peripheral sensory and information-processing impairments and strengths are noted. (2) Candidates for the battery are selected from the tests in Part III to answer the referral question and to assess the major areas of cognitive functioning. (3) The Presentation Modalities subsections of the test discussions are consulted to determine which tests do not require the patient's peripherally impaired sensory or information-processing ability. (4) Tests are then selected that both address the pertinent issues of the neuropsychological evaluation and avoid dependence on peripherally impaired areas of sensory functioning or information processing. If tests dependent on the impaired area of functioning must be used, this dependence can be clearly recognized, and the neuropsychologist can take it into account when interpreting the test results.

For patients with multiple sensorimotor impairments, the Response Modalities and Presentation Modalities subsections may be used in combination to assist in construction of an appropriate battery of tests for a given patient.

LNNB

Golden *et al.* (1985) have described numerous ways in which variations can be made in instructions and presentation of materials to accommodate patients with impaired sensorimotor functioning. Adjustments such as pointing out the missed stimuli or allowing the patient to redo the items have been suggested for patients with unilateral neglect. For some items (i.e., C4-Visual Functions), instructions and responses may be signed or written instead of spoken.

Moses (1984) classified an unselected sample of brain-damaged patients on the basis of presence or absence of sensorimotor and presence or absence of cognitive deficits. Analyses of group profiles revealed large group separations of mean LNNB profiles for groups that differed in the presence or absence of cognitive impairment, regardless of the presence or absence of sensorimotor impairment.

Golden (1989) has developed an abbreviated version of the LNNB for use with severely impaired patients. Intercorrelations between the abbreviated and regular forms exceeded 0.93 for all the basic and localization scales.

REFERENCES

Golden, C. J. (1989). Abbreviating administration of the LNNB in significantly impaired patients. *International Journal of Clinical Psychology, 11,* 177–181.

Golden, C. J., Purisch, A. D., & Hammeke, T. A. (1985). *Luria–Nebraska Neuropsychological Battery: Forms I and II.* Los Angeles: Western Psychological Services.

Heaton, S. K., & Heaton, R. K. (1981). Testing the impaired patient. In S. B. Filskov & T. J. Boll (Eds.), *Handbook of clinical neuropsychology,* Volume 1 (pp. 526–544). New York: Wiley.

Kaplan, E., Fein, D., Morris, R., & Delis, D. C. (1991). *WAIS-R (NI): Manual.* San Antonio: Psychological Corporation.

Moses, J. A. (1984). The effects of cognitive and sensorimotor deficits on Luria–Nebraska Neuropsychological Battery performance in a brain damaged population. *International Journal of Clinical Neuropsychology, 6,* 8–12.

Reitan, R. M., & Wolfson, D. (1993). *The Halstead–Reitan Neuropsychological Test Battery: Theory and Clinical Interpretation* (2nd ed.). Tucson: Neuropsychology Press.

Swiercinsky, D. P. (1987). Neuropsychological assessment of sensory and physically impaired patients. In L. C. Hartlage, M. J. Asken, & J. L. Hornsby (Eds.), *Essentials of neuropsychological assessment* (pp. 197–212). New York: Springer.

Handedness

Handedness is defined as the preferred hand used for a motor activity (manual preference) or the hand most skillful at performing a task (manual proficiency) (Fennell, 1986; Henninger, 1992). Approximately 90–95% of the population is right-handed (dextral) (Annett, 1970; Porac & Coren, 1978). The remainder are left-handed (sinistral) or mixed-handed. Left-handedness decreases with age and has been reported to vary with culture (Fennel, 1986). An increased incidence of left-handedness has been reported in a variety of groups, including individuals with epilepsy (Bolin, 1953), alcoholism (Bakan, 1953), learning disabilities (Geschwind & Behan, 1982), and mental retardation (DeSilva & Satz, 1979; Hicks & Barton, 1975). It has also been reported among specific groups not suffering from disorders (Fennell, 1986).

It is important to assess hand preference in a neuropsychological evaluation. Knowledge of hand preference is essential for interpretation of performance on motor and sensory tasks such as the FTT, GS, GP, and TPT. The dominant hand is expected to perform better than the nondominant hand. Hand dominance, prior to injury or illness, must be assessed to determine whether a functional deficit exists. Once premorbid dominance has been established, norms provided for the dominant and nondominant hands (Heaton et al., 1991) may be utilized. If impairment due to peripheral injury has been ruled out, impaired unimanual performance may suggest dysfunction in the contralateral hemisphere.

Assessment of handedness is also essential when making inferences from impaired language functioning to lesion location. Handedness has been related to cerebral organization and lateralization of function. There is a higher incidence of right hemisphere or bilateral representation of speech and language in left-handers. Support for this claim has been found in sodium Amytal studies (Rasmussen & Milner, 1977), unilateral electroconvulsive therapy (Warrington & Pratt, 1973), and laterality differences among groups of normal left-handers (Satz et al., 1967). There is twice the incidence of language impairment following a lesion of the right hemisphere in left-handers that there is in right-handers (Kertesz, 1979). Familial sinistrality has been found to be associated with bilateral representation of language functions (Hecaen et al., 1981). For this reason, in addition to assessing hand preference, it is important to collect information on sinistrality in parents, grandparents, and siblings.

Left-handers may perform less well on spatial tasks than right-handers (Filskov & Catanese, 1986; Levy, 1969), but this finding is controversial. Gregory and Paul (1980) found left-handers with inverted writing style to be impaired on the Vocabulary subtest of WAIS-R (V-WAIS-R), PC-WAIS-R, and TMTB.

Due to the possibility of right hemisphere or bilateral representation of speech in left-handers, inferences from impaired language functioning to left hemisphere dysfunction must be made with great care. Converging, corroborative data from a variety of sources should be obtained. It should be noted that the vast majority of the studies cited for the *Localization* subsections in Part III of this book used either right-handed subjects only or a mixture of subjects, with most being right-handed. Therefore, the results of these studies may be of limited relevance to left-handed patients.

Hand preference is sometimes assessed by simply asking the patient whether he or she is right- or left-handed. A variety of self-report instruments are available to provide a more detailed and precise evaluation of hand preference. The Annett Handedness Questionnaire (Annett, 1967, 1970) consists of 12 items: writing, throwing a ball, holding a racket, holding a match to strike, cutting with scissors, guiding thread through a needle, top hand on a broom, top hand on a shovel, dealing cards, hammering a nail, using a toothbrush, and unscrewing a jar lid. In one version, the patient is asked to indicate the hand habitually used. In a second version, the patient is asked simply to indicate the hand used. Responses are left, right, or either. The Edinburgh Handedness Inventory (Oldfield, 1971) consists of 10 items: writing, drawing, throwing, using a scissors, holding a toothbrush, cutting with a knife, using a spoon, upper hand on a broom, holding a match to strike, and opening a box. Responses are left, right, or both. Reliability and validity studies for these questionnaires have been reviewed by Fennell (1986). A number of other questionnaires are available (Briggs & Nebes, 1975; Crovitz & Zener, 1962; Steenhuis *et al.*, 1990). Studies have suggested that the relationship between hand preference and performance on unimanual tasks, such as finger-tapping, depends on the task and on the speed, accuracy, and dexterity required. Strength relates more weakly to handedness than skill. Left-handers exhibit more variability in the correlation of hand preference with performance (Fennell, 1986). Self-report inventories are also available that assess foot, eye, and ear preference as well as hand preference (Porac & Coren, 1981; Coren *et al.*, 1979). Strauss & Wada (1988) found that speech dominance as determined by carotid Amytal testing was predicted best using a combination of tests of hand preference (hand-preference items from Porac and Coren's inventory) and proficiency [GS, Purdue Pegboard Test (PPT)].

REFERENCES

Annett, M. (1967). The binomial distribution of right, mixed, and left handedness. *Quarterly Journal of Experimental Psychology, 19,* 327–333.

Annett, M. (1970). A classification of hand preference by association analysis. *British Journal of Psychology, 61,* 303–321.

Bakan, P. (1953). Left-handedness and alcoholism. *Perceptual and Motor Skills, 36,* 514.

Bolin, B. J. (1953). Left-handedness and stuttering as signs diagnostic of epileptics. *Journal of Mental Sciences, 99,* 483–488.

Briggs, G. G., & Nebes, R. D. (1975). Patterns of hand preference in a student population. *Cortex, 11,* 230–238.

Coren, S., Porac, C., & Duncan, P. (1979). A behaviorally validated self-report inventory to assess four types of lateral preference. *Journal of Clinical Neuropsychology, 1,* 55–64.

Crovitz, H. F., & Zener, K. (1962). A group-test for assessing hand- and eye-dominance. *American Journal of Psychology, 75,* 271–276.

DeSilva, D. A., & Satz, P. (1979). Pathological left-handedness: Evaluation of a model. *Brain and Language, 7,* 8–16.

Fennell, E. B. (1986). Handedness in neuropsychological research. In H. J. Hannay (Ed.), *Experimental techniques in human neuropsychology* (pp. 15–44). New York: Oxford University Press.

Filskov, S. B., & Catanese, R. A. (1986). Effects of sex and handedness on neuropsychological testing. In S. B. Filskov & T. J. Boll (Eds.), *Handbook of clinical neuropsychology,* Volume 2 (pp. 198–212). New York: Wiley.

Geschwind, N., & Behan, P. (1982). Left-handedness: Association with immune disease, migraine and developmental learning disorder. *Proceedings of the National Academy of Sciences, 79,* 5097–5100.

Gregory, R., & Paul, J. (1980). The effects of handedness and writing posture on neuropsychological test results. *Neuropsychologia, 18,* 231–235.

Heaton, R. K., Grant, I., & Matthews, C. G. (1991). *Comprehensive norms for an expanded Halstead–Reitan Battery: Demographic corrections, research findings, and clinical applications.* Odessa, FL: Psychological Assessment Resources.

Hecaen, H., DeAgostini, M., & Monzon-Montes, J. (1981). Cerebral organization in left handers. *Brain and Language, 12,* 261–284.

Henninger, P. (1992). Handedness and lateralization. In A. E. Puente & R. J. McCaffrey (Eds.), *Handbook of neuropsychological assessment: A biopsychosocial perspective* (pp. 141–179). New York: Plenum Press.

Hicks, R. E., & Barton, A. K. (1975). A note on left-handedness and severity of mental retardation. *Journal of Genetic Psychology, 127,* 323–324.

Kertesz, A. (1979). *Aphasia and associated disorders.* New York: Grune & Stratton.

Levy, J. (1969). Possible basis for the evolution of lateral specialization of the human brain. *Nature, 224,* 614–615.

Oldfield, R. C. (1971). The assessment and analysis of handedness: The Edinburgh Inventory. *Neuropsychologia, 9,* 97–113.

Porac, C., & Coren, S. (1978). Relationships among lateral preference behaviors in human beings. *Behavioral and Brain Sciences, 2,* 311–312.

Porac, C., & Coren, S. (1981). *Lateral preferences and human behavior.* New York: Springer-Verlag.

Rasmussen, T., & Milner, B. (1977). The role of left-brain injury in determining lateralization of cerebral speech functions. *Annals of the New York Academy of Sciences, 299,* 355–369.

Satz, P., Achenbach, K., & Fennel, E. (1967). Correlations between assessed manual laterality and predicted speech laterality in a normal population. *Neuropsychologia, 15,* 341–344.

Steenhuis, R. E., Bryden, M. P., Schwartz, M., & Lawson, S. (1990). Reliability of hand preference items and factors. *Journal of Clinical and Experimental Neuropsychology, 12,* 921–930.

Strauss, E., & Wada, J. (1988). Hand preference and proficiency and cerebral speech dominance determined by carotid Amytal test. *Journal of Clinical and Experimental Neuropsychology, 10,* 169–174.

Warrington, E. K., & Pratt, R. T. C. (1973). Language laterality in left handers assessed by unilateral ECT. *Neuropsychologia, 11,* 423–428.

Aging

An increase in the absolute numbers of older people is occurring throughout the world (Butler *et al.*, 1991). In the United States, 12% of the population was age 65 or older, in 1986. It is estimated that 20% of the population will be 65 or older by the year 2030. The 75-plus and 85-plus age groups are the fastest-growing age segments of the United States population.

BRAIN CHANGES IN NORMAL AGING

A decrease in brain weight and increase in ventricle size occur in normal aging (Albert & Stafford, 1988). Ischemic changes are observed and appear as low attenuation in the white matter on computed tomography scans (London *et al.*, 1986) or as high signal intensities on T2-weighted magnetic resonance imaging (Salgado *et al.*, 1986). Loss or degeneration of neurons also occurs in aging. An increase in granulovacuolar degeneration, plaques, and neurofibrillary tangles has been reported (Van Gorp & Mahler, 1990).

NEUROPSYCHOLOGICAL ASSESSMENT OF THE GERIATRIC PATIENT

Assessment of cognitive functioning in the elderly is often complicated due to sensorimotor impairments, systemic illnesses, and greater variability in cognitive abilities even among optimally healthy individuals (Valdois *et al.*, 1990; Williams, 1987).

Changes in the elderly include presbyopia, presbycusis, decreased sense of smell, slowed reaction time, limited upward gaze, decreased vibratory sense in the toes and feet, narrowed compass of perception, impairment of fine coordination and agility, reduced muscular power, and decrease in neuromuscular control, especially of the lower extremities. Reduced hepatic and renal functioning may affect the pharmacokinetics of drugs (Spar & Rue, 1990).

Diseases that are more common in the elderly include neoplasia, vascular diseases, fractures (e.g., hip), infections (e.g., pulmonary), and Alzheimer's disease (Adams & Victor, 1989). The evaluation commonly requires that the relative contributions of systemic diseases and other factors to the patient's cognitive profile be dissociated (Franzen & Rasmussen, 1990; Wedding & Cody, 1990). Obviously, a patient who exhibits cognitive impairments, but who has not had an appropriate physical examination, should be referred to a physician. This referral is particularly important for geriatric patients.

Longer neuropsychological batteries are often inappropriate for evaluating elderly patients. Mental status examinations or brief batteries may be used. Tests such as the Dementia Rating Scale (Mattis, 1988) and the Fuld Object-Memory Evaluation (Fuld, 1977, 1980) have been specifically designed for use with the elderly. Erickson *et al.* (1992) have published a bibliography of normative articles on cognition tests for older adults. La Rue (1992) has provided a thorough review of neuropsychological assessment of the elderly.

The Dementia Rating Scale (DRS) (Mattis, 1988) assesses digit span, following command, imitation, categorical word fluency, naming, verbal perseveration, performance of alternating movements, copying, similarities, differences, analogies, and verbal and visual memory. On some tasks, if a screening item is passed, the examiner proceeds to the next task; if not, a set of easier items is attempted. Scales are labeled as follows: Attention, Initiation and Perseveration, Construction, Conceptualization, and Memory. Norms extend from 65 to 81 years old.

In the Fuld Object-Memory Evaluation (Fuld, 1977, 1980; Fuld et al., 1990; La Rue, 1989), the patient is requested to reach into a cloth bag and feel and name objects. The patient then pulls each object from the bag and names it. Five recall trials are then conducted using a procedure similar to the Selective Reminding Test. Verbal fluency tests precede each request for recall. Finally, a recognition trial is administered.

WAIS and WAIS-R

The PIQ subtests are more affected by aging than the VIQ subtests. The decrement on PIQ tasks cannot be explained solely in terms of their being timed, but may be due in part to the fluid quality of the tasks. For the WAIS-R, Kaufman (1990) reported that age accounted for the greatest amount of variance for DSym, followed by Object Assembly (OA), PA, BD, PC, Comprehension (C), and Similarities (S). For the WAIS, Heaton et al. (1986) reported the greatest age-related effects for DSym, followed by PA, BD, OA, PC, and S. Of course, age-adjusted scaled scores, VIQ, PIQ, and FSIQ take age into account (Wechsler, 1981). The original WAIS norms (Wechsler, 1955) are obsolete. Heaton et al. (1991) have provided more contemporary norms.

HRNB

Heaton et al. (1986) found that a significant amount of variance for HRNB tests was accounted for by age with the exception of GS. Norms for the HRNB tests for different age groups may be found in Heaton et al. (1991).

LNNB

On the LNNB, age is taken into account in calculating the critical level that is used as a cutoff value in determining whether performance is impaired on the LNNB scales. Marvel et al. (1979) found significant age effects on all scales except Writing (C7), Reading (C8), and Arithmetic (C9). Vannieuwkirk and Galbraith (1985) found age effects on all scales except Rhythm (C2), C7–9, and Intellectual Processes (C11). A short form (141 items) of the LNNB has been recommended for use with the impaired elderly (McCue et al., 1985, 1989).

COGNITIVE CHANGES IN NORMAL AGING

Impairment Indexes

Halstead Impairment Index (HII) and Average Impairment Rating (AIR) have been found to exhibit aging main effects (Heaton et al., 1986).

Attention

DS is relatively insensitive to changes in age (Albert, 1988). Simple visual reaction time has been reported to decrease in the elderly (Bleecker et al., 1987).

Memory

Large age-related differences are found in delayed free recall. Decrements are greater on recall than on recognition tasks (Albert, 1988). Nonverbal recall [e.g., Benton Visual Retention Test (BVRT) (Shichita *et al.*, 1986)] tends to show more of a decrement with age than verbal recall, although some impairment has been noted in Logical Memory and Paired Associate Learning (Benton *et al.*, 1981). Bak and Greene (1980) reported relatively impaired performance on Visual Reproduction and Delayed Visual Reproduction. Serial Digit Learning has been reported impaired (Benton *et al.*, 1981).

Speech/Language

Phonological abilities and the lexicon are preserved (Bayles & Kazniak, 1987). Syntactic abilities generally remain intact (Albert, 1988). Semantic aspects of word retrieval may be impaired. Confrontation naming [Boston Naming Test (BNT)] decreases with age (Borod *et al.*, 1980). Verbal fluency for words beginning with a particular letter or for things in a particular category decreases with age (Obler & Albert, 1981). Aging main effects have been reported for the AST, SSPT, and SR (Heaton *et al.*, 1986). V-WAIS-R and Information (I-WAIS-R) generally do not decline and in many cases increase in older age.

Visuospatial Functioning

As noted above, a decrement has been found for the Performance subtests of the WAIS and WAIS-R. Impairment relative to younger age groups has been reported for Facial Recognition (FR) and Judgment of Line Orientation (JLO) (Benton *et al.*, 1981; Mittenberg *et al.*, 1989).

Sensory Functioning

TPT Time, Location, and Memory are affected by aging (Heaton *et al.*, 1986). Aging main-effects have been reported for the RKSPE.

Motor Functioning

Decrements with age have been reported on the PPT (Agnew *et al.*, 1988), GP, and FTT (Heaton *et al.*, 1986).

Executive Functioning

Halstead CT and TMTB performance has been reported to decrease with age (Bak & Greene, 1980; Heaton *et al.*, 1986). Design Fluency may exhibit a decrement (Mittenberg *et al.*, 1989).

Personality

Personality traits are generally stable throughout the adult life-span (McCrae & Costa, 1990). Nevertheless, individuals may experience stress, depression, and anxiety at various times in their lives. Major depression occurs in about 1–4% of individuals over 65 years old (Blazer & Williams, 1980). "Many elderly people who are depressed have experienced three or more losses of family or close friends by death or by moving away. Major illness and surgery may also be a precipitating factor for a depression" (Knight, 1986, p. 80). The Geriatric Depression Scale may be useful for evaluating depression in the elderly (Yesavage, 1986). Anxiety may also be a problem. Among community-residing older individuals, 17%

take tranquilizers that can result in cognitive and memory impairment (Knight, 1986). Paranoid thinking may sometimes be due to confusion resulting from impaired sensory processing (e.g., hearing) and impaired memory.

PSYCHOSOCIAL RESOURCES

Behavior Therapy

Behavioral problems in eating, bathing, sleeping, toileting, and other activities of daily living (ADLs) may respond to behavior modification (Pinkston & Linsk, 1984).

Psychotherapy

Therapy may focus on issues such as chronic illness and disability, adjustment to limitations, death and dying, grief for the loss of others, love, marriage, and sexuality. Therapy may assist the patient in developing greater empowerment and in enlarging his or her scope of activities and enjoyment (Knight, 1986). The therapist should be alert to the possibility of elder abuse. Many states have instituted reporting laws (Kosberg, 1983).

Resources

An extensive list of United States programs can be located in *Aging and Mental Health: Positive Psychosocial and Biomedical Approaches* (Butler *et al.,* 1991). Senior citizen programs are available in many localities.

REFERENCES

Adams, R. D., & Victor, M. (1989). *Principles of neurology* (4th ed.). New York: McGraw-Hill.

Agnew, J., Bolla-Wilson, K., Kawas, C. H., & Bleecker, M. L. (1988). Purdue Pegboard age and sex norms for people 40 years old and older. *Developmental Neuropsychology, 4,* 29–35.

Albert, M. S. (1988). Cognitive function. In M. S. Albert & M. B. Moss (Eds.), *Geriatric neuropsychology* (pp. 33–53). New York: Guilford Press.

Albert, M. S., & Stafford, J. L. (1988). Computed tomography studies. In M. S. Albert & M. B. Moss (Eds.), *Geriatric neuropsychology* (pp. 211–227). New York: Guilford Press.

Bak, J. S., & Greene, R. L. (1980). Changes in neuropsychological functioning in an aging population. *Journal of Consulting and Clinical Psychology, 48,* 395–399.

Bayles, K. A., & Kaszniak, A. W. (1987). *Communication and cognition in normal aging and dementia.* Boston: Little, Brown.

Benton, A. L., Eslinger, P. J., & Damasio, A. R. (1981). Normative observations on neuropsychological test performances in old age. *Journal of Clinical Neuropsychology, 3,* 33–42.

Blazer, D., & Williams, C. (1980). Epidemiology of dysphoria and depression in an elderly population. *American Journal of Psychiatry, 137,* 439–444.

Bleecker, M. L., Bolla-Wilson, K., Agnew, J., & Meyers, D. A. (1987). Simple visual reaction time: Sex and age differences. *Developmental Neuropsychology, 3,* 165–172.

Borod, J., Goodglass, H., & Kaplan, E. (1980). Normative data on the Boston Diagnostic Aphasia Examination, parietal lobe battery, and Boston Naming Test. *Journal of Clinical Neuropsychology, 2,* 209–215.

Butler, R. N., Lewis, M. I., & Sunderland, T. (1991). *Aging and mental health: Positive psychosocial and biomedical approaches* (4th ed.). New York: Maxwell Macmillan.

Erickson, R. C., Eimon, P., & Hebben, N. (1992). A bibliography of normative articles on cognition tests for older adults. *The Clinical Neuropsychologist, 6,* 98–102.

Franzen, M. D., & Rasmussen, P. R. (1990). Clinical neuropsychology and older populations. In A. W. Horton, Jr. (Ed.), *Neuropsychology across the life-span* (pp. 81–102). New York: Springer.

Fuld, P. A. (1977). *Fuld Object-Memory Evaluation.* Wood Dale, IL: Stoelting.

Fuld, P. A. (1980). Guaranteed stimulus-processing in the evaluation of memory and learning. *Cortex, 16,* 255–271.

Fuld, P. A., Masur, D. M., Blau, A. D., Crystal, H., & Aronson, M. K. (1990). Object-Memory Evaluation for prospective detection of dementia in normal functioning elderly: Predictive and normative data. *Journal of Clinical and Experimental Neuropsychology, 12,* 520–528.

Heaton, R. K., Grant, I., & Matthews, C. G. (1986). Differences in neuropsychological test performance associated with age, education, and sex. In I. Grant & K. M. Adams (Eds.), *Neuropsychological assessment of neuropsychiatric disorders* (pp. 100–120). New York: Oxford University Press.

Heaton, R. K., Grant, I., & Matthews, C. G. (1991). *Comprehensive norms for an expanded Halstead–Reitan Battery: Demographic corrections, research findings, and clinical applications.* Odessa, FL: Psychological Assessment Resources.

Kaufman, A. S. (1990). *Assessing adolescent and adult intelligence.* Boston: Allyn & Bacon.

Knight, B. (1986). *Psychotherapy with older adults.* Newbury Park, CA: Sage.

Kosberg, J. I. (1983). *Abuse and maltreatment of the elderly: Causes and interventions.* Boston: John Wright.

La Rue, A. (1989). Patterns of performance on the Fuld Object Memory Evaluation in elderly inpatients with dementia or depression. *Journal of Clinical and Experimental Neuropsychology, 11,* 409–422.

La Rue, A. (1992). *Aging and neuropsychological assessment.* New York: Plenum Press.

London, E., de Leon, M. J., George, A. E., Englund, E., Ferris, S., Gentes, C., & Reisberg, B. (1986). Periventricular lucencies in the CT scans of aged and demented. *Biological Psychiatry, 21,* 960–962.

Marvel, G. A., Golden, C. J., Hammeke, T., Purisch, A., & Osmon, D. (1979). Relationship of age and education to performance on a standardized version of Luria's neuropsychological tests in different patient populations. *International Journal of Neuroscience, 9,* 63–70.

Mattis, S. (1988). *Dementia Rating Scale.* Odessa, FL: Psychological Assessment Resources.

McCrae, R. R., and Costa, P. T. (1990). *Personality in adulthood.* New York: Guilford Press.

McCue, M., Shelly, C., & Goldstein, G. (1985). A proposed short form of the Luria–Nebraska Neuropsychological Battery oriented toward assessment of the elderly. *International Journal of Clinical Neuropsychology, 7,* 96–101.

McCue, M., Goldstein, G., & Shelly, C. (1989). The application of a short form of the Luria–Nebraska Neuropsychological Battery to discriminate between dementia and depression in the elderly. *International Journal of Clinical Neuropsychology, 11,* 21–29.

Mittenberg, W., Seidenberg, M., O'Leary, D. S., & DiGiulio, D. V. (1989). Changes in cerebral functioning associated with normal aging. *Journal of Clinical and Experimental Neuropsychology, 11,* 918–932.

Obler, L. K., & Albert, M. L. (1981). Language and aging: A neurobehavioral analysis. In D. S. Beasley & G. A. Davis (Eds.), *Aging: Communication processes and disorders* (pp. 107–121). New York: Grune & Stratton.

Pinkston, E. M., & Linsk, N. L. (1984). *Care of the elderly: A family approach.* New York: Pergamon Press.

Salgado, E. D., Weinstein, M., Furlan, A. J., Modic, M. T., Beck, G. J., Estes, M., Awad, I., & Little, J. R. (1986). Proton magnetic resonance imaging in ischemic cerebrovascular disease. *Annals of Neurology, 20,* 502–507.

Shichita, K., Hatano, S., Ohashi, Y., Shibata, H., & Matuzaki, T. (1986). Memory changes in the Benton Visual Retention Test between ages 70 and 75. *Journal of Gerontology, 41,* 385–386.

Spar, J. E., & La Rue, J. E. (1990). *A concise guide to geriatric psychiatry.* Washington, DC: American Psychiatric Association Press.

Valdois, S., Joanette, Y., Poissant, A., Ska, B., & Dehaut, F. (1990). Heterogeneity in the cognitive profile of the elderly. *Journal of Clinical and Experimental Neuropsychology, 12,* 587–596.

Van Gorp, W. G., & Mahler, M. (1990). Subcortical features of normal aging. In J. L. Cummings (Ed.), *Subcortical dementia* (pp. 231–250). New York: Oxford University Press.

Vannieuwkirk, R. R., & Galbraith, G. G. (1985). The relationship of age to performance on the Luria–Nebraska Neuropsychological Battery. *Journal of Clinical Psychology, 41,* 527–532.

Wechsler, D. (1955). *Wechsler Adult Intelligence Scale.* New York: Psychological Corporation.

Wechsler, D. (1981). *Wechsler Adult Intelligence Scale—Revised.* New York: Psychological Corporation.

Wedding, D., & Cody, S. (1990). Neurological disorders in the elderly. In A. W. Horton, Jr. (Ed.), *Neuropsychology across the life-span* (pp. 65–79). New York: Springer.

Williams, J. M. (1987). Brief and extended neuropsychological assessment of the geriatric patient. In L. C. Hartlage, M. J. Asken, & J. L. Hornsby (Eds.), *Essentials of neuropsychological assessment* (pp. 163–174). New York: Springer.

Yesavage, J. A. (1986). The use of self-rating scales of depression in the elderly. In L. W. Poon (Ed.), *Handbook for clinical memory assessment of older adults* (pp. 213–217). Washington, DC: American Psychological Association.

Education, Gender, and Ethnicity

EDUCATION

Education has been found to be significantly related to performance on the majority of neuropsychological tests that have been assessed for this effect. Stanton *et al.* (1984) reported a significant effect on the TMT and the Logical Memory (LM) and VR subtests of the WMS. Shichita *et al.* (1986) found a significant effect for education on BVRT performance.

WAIS and WAIS-R

A substantial relationship exists between education and WAIS-R IQs. For the 16- to 74-year age spectrum of the WAIS-R standardization sample, for 16+ years of education, the mean FSIQ is 115; for 13–15 years, FSIQ = 107; for 12 years, FSIQ = 100; for 9–11 years, FSIQ = 96; for 8 years, FSIQ = 91; and for 0–7 years, FSIQ = 82 (Reynolds *et al.*, 1987). According to Kaufman (1990), the 33-point difference in FSIQ between college graduates and those with minimal formal education exceeds 2 standard deviations and is a larger range than was found for any other WAIS-R stratification variable. Obviously, the clinical interpretation of a specific IQ score would be considerably different for an individual who has 6 years of education from that for one who has a college education. Education accounts for about one third of the variance in WAIS-R FSIQ.

Kaufman (1990) found all scaled score subtest comparisons to reach a level of significance of 0.001 except for OA and DSym at ages 16–19. In order of decreasing correlation with education, the subtests were V, I, C, S, A, DSym, DS, BD, PC, PA, and OA.

Heaton *et al.* (1986) found education to account for the greatest amount of the V-WAIS subtest variance followed by I, S, C, A, DSym, BD, PC, DS, PA, and OA.

HRNB

Heaton *et al.* (1986) reported education to account for the greatest amount of the TMTB variance, followed by SSPT, Aphasia, Halstead CT, TPT Time/Block, RKSPE, FTT, Tactile Form Recognition, TPT Location, and GS.

LNNB

Education is taken into account in the calculation of the critical level (Golden *et al.*, 1985).

GENDER

Research has suggested that some spatial abilities of males are better than those of females, while the reverse is true for some verbal abilities (Maccoby & Jacklin, 1974). These differences have not always been observed in studies of gender differences on neuropsychological tests. For example, studies generally have not found significant differences between males and females on the Time, Memory, or Location scores of the TPT (Dodrill, 1979; Yeudall et al., 1987). However, Heaton et al. (1986) found that males performed significantly better than females on TPT Total Time.

WAIS-R

Kaufman (1990) has reported that males in the WAIS-R standardization sample obtained slightly but not significantly higher IQs than females. They were about 2 points higher on VIQ, $1\frac{1}{2}$ points higher on PIQ, and 2 points higher on FSIQ. On the subtests, significant differences favoring males were found for age groups in the range 20–74 years on I and A and for age groups in the range 16–54 years on BD. Females outperformed males on DSym across all age groups. Kaufman concluded that "adult males are superior to adult females in the skills assessed by Block Design and Arithmetic, and that females clearly outstrip males in the ability measured by Digit Symbol" (Kaufman, 1990, p. 157).

Research has suggested the possibility that males have different VIQ and PIQ profiles after lateralized brain damage (Matthews, 1992). Although the results of research have been mixed (Bornstein & Matarazzo, 1984; McGlone, 1977), Kaufman (1990) has determined by combining the data from eight studies that the mean PIQ > VIQ difference for males with left lesions was 6.2 points, but was 1.6 for females with left lesions. For males with right lesions, the VIQ > PIQ difference was 12 points, and for females with right lesions, $6\frac{1}{2}$ points.

HRNB

Gender differences have been found on the FTT and GS (Heaton et al., 1986). Norms taking into account age, education, and gender may be found in Heaton et al. (1991).

LNNB

Vannieuwkirk and Galbraith (1985) found the performance of males on the Motor Functions (C1) and Visual Functions (C4) of the LNNB to be significantly better than that of females.

ETHNICITY

Research on the effect of culture, ethnicity, or race on neuropsychological tests has been minimal. Puente (1990) has noted that culture, ethnicity, and race are not addressed in three of the most prominent neuropsychology textbooks. Spanish versions of the WAIS-R, LNNB, and HRNB have been developed (Puente, 1990), but few comparative studies have been reported. A Spanish version of the BDAE has also been developed and normed (Rosselli et al., 1990). Rosselli and Ardila (1991) have reported ROCFT norms for ages 56 to greater than 75 years for Spanish-speaking residents of Columbia.

Chinese versions have been developed for the WAIS-R (Dai *et al.,* 1990, 1991), LNNB (Yun *et al.,* 1987), and HRNB (Doerr & Storrie, 1981; Yao-Xian, 1986).

Numerous studies have suggested that the performance of Japanese subjects is significantly better than that of American subjects on certain visuoconstructional tasks (Lynn, 1982; Porteus, 1959; Saeki *et al.,* 1985). Lee *et al.* (1991), however, found no differences between Japanese and Americans on Three-Dimensional Block Construction (TDBC). Their results with brain-damaged patients did not uncover any differences and did not confirm the hypothesis that Japanese and Americans differ in their cerebral organization.

The mean WAIS-R FSIQ of whites is approximately $14\frac{1}{2}$ points higher than that of African-Americans (Kaufman, 1990). Differences are smallest for individuals with 0–8 years of education. A breakdown by age, gender, education, and occupation may be found in Kaufman (1990). For subtests, the differences were greatest for BD and V, followed by C, I, A, OA, PC, S, DSym, PA, and DS.

REFERENCES

Bornstein, R. A., & Matarazzo, J. D. (1984). Wechsler VIQ versus PIQ differences in cerebral dysfunction: A literature review with emphasis on sex differences. *Journal of Clinical Neuropsychology, 4,* 319–334.

Dai, X., Gong, Y., & Zhong, L. (1990). Factor analysis of the Mainland Chinese version of the Wechsler Adult Intelligence Scale. *Psychological Assessment, 2,* 31–34.

Dai, X., Ryan, J. J., Paolo, A. M., & Harrington, R. G. (1991). Sex differences on the Wechsler Adult Intelligence Scale—Revised for China. *Psychological Assessment, 3,* 282–284.

Dodrill, C. B. (1979). Sex differences on the Halstead–Reitan Neuropsychological Battery and on other neuropsychological measures. *Journal of Clinical Psychology, 35,* 236–241.

Doerr, H. O., & Storrie, M. C. (1981). Neuropsychological testing in the People's Republic of China: The Halstead–Reitan Seattle/Changsha Project. *Clinical Neuropsychology, 4,* 49–51.

Golden, C. J., Purisch, A. D., & Hammeke, T. A. (1985). *Luria–Nebraska Neuropsychological Battery: Forms I and II.* Los Angeles: Western Psychological Services.

Heaton, R. K., Grant, I., & Matthews, C. G. (1986). Differences in neuropsychological test performance associated with age, education, and sex. In I. Grant & K. M. Adams (Eds.), *Neuropsychological assessment of neuropsychiatric disorders* (pp. 100–120). New York: Oxford University Press.

Heaton, R. K., Grant, I., & Matthews, C. G. (1991). *Comprehensive norms for an expanded Halstead–Reitan Battery: Demographic corrections, research findings, and clinical applications.* Odessa, FL: Psychological Assessment Resources.

Kaufman, A. S. (1990). *Assessing adolescent and adult intelligence.* Boston: Allyn & Bacon.

Lee, G. P., Sasanuma, S., Hamsher, K., & Benton, A. L. (1991). Constructional praxis performance of Japanese and American, normal and brain-damaged patients. *Archives of Clinical Neuropsychology, 6,* 15–25.

Lynn, R. (1982). IQ in Japan and the United States shows a growing disparity. *Nature, 297,* 222–223.

Maccoby, E. E., & Jacklin, C. N. (1974). *The psychology of sex differences.* Stanford, CA: Stanford University Press.

Matthews, J. R. (1992). Sex and gender. In A. E. Puente & R. J. McCaffrey (Eds.), *Handbook of neuropsychological assessment* (pp. 121–138). New York: Plenum Press.

McGlone, J. (1977). Sex differences in the cerebral organization of verbal functions in patients with unilateral brain lesions. *Brain, 100,* 775–793.

Porteus, S. D. (1959). *The maze test and clinical psychology.* Palo Alto: Pacific Books.

Puente, A. E. (1990). Psychological assessment of minority group members. In G. Goldstein & M. Hersen (Eds.), *Handbook of psychological assessment* (2nd ed.) (pp. 505–520). New York: Pergamon Press.

Reynolds, C. R., Chastain, R. I.., Kaufman, A. S., & McLean, J. E. (1987). Demographic characteristics and IQ among adults: Analysis of the WAIS-R standardization sample as a function of the stratification variables. *Journal of School Psychology, 25,* 323–342.

Rosselli, M., & Ardila, A. (1991). Effects of age, education, and gender on the Rey–Osterrieth Complex Figure. *The Clinical Neuropsychologist, 5,* 370–376.

Rosselli, M., Ardila, A., Florez, A., & Castro, C. (1990). Normative data on the Boston Diagnostic Aphasia

Examination in a Spanish-speaking population. *Journal of Clinical and Experimental Neuropsychology, 12,* 313–322.

Saeki, K., Clark, F. A., & Azen, S. P. (1985). Performance of Japanese and Japanese-American children on the motor accuracy–revised and design copying tests of the Southern California Sensory Integration Tests. *American Journal of Occupational Therapy, 39,* 103–109.

Shichita, K., Hatano, S., Ohashi, Y., Shibata, H., & Matuzaki, T. (1986). Memory changes in the Benton Visual Retention Test between ages 70 and 75. *Journal of Gerontology, 41,* 385–386.

Stanton, B. A., Jenkins, C. D., Savageau, J. A., Zyzanski, S. J., & Aucoin, R. (1984). Age and education differences on the Trail Making Test and Wechsler Memory Scales. *Perceptual and Motor Skills, 58,* 311–318.

Vannieuwkirk, R. R., & Galbraith, G. G. (1985). The relationship of age to performance on the Luria–Nebraska Neuropsychological Battery. *Journal of Clinical Psychology, 41,* 527–532.

Yao-Xian, G. (1986). The Chinese revision of the Halstead–Reitan Neuropsychological Test Battery for adults. *Acta Psychologica Sinica, 18,* 433–442.

Yeudall, L., Reddon, J., Gill, D., & Stefanyk, W. (1987). Normative data for the Halstead–Reitan neuropsychological tests stratified by age and sex. *Journal of Clinical Psychology, 43,* 346–367.

Yun, X., Yao-Xian, G., & Matthews, J. R. (1987). The Luria–Nebraska Neuropsychological Battery revised in China. *International Journal of Clinical Neuropsychology, 9,* 97–101.

Anxiety, Amotivation, and Fatigue

ANXIETY

Anxiety may adversely influence test performance. The inverted-U function of performance vs. arousal is a well-known phenomenon in psychology (Hebb, 1958). Performance on other than extremely simple tasks is generally impaired at states of low and high arousal and is optimal at midlevels. Test anxiety can impair test performance (Sarason, 1984). Little research has been conducted on the influence of anxiety specifically on performance on neuropsychological tests. The research that has been performed has often yielded mixed or inconclusive results.

Hodges and Spielberger (1969) reported a statistically significant decrement in DS performance for high-A-state individuals. King et al. (1978) found that for women only, high A-Trait anxiety had a deleterious effect on FTT and TPT-Time. Chavez et al. (1983) did not find test anxiety to affect performance of TMTA&B, FFT, DS, or DSym. The results of these studies are of questionable relevance to clinical practice, since none of the studies used patients clinically diagnosed as suffering from anxiety.

Anxiety may be assessed by self-report inventories such as the State–Trait Anxiety Inventory (STAI) (Spielberger et al., 1983), the Taylor Manifest Anxiety Scale (Taylor, 1953), or the Self-Rating Anxiety Scale (Zung, 1971). Global ratings can be taken on the 0–100 (SUDS) scale. Electromyographic (EMG) and galvanic skin response (GSR) readings may provide an additional "window" on anxiety (Rice & Blanchard, 1982).

AMOTIVATION

Anyone who has tested patients can attest to the importance of motivation in performance on neuropsychological tests. Manuals for many neuropsychological tests instruct the examiner to "encourage the unmotivated examinee to provide a response" (Kaplan et al., 1991, p. 13), to make every effort "to encourage the subject to perform as well as his/her brain will permit" (Reitan & Wolfson, 1993, p. 40), or to provide "constant encouragement" (Golden et al., 1985, p. 7) if necessary. Despite these exhortations to motivate patients, research on the effect of motivation on neuropsychological testing is virtually nonexistent. A literature search of PsychLIT (1/83–12/91) revealed only one relevant publication. Richards and Ruff (1989) reported that when depressed and nondepressed individuals were compared under two conditions of motivation, depression but not motivation yielded an effect. Further research is needed in this area.

FATIGUE AND SLEEP DISORDERS

Sleepiness and fatigue may affect alertness and performance (Anderson & Bremer, 1987; Borland *et al.*, 1986). Performance on auditory vigilance tasks has been shown to be impaired by sleep deprivation (Glenville *et al.*, 1978). Reaction time (Wilkinson & Houghton, 1975) and memory (Williams *et al.*, 1966) may be impaired. It has been suggested that the impairments noted on vigilance and reaction time tests has been due to lapses or gaps—nonresponse periods of approximately 1 sec. (Broughton, 1982). Herscovitch *et al.* (1980) found greater perseveration on the WCST with sleep loss. During the period over which sleep time was being regained, WCST performance was characterized by increased nonperseverative errors.

Neuropsychological aspects of sleep disorders have been extensively reviewed by Pegram *et al.* (1985). Kelly *et al.* (1990) have reviewed neuropsychological aspects of sleep apnea syndrome. They reported that neuropsychological studies of persons with sleep apnea syndrome have revealed moderate cognitive deficits similar to those of persons who have experienced more prolonged hypoxia. The reader is referred to Chapter 47 of this book. Kelly *et al.* (1990, p. 334) also stated that "apneics typically perform worse on neuropsychological tests than do those individuals with other sleep disorders or healthy controls, substantiating the relationship between hypoxic events and cortical dysfunction." It should be noted, however, that Bedard *et al.* (1991) were able to distinguish a contribution of vigilance impairment from respiratory impairment. Moderate apneics differed from controls on the ROCFT:M (Immediate), PA-WAIS-R, Wechsler Intelligence Scale for Children—Revised (WISC-R) Mazes, and PPT. Severe apneics differed on these measures plus WAIS-R FSIQ, WAIS-R PIQ, DSym-WAIS-R, Letter Cancellation Test (LCT), ROCFT:M (Delayed), WMS Delayed Logical Memory, verbal fluency, ROCFT:C, BD-WAIS-R, OA-WAIS-R, and TMTB. Differences were not found for WAIS-R VIQ, HVOT, Thurstone Visual Matching Test, WMS Immediate Logical Memory, C-WAIS-R, or S-WAIS-R. Bedard *et al.* (1993) found that most cognitive impairments improved with continuous positive-airway-pressure treatment. Residual impairments were noted on mazes and the PPT.

Valley and Broughton (1983) found that narcoleptics performed significantly worse than controls on tests of vigilance and choice serial reaction, but not on the PASAT or DS. Aguirre *et al.* (1985) found no impairments for narcoleptics on DS, Knox Cubes, Recurring Figures-Nonverbal and Verbal, WMS-Logical Memory, WMS-Visual Reproduction, WMS-Paired Associate Learning, a naming test, and a verbal fluency test.

The Stanford Sleepiness Scale (SSS) (Hoddes *et al.*, 1972) may be useful for evaluating the patient's self-reported sleepiness. Level of sleepiness is reported on a 7-point Likert-type scale.

REFERENCES

Aguirre, M., Broughton, R., & Stuss, D. (1985). Does memory impairment exist in narcolepsy–cataplexy? *Journal of Clinical and Experimental Neuropsychology, 7,* 14–24.

Anderson, R. M., & Bremer, D. A. (1987). Sleep duration at home and sleepiness on the job in rotating twelve-hour shift workers. *Human Factors, 29,* 477–481.

Bedard, M., Montplaisir, J., Richer, F., Rouleau, I., & Malo, J. (1991). Obstructive sleep apnea syndrome: Pathogenesis of neuropsychological deficits. *Journal of Clinical and Experimental Neuropsychology, 13,* 950–964.

Bedard, M., Montplaisir, J., Malo, J., Richer, F., & Rouleau, I. (1993). Persistent neuropsychological deficits and vigilance impairment in sleep apnea syndrome after treatment with continuous positive airways pressure (CPAP). *Journal of Clinical and Experimental Neuropsychology, 15,* 330–341.

Borland, R. G., Rogers, A. S., Nicholson, A. N., Pascoe, P. A., & Spencer, M. B. (1986). Performance overnight in shiftworkers operating a day–night schedule. *Aviation Space and Environmental Medicine, 57,* 241–249.

Broughton, R. (1982). Human consciousness and sleep/waking rhythms: A review and some neuropsychological considerations. *Journal of Clinical Neuropsychology, 4,* 193–218.

Chavez, E. L., Brandon, A., Trautt, G. M., & Steyaert, J. (1983). Effects of test anxiety and sex of subject on neuropsychological test performance: Finger Tapping, Trail Making, Digit Span, and Digit Symbol Tests. *Perceptual and Motor Skills, 56,* 923–929.

Glenville, M., Broughton, R., Wing, A. M., & Wilkinson, R. T. (1978). Effects of sleep deprivation on short duration performance measures compared to the Wilkinson Auditory Vigilance Task. *Sleep, 1,* 169–176.

Golden, C. J., Purisch, A. D., & Hammeke, T. A. (1985). *Luria–Nebraska Neuropsychological Battery: Forms I and II.* Los Angeles: Western Psychological Corporation.

Hebb, D. O. (1958). *A textbook of psychology.* Philadelphia: W. B. Saunders.

Herscovitch, J., Stuss, D., & Broughton, R. (1980). Changes in cognitive processing following short-term cumulative partial sleep deprivation and recovery oversleeping. *Journal of Clinical Neuropsychology, 2,* 301–319.

Hoddes, E., Dement, W., & Zarcone, V. (1972). The development and use of the Stanford Sleepiness Scale (SSS). *Psychophysiology, 9,* 150.

Hodges, W. F., & Spielberger, C. D. (1969). Digit Span: An indicant of trait or state anxiety? *Journal of Consulting and Clinical Psychology, 33,* 430–434.

Kaplan, E., Fein, D., Morris, R., & Delis, D. C. (1991). *WAIS-R (NI) Manual.* San Antonio: Psychological Corporation.

Kelly, D. A., Claypoole, K. H., & Coppel, D. B. (1990). Sleep apnea syndrome: Symptomatology, associated features, and neurocognitive correlates. *Neuropsychology Review, 1,* 323–342.

King, G. D., Hannay, H. J., Masek, B. J., & Burns, J. W. (1978). Effects of anxiety and sex on neuropsychological tests. *Journal of Consulting and Clinical Psychology, 46,* 375–376.

Pegram, G. V., Connell, B. E., Gnadt, J., & Weiler, D. (1985). Neuropsychology and the field of sleep and sleep disorders. In S. B. Filskov & T. J. Boll (Eds.), *Handbook of clinical neuropsychology,* Vol. 2 (pp. 426–492). New York: Wiley-Interscience.

Reitan, R. M., & Wolfson, D. (1993). *The Halstead–Reitan Neuropsychological Test Battery: Theory and clinical interpretation* (2nd ed.). Tucson: Neuropsychology Press.

Rice, A., & Blanchard, E. (1982). Biofeedback and the treatment of anxiety disorders. *Clinical Psychology Review, 2,* 557–577.

Richards, P. M., & Ruff, R. M. (1989). Motivational effects on neuropsychological functioning: Comparison of depressed versus nondepressed individuals. *Journal of Consulting and Clinical Psychology, 57,* 396–402.

Sarason, I. G. (1984). Stress, anxiety, and cognitive interference: Reactions to tests. *Journal of Personality and Social Psychology, 46,* 929–938.

Spielberger, C. D., Gorsuch, R. L., & Lushene, R. E. (1983). *Manual for the State–Trait Anxiety Inventory (STAI).* Palo Alto, CA: Consulting Psychologist Press.

Taylor, J. (1953). A personality scale of manifest anxiety. *Journal of Abnormal and Social Psychology, 48,* 285–290.

Valley, V., & Broughton, R. (1983). The physiological (EEG) nature of drowsiness and its relation to performance deficits in narcoleptics. *Electroencephalography and Clinical Neurophysiology, 55,* 505–512.

Wilkinson, R. T., & Houghton, D. (1975). Portable four-choice reaction time test with magnetic tape memory. *Behavioral Research Methods and Instrumentation, 7,* 441–446.

Williams, H. L., Geiseking, C. F., & Lubin, A. (1966). Some effects of sleep loss on memory. *Perceptual and Motor Skills, 23,* 1287–1293.

Zung, W. (1971). A rating instrument for anxiety disorders. *Psychosomatics, 12,* 371–379.

Assessment Strategies and Instruments

Part III reviews the data-gathering methods and instruments used in a neuropsychological evaluation. The data-gathering methods include review of records, interview, behavioral observation, and formal testing. Many of the more popular tests are reviewed. The tests are organized according to their primary area of assessment. The areas are arranged as they might be in a neuropsychological report: Mental Status Evaluation, Orientation, Attention, Memory, Intelligence, General Knowledge, Social Understanding, Speech and Language, Arithmetic, Visual–Spatial Functioning, Tactile Functioning, Motor Functioning, Executive Functioning, Malingering, and Personality. Some of these categories of functioning are further broken down into subcategories. Within each category, the Wechsler and Halstead–Reitan Tests generally are reviewed first, followed by Benton and miscellaneous tests. The Luria–Nebraska scales are reviewed last. Each test is reviewed according to the outline presented below.

Test Title

Microdescription

This is a brief, one-sentence description of the test for quick reference. It may be suitable for use as a "macro" in a test-report word processor.

Primary Assessment Areas

This section lists primary areas of functioning assessed by the test. The listing is not necessarily in order of importance; some of the listings are simply different ways of referring to the same functioning. The lists were constructed on the basis of the area of functioning purported to be assessed by the test, validity studies, or—in some cases—an operational description of the test with the appearance of face validity. The lack of sufficient, in-depth validity studies for most neuropsychological tests (Franzen, 1989) prohibited the sole use of validity studies in determining the areas of functioning assessed by the tests. This heading may assist the practitioner in selecting tests to assess a particular area of functioning and in test interpretation.

Secondary Assessment Areas

Categories of functioning are listed that are not the primary areas of functioning purported to be assessed by the test but that may be required to perform adequately on the test.

Presentation Modalities

Modalities in which the test instructions and stimuli are presented are listed under this heading. Possible modalities include visual, auditory, or tactile. Each of these may involve verbal or nonverbal material. This information may assist the practitioner in either assessing these modalities or avoiding them in patients with severe impairments (see Chapter 6).

Response Modalities

This heading lists the motor or cognitive modalities or both required for a response. A test may be *timed* (i.e., a higher score is obtained for a faster time or greater production in a specific period of time), *time-limited* (i.e., a set time period is allowed for the completion of the task), *paced* (i.e., the responses must keep up with a set pace), or *untimed* (i.e., no time limit is placed on completion of the task). As with the Presentation Modalities, this information may assist the practitioner in either assessing these modalities or avoiding them in patients with severe impairments (see Chapter 6).

Description

The materials, method of administration, and scoring are briefly described. Since this description will often be a very brief and truncated summary, it will generally be inadequate for actual test administration and scoring. It should not be used in place of the test manual.

Localization

The sensitivity of the test to brain dysfunction and the ability of the test to localize brain lesions are reviewed.

Norms

Sources where norms may be obtained are listed. The breakdown of each normative sample by demographic group is noted.

Source

The company or publication where the instrument may be obtained is noted. Addresses for sources are in Appendix D.

REFERENCE

Franzen, M. (1989). *Reliability and validity in neuropsychological assessment.* New York: Plenum Press.

Records Review

A review of relevant records is an essential part of the information-gathering process of the neuropsychological evaluation. In addition to the physician's medical appraisal of the patient, a wealth of information about the patient's physical, cognitive, emotional, social, self-care, and community functioning is available in the reports and notes of the health professionals who treat the patient. Knowledge and understanding of these records are essential for the neuropsychologist who is a member of a hospital treatment team. Records about the patient's premorbid activities can assist in the estimation of premorbid functioning. If the patient has been injured, the circumstances of the accident and emergency care can assist in understanding the patient's condition.

PHYSICIAN'S EXAMINATION AND REPORT

The physician's history and physical can be a valuable source of information about the patient (Bates, 1979). Of special interest are the chief complaints, history, medications, neurological examination, reports of laboratory test abnormalities, brain scans, EEGs, impression, plan, and diagnosis. The examination and report generally run as follows:

Identifying Data
Source of Referral
Chief Complaints

History

History of Present Illness. This is a chronological account of the problems for which the patient is seeking care.

Past Medical History. The patient's general state of health, childhood illnesses, immunizations, adult illnesses, operations, injuries, hospitalizations, and habits such as eating, sleeping, tobacco use, alcohol use, and drug use are reported.

Medications
Allergies
Family Medical History

Social History. Lifestyle, home situation, significant others, typical day, schooling, military service, job history, financial situation, and recreation are described.

Physical Examination

The physical systems are reviewed.

General Appearance. Stature, dress, grooming, weight, posture, gait, and manner are reported.

Vital Signs. Pulse, respiratory rate, blood pressure, and temperature are recorded.

Skin. The color, vascularity, lesions, edema, and moisture of the skin are noted.

HEENT. Evaluation of the head, eyes, ears, nose, and throat is reported.

Neck

Thorax and Lungs

Heart

Extremities. The musculoskeletal system is examined and abnormalities are noted.

Neurological Examination. Cranial nerves, motor exam, sensory exam, and cerebellar exam are included in this category. This exam is described in more detail below.

Laboratory Tests and Scans. Routine laboratory tests include a urinalysis, complete blood cell count (CBC), and blood chemistries (Byrne *et al.,* 1986; Ravel, 1984). The blood chemistries may include measures of electrolytes, liver function, and kidney function such as blood urea nitrogen (BUN) and creatinine. Indices related to impaired protein synthesis (prothrombin time, partial thromboplastin time, and serum albumin) have been found to be related to the presence of deficiencies in language efficiency, perception, and psychomotor performance seen in subclinical hepatic encephalopathy (Moss *et al.,* 1992). BUN and blood ammonia have been found to be related to visual–spatial impairment. X rays and various scans may be reported. Tests of special relevance to neurological functioning are reviewed below.

Assessment/Impression

Treatment Plan

Diagnosis

Neurological Examination

A neurological evaluation will involve taking a history and conducting a physical, but will, of course, focus on neurological impairments. It generally runs as follows (Bickerstaff & Spillane, 1989; DeMyer, 1980):

Handedness, level of consciousness, orientation, and degree of cooperation are recorded. Neck stiffness is assessed, followed by evaluation of the cranial nerves.

Cranial Nerves. The first cranial nerve (olfactory nerve) is assessed via the presentation of odors. Assessment of the visual pathway and the second cranial nerve (optic nerve) involves testing of visual acuity, visual fields, and examination of fundi. The third (oculomotor), fourth (trochlear), and sixth (abducent) cranial nerves are evaluated by examining pupils and ocular movements and testing for nystagmus. Assessment of the fifth cranial nerve (trigeminal) includes testing of superficial, facial skin sensation, corneal reflexes, jaw jerk reflex, and temporal muscles and masseters. The seventh cranial nerve (facial) is evaluated by examining facial muscles and taste. Testing of the eighth cranial nerve (auditory) is accomplished by examining hearing, by tests utilizing the placement of tuning forks (Rinne's test and Weber's test), and by tests of vestibular functioning. The ninth (glossopharyngeal) and tenth (vagus) cranial nerves are assessed by examining the gag reflex, the muscles of the palate, and the vocal cords. Testing of the eleventh cranial nerve (accessory) is accomplished by assessing trapezius and sternomastoid muscles. The twelfth cranial nerve (hypoglossal) is evaluated by exam observing tongue protrusion.

Motor System. The motor system (arms, trunk, and legs) is evaluated for deformities, wasting, fasciculation, involuntary movements, loss of tone, and weakness.

Sensory System. Sensitivity to pain, temperature, light touch, position, and vibration is evaluated. Stereognosis, graphesthesia, and two-point discrimination are assessed.

Reflexes. These include biceps jerk, supinator jerk, triceps jerk, finger jerk, abdominal reflexes, knee jerk, ankle jerk, and plantar reflexes.

Coordination, stance, gait, leg-raising, carotid pulses, skull, and spine are also assessed. A neurological evaluation will generally contain an extended mental status evaluation with some brief tests of areas of cognitive functioning (Strub & Black, 1985).

Electroencephalography (EEG)

Fluctuations in the electrical activity of the brain are recorded via 8, 16, or more scalp electrodes (Adams & Victor, 1989; Fisch, 1991). Amplified potentials move pens that reproduce the waveform of the brain electrical activity on a moving roll of paper. The resultant graph of pattern or voltage vs. time is called the electroencephalogram (EEG). A resting EEG may be taken with the patient relaxed and with eyes closed. Activating procedures may be carried out to reveal abnormalities: (1) breathing 20 times/min for 3 min, (2) a strobe light flashing at 1–20 times/sec, and (3) sleep. Delta waves occur at less than $f = 4$/sec and have an amplitude of $V = 50$–$350 \, \mu$V. For theta waves, $f = 4$–7/sec and $V = 50$–$350 \, \mu$V; for alpha waves, $f = 8$–13/sec and $V \approx 50 \, \mu$V; and for beta waves, $f > 13$/sec and $V = 10$–$20 \, \mu$V. Higher-voltage, faster waves are termed "spikes." The EEG is commonly used to assist in the diagnosis of seizure disorders, but abnormalities may be noted in a variety of neurological disorders.

Evoked Responses

Brainstem Auditory Evoked Response (BAER). A series of clicks is introduced through earphones. The electrical response to each click is measured via surface electrodes as it travels through the synaptic connections at brainstem nuclei. The latencies between peaks at each brainstem level are recorded. BAER testing is useful in assessing the integrity of the brainstem (Adams & Victor, 1989).

Visual Evoked Response (VER). A light is flashed on the retina. The electrical response is measured as impulses traverse the optic pathway. This technique may reveal lesions in the visual system (Adams & Victor, 1989).

Somatosensory Evoked Potential (SEP or SSEP). Painless electrical stimuli at 5/sec are applied over peripheral nerves and are recorded en route to and at the contralateral parietal cortex. Delays between various points may suggest dysfunction (Adams & Victor, 1989).

Computed Tomography (CT)

In CT of the head, a thin beam of X rays is passed through the head to a receptor (Rutledge, 1989). The device rotates around the subject, and a computer algorithm constructs a two-dimensional image. A series of two-dimensional images or sections is produced. The greatest attenuation of X rays is represented as white and the least as black. Therefore, bone is white, water is gray, and air is black. CT permits visual separation of cerebrospinal fluid (CSF), blood, brain parenchyma, and blood clots (Reitan & Wolfson, 1985). CT scan with contrast enhancement involves the injection of a contrast medium and may improve the visualization of some structures.

Magnetic Resonance Imaging (MRI)

MRI capitalizes on the fact that nuclei spin and create magnetic fields and orient when placed in a magnetic field (Rutledge, 1989). When sections of the organ to be imaged are stimulated with radiofrequency waves, the nuclei absorb energy and change orientation. When the radiofrequency source is turned off, the energy is released as radiofrequency signals that may be detected and processed into images. Different characteristics of the signals yield T1-weighted and T2-weighted images. In T1-weighted images, fat or subacute hemorrhage appears white and fluid such as CSF appears black. In T2-weighted images, fat appears gray, iron appears black, and fluid appears white. A more thorough but accessible explanation of MRI can be found in *Understanding MRI* (Newhouse & Weiner, 1991).

Lumbar Puncture

In lumbar puncture, a needle is advanced between the lumbar vertebrae into the lumbar interspace and into the subarachnoid space. Lumbar puncture may be performed to obtain pressure measurements and to obtain a sample of CSF for cellular, chemical, and bacteriological examination (Adams & Victor, 1989). Lumbar puncture carries an added risk when CSF pressure is high. The possibility of brain herniation is increased. An examination of the fluid provides information as to whether there are abnormal amounts of red or white blood cells, proteins, glucose, and other constituents. Normal values and disorders associated with abnormal values may be found in Adams and Victor (1989).

Skull X Rays

Plain X-ray films of the skull may reveal fractures, but the use of simple X rays is dwindling due to increased use of the much more informative CT and MRI scans.

Angiography

A radiopaque contrast medium is introduced and injected to visualize the arch of the aorta and the origins of the carotid and vertebral systems. Angiography is used primarily to diagnose vascular disorders such as aneurysms, vascular malformations, and occluded arteries and veins. There is some risk to the procedure. Adams and Victor (1989) reported that approximately 1% of their patients had a worsening of their condition or even a frank ischemic lesion in the territory of the catheterized artery. Vascular spasm and occlusion may occur and clots may form on the catheter tip and embolize the artery.

Myelography

A radiopaque substance is introduced through a lumbar puncture needle, and the patient is tipped on a tilt table. The spinal subarachnoid space may be visualized.

Ultrasound

Ultrasound at frequencies of 4–8 MHz is used to generate an image (Matthews & Arnold, 1991). At interphases between two tissues, a portion of the beam is reflected or echoed. Denser structures result in greater reflection. Ultrasound is used to image the carotid arteries and, using the Doppler effect, blood flow.

Positron Emission Tomography (PET)

PET uses neutron-deficient radioisotopes of carbon, oxygen, nitrogen, or fluorine. The isotopes emit positrons that collide with electrons and produce two detectable photons. PET scanners produce pseudocolor-coded tomographic images of the radioactivity distributions after the isotopes have been introduced into the brain. An advantage of PET is that it allows imaging of the cerebral metabolic rate for glucose, regional cerebral blood flow (rCBF), and oxygen consumption (Pawlik & Heiss, 1989). Since the radioisotopes used for PET decay rapidly, they must be produced by a nearby cyclotron. PET is not available in most hospitals.

Single Photon Emission Computed Tomography (SPECT)

Gamma-emitting ^{123}I-labeled amines may be imaged using transaxial tomographic technology with a standard gamma camera. A representation of cerebral blood flow may be produced using this technology. Emission is greatest, and appears dark in a black and white image, in the cortical gray matter, which has four times the blood flow of the white matter. Emission is also greater in the basal ganglia and thalamus. Areas of decreased blood flow are white and appear as "cold spots" (Orrison, 1989).

Brain Electrical Activity Mapping (BEAM)

In BEAM, 20 electrodes are attached to the surface of the scalp, and the information obtained is used to estimate the electrical potentials at areas not directly measured by the electrode as well as that at the electrode site (Desmedt, 1986). A multicolored topographic map of electrical brain activity is the ultimate product of the procedure. The data that are mapped may be raw EEG data, spectrally analyzed data, or evoked potential data (Duffy, 1986).

NURSING EVALUATION AND REPORT

The nursing evaluation and report will generally contain information on vital signs, bowel and bladder function, skin integrity, mental status, and self-care skills (Pires & Kelly-Hayes, 1990). The mental status and self-care skills or activities of daily living (ADLs) information of the report is most useful to the neuropsychologist. In trauma and neurological units, nurses often perform neurochecks and track mental status. For head-injury patients, this monitoring often provides a picture of the patient emerging from coma. The self-care portion of the nursing report contains information on the degree and type of assistance needed for hygiene, washing, dressing, and ambulation. A judgment is made about the patient's ability to self-administer his or her medication. The inpatient nursing staff are continually interacting with the patient. The nursing notes and reports about the patient's behavior may contain valuable behavioral observations. Notes made during the evening when there are fewer structured activities and families may be present may be especially helpful.

SOCIAL WORK EVALUATION AND REPORT

The social work evaluation may contain a social history and an accounting of the social, financial, and institutional resources available to the patient. It may also address family dynamics and problems.

SPEECH THERAPY EVALUATION AND REPORT

The speech therapy report may contain a comprehensive evaluation of speech/language functioning (Simmons, 1990). The report may contain information on attention, memory, thinking, and judgment. An assessment of oral–motor functioning and swallowing to rule out dysphagia may be performed and reported when appropriate.

OCCUPATIONAL THERAPY EVALUATION AND REPORT

The occupational therapy evaluation may contain information on upper extremity sensorimotor functioning, self-care skills, basic ability to communicate and use the telephone, homemaking abilities, money management, ability to use transportation, basic cognition–orientation, and visuospatial skills. Occupational therapists may also evaluate specialized occupational abilities and driving ability. The patient's goals will also be in the report.

PHYSICAL THERAPY EVALUATION AND REPORT

The physical therapy evaluation usually contains information about ambulation, the ability of the patient to transfer, bed mobility, and strength. Observations of the patient's general cognitive functioning, safety awareness, and impulsivity may be recorded.

THERAPEUTIC RECREATION EVALUATION AND REPORT

The therapeutic recreation report and notes may contain observations on the patient's cognitive and emotional status and his or her ability to interact meaningfully with others and participate in group activities (Humphrey, 1990). Observations of the appropriateness of the patient's behavior on therapeutic recreation community outings may be especially valuable.

ADDITIONAL RECORDS

It is important to obtain records regarding the patient's premorbid activities and level of functioning. Due to the nature of the referral question and time constraints, it may not always be necessary or feasible to do so. If the patient has been in an accident, it may also be useful to obtain police, ambulance, and emergency room reports. For a forensic neuropsychological evaluation, it is essential to obtain all this information.

School Records

If possible, educational records should be obtained to supplement, and with the hope of corroborating, the reports of the patient and family. In addition to grades, the records may contain the results of standardized testing that may be helpful in determining the patient's premorbid level of functioning.

Employment Records

Work records provide independent information about the patient's performance on the job and the requirements of the patient's work. This information can be helpful in determining the patient's premorbid level of functioning, in making a judgment about readiness to return to work, and in planning a remediation program to prepare the patient for return to work.

Police and Ambulance Records

If the patient has been in an accident, it may also be useful to obtain police, ambulance, and emergency room reports. These documents can assist the examiner in determining the circumstances of the accident and the severity of any initial mental status changes such as loss of consciousness, GCS ratings, and others.

REFERENCES

Adams, R. D., & Victor, M. (1989). *Principles of neurology* (4th ed.). New York: McGraw-Hill.

Bates, B. (1979). *A guide to physical examination* (2nd ed.). Philadelphia: Lippincott.

Bickerstaff, E. R., & Spillane, J. A. (1989). *The neurological examination in clinical practice.* Oxford: Blackwell Scientific Publications.

Byrne, C. J., Saxton, D. F., Pelikan, P. K., & Nugent, P. M. (1986). *Laboratory tests: Implications for nursing care.* Reading, MA: Addison-Wesley.

DeMyer, W. (1980). *Technique of the neurologic examination* (3rd ed.). New York: McGraw-Hill.

Desmedt, J. E. (1986). Color imaging of scalp somatosensory evoked potential fields. In F. H. Duffy (Ed.), *Topographic mapping of brain electrical activity* (pp. 1–6). Boston: Butterworths.

Duffy, F. H. (1986). Brain electrical activity mapping: Issues and answers. In F. H. Duffy (Ed.), *Topographic mapping of brain electrical activity* (pp. 401–417). Boston: Butterworths.

Fisch, B. J. (1991). *Spehlmann's EEG primer* (2nd ed.). Amsterdam: Elsevier.

Humphrey, F. (1990). Therapeutic recreation. In D. A. Umphred (Ed.), *Neurological rehabilitation* (2nd ed.) (pp. 811–821). St. Louis: C. V. Mosby.

Matthews, P. M., & Arnold, D. L. (Eds.). (1991). *Diagnostic tests in neurology.* New York: Churchill-Livingston.

Moss, H. B., & Tarter, R. E., Yao, J. K., & Van Thiel, D. H. (1992). Subclinical hepatic encephalopathy: Relationship between neuropsychological deficits and standard laboratory tests assessing hepatic status. *Archives of Clinical Neuropsychology, 7,* 419–429.

Newhouse, J. H., & Weiner, J. I. (1991). *Understanding MRI.* Boston: Little, Brown.

Orrison, Jr., W. W. (1989). *Introduction to neuroimaging.* Boston: Little, Brown.

Pawlik, G., & Heiss, W. D. (1989). Positron emission tomography and neuropsychological function. In E. D. Bigler, R. A. Yeo, & E. Turkenheimer (Eds.), *Neuropsychological function and brain imaging* (pp. 65–138). New York: Plenum Press.

Pires, M., & Kelly-Hayes, M. (1990). Collaborative nursing therapies for clients with neurological dysfunction. In D. A. Umphred (Ed.), *Neurological rehabilitation* (2nd ed.) (pp. 791–810). St. Louis: C. V. Mosby.

Ravel, R. (1984). *Clinical laboratory medicine: Clinical application of laboratory data* (4th ed.). Chicago: Year Book Medical Publishers.

Reitan, R. M., & Wolfson, D. (1985). *Neuroanatomy and neuropathology: A clinical guide for neuropsychologists.* Tucson: Neuropsychology Press.

Rutledge, J. N. (1989). Neuroanatomy and neuropathology: Computed tomography and magnetic resonance imaging correlates. In E. D. Bigler, R. A. Yeo, & E. Turkenheimer (Eds.), *Neuropsychological function and brain imaging* (pp. 13–46). New York: Plenum Press.

Simmons, N. N. (1990). Disorders in oral, speech, and language functions. In D. A. Umphred (Ed.), *Neurological rehabilitation* (2nd ed.) (pp. 683–703). St. Louis: C. V. Mosby.

Strub, R. L., & Black, F. W. (1985). *The mental status examination in neurology* (2nd ed.). Philadelphia: F. A. Davis.

12

Interview

An extensive interview of the patient and significant others is an essential part of the neuropsy-chological evaluation. A suggested Neuropsychological Interview Form is outlined in Appendix B. The form lists categories of information to be obtained from interviewees or from records. It may be helpful to use different color inks to identify the source of each piece of information. By obtaining the same type of information from sources other than the patient, the patient's reliability, remote memory, and self-knowledge may be assessed.

The patient is generally asked about his or her symptoms and medical condition. The last clear memory before injury and the first continuous memory after injury are solicited in order to determine the existence and duration of retrograde and posttraumatic amnesia, respectively. Pre- vs. postinjury levels of functioning are determined. Developmental, educational, occupational, military, recreational, substance use, family, and marital histories are obtained.

A form for history-taking may also be found in Spreen and Strauss (1991). The *Neuropsy-chological Status Examination* is an interview form published by Psychological Assessment Resources (1983a). The *Neuropsychological Symptom Checklist,* to be filled out by the patient, is also available (Psychological Assessment Resources, 1983b). The interview may be supplemented by formal instruments such as the Vineland Adaptive Behavior Scales (Sparrow *et al.,* 1984), a semistructured interview administered to the patient's significant other or primary care-taker and used to assess adaptive abilities. Wolfson (1985) has authored the *Neuropsychological History Questionnaire,* which is completed by the patient or a significant other. Berent (1991) has provided a neuropsychological interview information form. The *Cognitive Behavior Rating Scales* (Williams, 1987) are filled out by someone who knows the patient well on the basis of his or her observations of the patient. Scales include Language Deficit, Apraxia, Disorientation, Agitation, Need for Routine, Depression, Higher Cognitive Deficits, Memory Disorder, and Dementia.

REFERENCES

Berent, S. (1991). Modern approaches to neuropsychological testing. In D. Smith, Treiman, D. M. & M. Trimble (Eds.), *Advances in neurology,* Volume 55 (pp. 423–437). New York: Raven Press.

Psychological Assessment Resources (1983a). *Neuropsychological Status Examination (NSE).* Odessa, FL: Psychological Assessment Resources.

Psychological Assessment Resources (1983b). *Neuropsychological Symptom Checklist (NSC).* Odessa, FL: Psychological Assessment Resources.

Sparrow, S. S., Balla, D. A., & Cicchetti, D. V. (1984). *Vineland Adaptive Behavior Scale*. Circle Pines, MN: American Guidance Service.

Spreen, O., & Strauss, E. (1991). *A compendium of neuropsychological tests: Administration, norms, and commentary*. New York: Oxford University Press.

Williams, J. M. (1987). *Cognitive Behavior Rating Scales: Manual*. Odessa, FL: Psychological Assessment Resources.

Wolfson, D. (1985). *Neuropsychological History Questionnaire*. Tuscon: Neuropsychology Press.

Behavioral Observations

Behavioral observations are an important source of information in a neuropsychological evaluation. If the patient is an outpatient, observation begins with the patient's arrival at the appointment. Pertinent questions include: (1) Is the patient accompanied or did he or she come to the appointment alone? (2) If alone, what mode of transportation was used? (3) Did the patient arrive on time? The answers to these and similar questions may provide information about the patient's ability to function independently. The patient's general physical presentation should be noted. This presentation may include his or her physical build, grooming, dress, and ambulation. Careful observation should be made of speech, including rate, tone, volume, prosody, and quantity. The quality of speech should be evaluated for content and relevancy. Of course, errors suggestive of dysarthria or dysphasia should be recorded. The patient's ability to relate to the interviewer and participate in the interview process should be noted. Appropriate notes may include observations of the patient's body language, eye contact, interpersonal warmth, and cooperativeness.

Behavioral observations should be made throughout neuropsychological testing. The patient's level of motivation, including variations during the testing, should be noted. Speed of performance, ability to follow instructions, cooperativeness, ability to attend and concentrate, and perseverance in the face of difficulty or failure should be observed. The effect of encouragement on the patient's performance should be noted. Disruptions that occur during the testing should be recorded, as should any nonstandard administrations of tests that are performed.

Mental Status Evaluation

The mental status examination takes many forms. In psychiatry, the mental status examination may involve an appraisal of the patient's appearance, observations of motor behavior, attitude toward the examiner, speech, and thought process, and assessment of mood, feelings, and affect (Kaplan & Sadock, 1981). Orientation, memory, judgment, and insight are also assessed. A neurologically focused mental status examination may involve a more extended assessment of areas of cognitive functioning. A description of one such evaluation may be found in *The Mental Status Examination in Neurology* (Strub and Black, 1985).

The term "mental status examination" is also used to refer to brief evaluations of cognitive functioning. Numerous tests have been developed: Mini-Mental State Examination (MMSE) (Folstein *et al.*, 1975), Neurobehavioral Cognitive Status Examination (NCSE) (Northern California Neurobehavioral Group, 1988), Short Portable Mental Status Questionnaire (Pfeiffer, 1975), Cognitive Capacity Screening Examination (CCSE) (Jacobs *et al.*, 1977), and Modified Mini-Mental State Examination (3MS) (Teng & Chui, 1987). The MMSE and the NCSE are described below.

MINI-MENTAL STATE EXAMINATION (MMSE)

The MMSE is a cognitive screening test that consists of 11 items and requires 5–10 min to administer. The items involve orientation, repetition of three objects, serial sevens or spelling the word "world" backward, recall of three objects, object-naming, sentence repetition, following a three-stage command, reading and obeying "close your eyes," writing a sentence, and copying a design (Folstein *et al.*, 1975). A maximum score of 30 points is possible.

The MMSE has commonly been used as a screening instrument for delirium or dementia. It is routinely included by some neuropsychologists in their assessments (Orsini *et al.*, 1988). Nelson *et al.* (1986), in their review of ten studies with the MMSE, reported that patients with clinically diagnosed delirium or dementia will have scores of less than 24 at least 75% of the time. Nonpsychotic psychiatric inpatients without diagnosed organic mental disorders usually obtain scores of 20 or higher. Depression with cognitive impairment resulted in scores of less than 24 but greater than 10. Studies generally revealed that 25–50% of patients with radiologically diagnosed cerebral disease may obtain scores of 24 or higher—a high false-negative rate. Nelson *et al.* (1986) have suggested that cognitive screening instruments such as the MMSE are not sufficiently sensitive to reliably detect cognitive deficits that are not obvious clinically.

A high false-positive rate has been observed in some populations. Anthony *et al.* (1982) reported that all false-positive scores in a medical inpatient population had no more than 8 years of education. Age was also found to affect test results. Cavanaugh and Wettstein (1983) found main effects for race and socioeconomic status on MMSE scores. These results suggest that correction factors for variables such as age and education might increase diagnostic utility. Spencer and Folstein (1987) have reported 5th percentile scores for several populations: 18–44 years = 26, 45–64 years = 22, 65 and over = 17; 0–8 years education = 17 and 9 or more years education = 26. Crum *et al.* (1993) have published norms for ages 18 through 85 or older at 5-year intervals crossed with education.

NEUROBEHAVIORAL COGNITIVE STATUS EXAMINATION (NCSE)

The NCSE is a brief cognitive screening test that provides a profile of cognitive functioning (Kiernan *et al.,* 1987; Northern California Neurobehavioral Group, 1988). The NCSE uses independent tests to assess orientation, attention, comprehension, repetition, naming, constructions, memory, calculations, similarities, and judgment. In each subtest, the patient is first presented with a difficult screening item that, if passed, grants the maximal score or near the maximal score for the subtest. If the screen is failed, a ''metric'' or series of items of graded difficulty is presented.

The subtests are as follows: *Orientation* is assessed in the usual manner for person, place, and time. *Attention* is evaluated with digit repetition forward. Oral language, *Comprehension,* and complex motor praxis are evaluated with one- to three-step commands. In the *Repetition* subtest, the patient is required to repeat orally presented phrases and sentences. *Naming* is assessed by requiring the patient to name parts of an object or line drawings of objects. *Constructions* requires the patient to draw geometric figures immediately after presentation or to copy colored designs using flat red and white pieces. For *Memory,* the patient is required to repeat four words and subsequently either recall them without cuing, recall them with a categorical cue, or recognize them when presented with two foils. *Calculations* are assessed via orally presented arithmetic problems. On the *Similarities* subtest, the patient is asked to state in what way two concepts are alike. ''What would you do if . . .'' questions are asked in the *Judgment* subtest. Administration time is from 5 to 20 min.

Cutoff scores for each subtest may be found in the *NCSE Manual* (Northern California Neurobehavioral Group, 1988). A patient is impaired in an area of cognition if he or she scores below the cutoff value for that area. Schwamm *et al.* (1987) found 28 of 30 neurosurgical patients to be impaired using this criterion. They found the NCSE to be more sensitive to brain damage than the MMSE or the CCSE.

Anderson (1991) found cognitive impairment on the NCSE in 29 of 32 closed head-injury patients. A factor analysis yielded four factors. Orientation, Constructions, Memory, and Similarities loaded most heavily on Factor 1, which was labeled *Memory.* Calculations and Attention loaded negatively on Factor 2—labeled *Distractibility.* Comprehension, Repetition, and Naming loaded negatively on Factor 3—labeled *Dysphasia.* Only Judgment loaded heavily on Factor 4—*Judgment.* Anderson (1991) concluded that the NCSE requires a minimal investment of clinician time and makes minimal demands on the patient, yet provides an informative profile of cognitive functioning.

REFERENCES

Anderson, R. M. (1991). Neurobehavioral Cognitive Status Examination: A factor analytic study of head-injury patients. *Journal of Clinical and Experimental Neuropsychology, 13,* 416.

Anthony, J. C., Le Resche, L., Niaz, U., Von Korff, M. R., & Folstein, M. F. (1982). Limits of the "Mini-Mental State" as a screening test for dementia and delirium among hospital patients. *Psychological Medicine, 12,* 397–408.

Cavanaugh, S. V., & Wettstein, R. M. (1983). The relationship between severity of depression, cognitive dysfunction, and age in medical inpatients. *American Journal of Psychiatry, 140,* 495–496.

Crum, R. M., Anthony, J. C., Bassett, S. S., & Folstein, M. F. (1993). Population-based norms for the Mini-Mental State Examination by age and education level. *JAMA, 269,* 2386–2391.

Folstein, M. F., Folstein, S. E., & McHugh, P. R. (1975). Mini-mental state: A practical method for grading the cognitive state of patients for the clinician. *Journal of Psychiatric Research, 12,* 189–198.

Jacobs, J. W., Bernhard, M. R., Delgado, A., & Strain, J. J. (1977). Screening for organic mental syndromes in the medically ill. *Annals of Internal Medicine, 86,* 40–46.

Kaplan, H. I., & Sadock, B. J. (1981). *Modern synopsis of comprehensive textbook of psychiatry/III* (3rd ed.). Baltimore: Williams & Wilkins.

Kiernan, R. J., Mueller, J., Langston, J. W., & Van Dyke, C. (1987). The Neurobehavioral Cognitive Status Examination: A brief but differentiated approach to cognitive assessment. *Annals of Internal Medicine, 107,* 481–485.

Nelson, A., Fogel, B. S., & Faust, D. (1986). Bedside cognitive screening instruments: A critical assessment. *Journal of Nervous and Mental Disease, 174,* 73–83.

Northern California Neurobehavioral Group (1988). *Neurobehavioral Cognitive Status Examination: Manual.* Fairfax, CA: Northern California Neurobehavioral Group.

Orsini, D. L., Van Gorp, W. G., & Boone, K. B. (1988). *The neuropsychology casebook.* New York: Springer-Verlag.

Pfeiffer, E. (1975). A short portable mental status questionnaire for the assessment of organic brain deficit in elderly patients. *Journal of the American Geriatric Society, 23,* 433–441.

Schwamm, L. H., Van Dyke, C., Kiernan, R. J., Merrin, E. L., & Mueller, J. (1987). The Neurobehavioral Cognitive Status Examination: Comparison with the Cognitive Capacity Screening Examination and the Mini-Mental State Examination in a neurosurgical population. *Annals of Internal Medicine, 107,* 486–491.

Spencer, M. P., & Folstein, M. F. (1987). The Mini-Mental State Examination. In P. A. Keller, & L. G. Ritt (Eds.), *Innovations in clinical practice: A source book,* Volume 2 (pp. 305–310). Sarasota, FL: Professional Resource Exchange.

Strub, R. L., & Black, F. W. (1985). *The mental status examination in neurology* (2nd ed.). Philadelphia: F. A. Davis.

Teng, E. L., & Chui, H. C. (1987). The Modified Mini-Mental State (3MS) Examination. *Journal of Clinical Psychiatry, 48,* 314–317.

Orientation

Orientation is knowledge of basic personal attributes (e.g., name, age, birth date) and of one's locus in space and time (Berrios, 1983; Strub & Black, 1985). Orientation is dependent on attention and memory (recent and remote) being at least minimally intact (Lezak, 1983).

After an insult to the brain, recovery of orientation generally occurs as follows: (1) orientation to person, (2) orientation to place, and (3) orientation to time (Daniel *et al.*, 1987). If knowledge of year is impaired, the year is usually displaced backward in time (Benson & Geschwind, 1967; Liddle & Crow, 1984). Time reorientation appears to proceed from past to present (Daniel *et al.*, 1987).

TEMPORAL ORIENTATION TEST (TOT)

Microdescription. Assesses knowledge of day, date, and time (Benton *et al.*, 1983).

Primary Assessment Areas. Temporal orientation.

Secondary Assessment Areas. (1) Verbal comprehension; (2) verbal expression; (3) memory.

Presentation Modalities. (1) Auditory–verbal; (2) adaptation: The test might be presented in the visual–verbal modality by allowing the examinee to read the test questions.

Response Modalities. (1) Speech; (2) writing; (3) untimed; (4) adaptation: The patient might be allowed to respond by *pointing* to the date on a calendar, the day in a list of days of the week, and the time on a clock face. The norms cited below may not apply.

Description. The patient is asked the date (month, day, and year), the day of the week, and the time. In scoring, 1 error point is scored for each day from the correct day of the week to a maximum of 3 and for each day from the correct day of the month to a maximum of 15. For each month from the correct month, 5 error points are scored. For each year from the correct year, 10 error points are scored to a maximum of 60. (For month and year, no error is scored if the date is within 15 days of the correct date.) For each 30 min from the correct time, 1 error point is scored to a maximum of 5. The patient's score is total error points. The test allows for an objective appraisal of temporal orientation via comparison with norms (Benton *et al.*, 1983).

Localization. A locus for this function has not been determined. There appears to be some relationship to nonspecific impairment of brain functioning (Benton *et al.*, 1964). Bilateral lesions may be suggested by significantly impaired performance on this test (Benton,

1968). Although schizophrenic patients may be impaired on the TOT, they are less likely to exhibit impairment than brain-damaged patients (Joslyn & Hutzell, 1979).

   Norms (Benton *et al.,* 1983)

                  3 = Borderline (exceeded by 93% of normative group)
            4–7 = Moderately defective (exceeded by 95% of normative group)
            >8 = Severely defective (exceeded by 99.4% of normative group)
  Frequent error = Miss day of the month by one or more days
               = Miss time of day by more than 30 min
  Infrequent error = Miss year or month

   Source. Oxford University Press.

INFORMATION AND ORIENTATION QUESTIONS (O-WMS-R)

   Microdescription. The patient must answer questions about orientation, basic biographical information, and general information.

   Primary Assessment Areas. (1) Orientation to person, place, and time; (2) knowledge of general information.

   Secondary Assessment Areas. (1) Verbal comprehension; (2) verbal expression; (3) recent and remote memory.

   Presentation Modalities. (1) Auditory–verbal for instructions and presentation of items.

   Response Modalities. (1) Speech; (2) untimed.

   Description. The patient is asked to provide basic biographical information: name, age, place of birth, mother's first name, handedness, and any sensory impairments. The patient is also asked to recall the name of the current and previous Presidents. The patient is asked to state the date, day of the week, time, place, and city (Wechsler, 1987).

   Localization. A specific locus has not been correlated with impaired performance on this test.

   Norms. See the WMS-R.

   Source. The Psychological Corporation.

GALVESTON ORIENTATION AND AMNESIA TEST (GOAT)

   Microdescription. Assesses orientation, anterograde amnesia, and retrograde amnesia.

   Primary Assessment Areas. (1) Orientation; (2) anterograde amnesia; (3) retrograde amnesia (Levin *et al.,* 1979).

Secondary Assessment Areas. (1) Verbal comprehension; (2) verbal expression.

Presentation Modality. Auditory–verbal.

Response Modalities. (1) Speech; (2) untimed.

Description. The patient is asked questions that assess orientation as to person, place, and time. Anterograde amnesia is assessed by asking the patient to report the *first* event he or she can recall *after* the injury and to describe the event in detail. Retrograde amnesia is assessed by asking the patient to report the *last* event he or she can recall *before* the injury and to describe the event in detail. Points are assigned to each question, and a summary score can be calculated. The serial summary scores can be plotted to track recovery from closed head injury (Levin *et al.,* 1979).

Localization. The GOAT has been shown to be sensitive to brain impairment resulting from closed head injury. Scores are related to severity of injury and predictive of long-term recovery (Levin *et al.,* 1979).

Norms. Statistics have been provided for a group of recovered mildly head-injured patients (Levin *et al.,* 1979).

Source. Levin *et al.* (1979, 1982) provide examples of test materials and administration protocols.

REFERENCES

Benson, D. F., & Geschwind, N. (1967). Shrinking retrograde amnesia. *Journal of Neurology, Neurosurgery, and Psychiatry, 30,* 539–544.

Benton, A. L. (1968). Differential behavioral effects in frontal lobe disease. *Neuropsychologia, 6,* 53–60.

Benton, A. L., Van Allen, M. W., & Fogel, M. L. (1964). Temporal orientation in cerebral disease. *Journal of Nervous and Mental Disease, 139,* 110–119.

Benton, A. L., Hamsher, K. deS., Varney, N. R., & Spreen, O. (1983). *Contributions to neuropsychological assessment.* New York: Oxford University Press.

Berrios, G. E. (1983). Orientation failures in medicine and psychiatry: Discussion paper. *Journal of the Royal Society of Medicine, 76,* 379–385.

Daniel, W. F., Crovitz, H. F., & Weiner, R. D. (1987). Neuropsychological aspects of disorientation. *Cortex, 23,* 169–187.

Joslyn, D., & Hutzell, R. R. (1979). Temporal disorientation in schizophrenic and brain damaged patients. *American Journal of Psychiatry, 136,* 1220–1222.

Levin, H. S., O'Donnell, V. M., & Grossman, R. G. (1979). The Galveston Orientation and Amnesia Test: A practical scale to assess cognition after head injury. *Journal of Nervous and Mental Disease, 167,* 675–684.

Levin, H. S., Benton, A. L., & Grossman, R. G. (1982). *Neurobehavioral consequences of closed head injury.* New York: Oxford University Press.

Lezak, M. (1983). *Neuropsychological assessment* (2nd ed.). New York: Oxford University Press.

Liddle, P. F., & Crow, T. J. (1984). Age-disorientation in chronic schizophrenics associated with global intellectual impairment. *British Journal of Psychiatry, 144,* 193–199.

Strub, R. L., & Black, F. W. (1985). *The mental status examination in neurology* (2nd ed.). Philadelphia: F. A. Davis.

Wechsler, D. A. (1987). *Wechsler Memory Scale—Revised.* New York: Psychological Corporation.

Attention

Attention may be defined as the capacity to perform a selective analysis of inputs (Glass & Holyoak, 1986). Several aspects of attention may be distinguished: *Focused attention* is the ability to focus on a task or a part of the environment and to ignore distracters (Van Zomeren & Brouwer, 1987). *Sustained attention* or vigilance is the capacity to sustain the focus for a significant period of time (Van Zomeren & Brouwer, 1987). *Divided attention* is the capacity to divide or share attention between different tasks or different parts of the environment (Van Zomeren & Brouwer, 1987). The ability to divide attention is closely related to information-processing capacity. *Cognitive flexibility* is the ability to shift attention appropriately and adaptively from one part of the environment to another.

The tests discussed in this chapter are classified under four headings: (1) memory span, (2) serial arithmetic, (3) symbol copying, and (4) vigilance.

MEMORY SPAN

Digit Span (DS-WAIS-R) [DS-WMS-R (NI)]

Microdescription. Requires the patient to repeat numbers forward and backward.

Primary Assessment Areas

Digits Forward: (1) Focused attention (Kaplan *et al.,* 1991); (2) immediate verbal memory.
Digits Backward: (1) Focused attention; (2) divided attention; (3) immediate verbal memory.

Secondary Assessment Areas

Digits Forward: (1) Speech; (2) verbal comprehension.
Digits Backward: (1) Speech; (2) verbal comprehension; (3) visual–spatial imagery (Weinberg *et al.,* 1972).

Presentation Modality. Auditory–verbal.

Response Modalities. (1) Speech; (2) untimed.

Description. The patient is read number sequences of increasing length. After each sequence, he or she is asked to repeat the sequence from memory. In Digits Forward, the sequences range from 3 to 8 in length. Two sequences are attempted at each length. In Digits Backward, the patient is asked to repeat the numbers in reverse order. The sequences range from 2 to 7 in length (Wechsler, 1981, 1987).

The WAIS-R NI Record Form allows for recording of raw score, scaled score, longest string given correctly, greatest number of digits recalled correctly but incorrectly sequenced, and percentage of total digits correctly recalled (Kaplan *et al.*, 1991). Errors of omission, addition, perseveration, substitution, and sequence can also be recorded.

Poorer performance on Digits Forward than on Digits Backward suggests that the patient may have exerted less effort on the simpler Digits Forward (Lezak, 1983).

Localization. DS Backward may be more sensitive to brain damage than DS Forward (Black, 1986; Costa, 1975). Neither DS Forward nor DS Backward is a reliable indicator of laterality (Black, 1986). Backward digit repetition is often depressed in patients with visual–spatial deficits regardless of locus of lesion (Black, 1986).

Norms. The WMS-R contains separate norms for DS Forward and DS Backward (Wechsler, 1987). Education may increase performance (Weinberg *et al.*, 1972), and anxiety may decrease performance (Pyke & Agnew, 1963). Cumulative percentages for longest Digit Span (Forward and Backward) by age group and cumulative percentages of the difference between the longest forward and backward spans are available in the *WAIS-R NI Manual* (Kaplan *et al.*, 1991).

Source. The Psychological Corporation.

Visual Memory Span (VMS-WMS-R) and Spatial Span (WAIS-R NI)

Microdescription. Requires the patient to tap a series of squares or blocks in a demonstrated order.

Primary Assessment Areas.

Tapping Forward and Spatial Span Forward: (1) Focused attention; (2) visuospatial attention; (3) immediate visual memory.
Tapping Backward and Spatial Span Backward: (1) Focused attention; (2) divided attention; (3) visuospatial attention; (4) immediate visual memory.

Secondary Assessment Areas. (1) Visuospatial perception; (2) upper extremity motor functioning; (3) verbal comprehension.

Presentation Modalities. (1) Visual–nonverbal; (2) auditory–verbal for instructions.

Response Modalities. (1) Simple upper extremity movements—pointing; (2) untimed.

Description

Tapping Forward: Materials consist of a card containing 9 red squares. The patient observes as the squares are tapped in sequences of increasing length. After each sequence, he or she attempts to repeat the tapping from memory. The sequences range in length from 2 to 8 taps, and there are two sequences at each length (Wechsler, 1987).

Spatial Span Forward: Materials consist of 10 blue blocks attached to a white Spatial Span Board. The procedure is similar to that for Tapping Forward (Kaplan *et al.,* 1991).

Tapping Backward: Materials consist of a card containing 9 green squares. The procedure is similar to that for Tapping Forward except that the patient is required to repeat the performance in reverse. The sequences range in length from 2 to 7 taps, and there are two sequences at each length.

Spatial Span Backward: The procedure is similar to that for Tapping Backward except that the Spatial Span Board is used and the maximum sequence length is 8.

Localization. Although there are few data on localization for this task, VMS: Tapping Forward appears to resemble Corsi's Block Tapping Test (Milner, 1971), which requires the patient to repeat series of taps on cubes as in Spatial Span, rather than squares. On this task, DeRenzi and Nichelli (1975) found that visual field defects tended to result in impaired performance regardless of lateralization.

Norms. See the WMS-R.

Source. The Psychological Corporation.

SERIAL ARITHMETIC

Mental Control (MC-WMS-R)

Microdescription. Requires the production of some numeric and alphabetic sequences.

Primary Assessment Areas. (1) Focused attention; (2) production of overlearned, automatic series; (3) serial addition.

Secondary Assessment Areas. (1) Speech; (2) verbal comprehension.

Presentation Modality. Auditory–verbal for instructions.

Response Modalities. (1) Speech; (2) time-limited.

Description. The patient is asked to count backward from 20 to 1, say the alphabet, and count by threes from 1 to 40 (Serial Threes). In Serial Threes, each incorrect addition is counted as an error (Wechsler, 1987).

Localization. Localization data are not available.

Norms. See the WMS-R.

Source. The Psychological Corporation.

Paced Auditory Serial Addition Test (PASAT)

Microdescription. Requires the addition of pairs of numbers at a predetermined rate.

Primary Assessment Areas. (1) Sustained attention (Spreen & Strauss, 1991); (2) divided attention (Van Zomeren & Brouwer, 1987); (3) immediate verbal memory; (4) addition; (5) inhibition of encoding of one's own response while attending to the next stimulus in a series (Spreen & Strauss, 1991).

Secondary Assessment Areas. (1) Verbal comprehension; (2) speech.

Presentation Modalities. (1) Auditory–verbal; (2) visual–verbal for examples.

Response Modalities. (1) Speech; (2) paced.

Description. A tape recording of a male voice reciting single digits at a predetermined rate is played. The patient is required to add each number to the one presented just before it and say the answer aloud. First, a demonstration is given using written numbers. Next, a practice list of 10 digits recorded at intervals of 2.4 sec is followed by four 61-digit lists recorded with intervals of 2.4, 2.0, 1.6, and 1.2 sec. For severely impaired patients, Spreen and Strauss (1991) have provided more extended instructions.

A short version containing 50 numbers instead of 61 has been developed by H. Levin (Brittain *et al.,* 1991).

Localization. The PASAT has been found to be sensitive to impairment following closed head injury (Gronwall & Wrightson, 1981; Gronwall, 1987).

Norms. Means and standard deviations for a control group are presented in Gronwall (1977). Norms are available for the age groups 16–19, 20–29, 30–39, 40–49, 50–59, and 60–69 (Stuss *et al.,* 1987, 1988). Education (Stuss *et al.,* 1987) and intelligence (Egan, 1988) have been found to significantly affect performance. There is a significant practice effect on retesting (Stuss *et al.,* 1987).

Norms for the Levin version of the PASAT are available for age groups with means of 19, 40, and 69 years (Roman *et al.,* 1991) and age groups less than 25, 25–39, 40–54, and greater than 54 years (Brittain *et al.,* 1991). Brittain *et al.* (1991) found a significant effect for age and IQ, but none for education or race.

Source. Administration is described in Gronwall (1977). Information on obtaining materials is available from Neuropsychology Laboratory, University of Victoria, PO Box 1700, Victoria, British Columbia V8W 3P5 Canada.

Subtracting Serial Sevens (SSS)

Microdescription. Requires the patient to repeatedly subtract 7s.

Primary Assessment Areas. (1) Focused attention; (2) immediate verbal memory; (3) serial subtraction.

Secondary Assessment Areas. (1) Verbal comprehension; (2) speech.

Presentation Modality. Auditory – verbal for instructions.

Response Modalities. (1) Speech; (2) untimed.

Description. The patient is required to count down from 100 by 7s (Strub & Black, 1985).

Localization. Smith (1967) found patterns of errors believed to be associated with psychiatric disorders or frontal lobe lesions in 12.1% of a group of normal adults with above-average education and socioeconomic status. He suggested that poor performances on SSS may frequently reflect premorbid capacities and have no pathological significance.

Norms. In his sample, Smith (1967) found that 42% made no errors, 19% made 1 error, 14% made 2 errors, 23% made 3–12 errors, and 2% abandoned the task.

Source. SSS is included in the MMSE (Folstein *et al.,* 1975). It is item 221 of the LNNB Form I (Golden *et al.,* 1985).

SYMBOL COPYING

Digit Symbol [DSym-WAIS-R (NI)]

Microdescription. Requires rapid copying of symbols corresponding to numbers.

Primary Assessment Areas. (1) Sustained attention (Lezak, 1983); (2) visuomotor coordination and speed (Lezak, 1983); (3) visual scanning (Kaplan *et al.,* 1991); (4) incidental learning (Kaplan *et al.,* 1991).

Secondary Assessment Areas. (1) Verbal comprehension; (2) learning of an unfamiliar task (Gregory, 1987); (3) upper extremity motor functioning.

Presentation Modalities. (1) Visual – verbal and nonverbal; (2) auditory – verbal for instructions.

Response Modalities. (1) Upper extremity movements — writing symbols; (2) timed.

Description. The test is administered only if the patient can use his or her dominant hand for writing (Kaplan *et al.,* 1991). A key is provided with nine numbers in boxes on the top and corresponding symbols on the bottom. The test sheet contains four rows of boxes with numbers on the top and empty spaces below — 100 items in all. The patient's task is to write the appropriate symbols under the numbers. After completing 7 practice items, the patient attempts to fill in the remaining spaces as rapidly as possible. Work is stopped at 90 sec (Wechsler, 1981).

In administering the WAIS-R NI, the examiner places a mark every 30 sec where the patient is working (Kaplan *et al.,* 1991). The place where the patient is working at 90 sec is used to determine the scaled score. If the patient has not begun the fourth row, he or she is allowed to finish the third row. A test of incidental learning of the symbols and symbol – number pairs is then administered. Symbol Copy, in which the patient simply copies symbols, may be administered later in the testing to avoid fatigue affects to assess perceptual and graphomotor speed.

Localization. DSym is more sensitive to brain damage than any other subtest of the WAIS-R. It may be affected regardless of the locus of the lesion and is of little use in lateralizing lesions (Lezak, 1983).

Norms. See the WAIS-R.

Source. The Psychological Corporation.

Symbol Digit Modalities Test (SDMT)

Microdescription. Requires the written (or oral) production of numbers corresponding to symbols.

Primary Assessment Areas. (1) Sustained attention; (2) visuomotor coordination and speed; (3) visual scanning; (4) incidental learning.

Secondary Assessment Areas. (1) Verbal comprehension; (2) memory; (3) learning of an unfamiliar task; (4) upper extremity motor functioning and/or (5) speech.

Presentation Modalities. (1) Visual–nonverbal and verbal; (2) auditory–verbal for instructions.

Response Modalities. (1) Upper extremity movements—writing; (2) speech; (3) timed.

Description. A key is provided with nine symbols in boxes on the top and corresponding numbers on the bottom. The test sheet contains eight rows of boxes with symbols on the top and empty spaces below—120 items in all. The patient's task is to write the appropriate numbers under the symbols or say the number corresponding to each symbol. After completing 10 practice items, the patient attempts to fill in the remaining spaces as rapidly as possible. Work is stopped at 90 sec (Smith, 1982). The oral version offers a convenient alternative method for testing patients with upper extremity motor impairment. It can also be used to corroborate the result of the written test.

Localization. The test is very sensitive to impairment of brain functioning. A score 1.5 standard deviations or more below the mean is indicative of possible brain damage (Smith, 1982). Since the test is sensitive to bilateral processing, it does not appear to be useful for localizing brain dysfunction.

Norms. Norms for both written and oral administrations are provided (Smith, 1982) for age group (18–24, 25–34, 35–44, 45–54, 55–64, 65+) crossed with education (≤12 years, ≥13 years). Although DSym-WAIS-R and SDMT are highly correlated, relative to the tests' normative populations, the SDMT may yield scores that are as much as 4–5 WAIS-R age-scaled points lower than DSym-WAIS-R scores (Morgan & Wheelock, 1992).

Source. Western Psychological Services.

VIGILANCE

Continuous Performance Test (CPT)

Microdescription. Requires the patient to rapidly respond to sequentially presented stimuli.

Primary Assessment Areas. (1) Sustained attention (Mirsky *et al.*, 1991); (2) reaction time.

Secondary Assessment Area. Verbal comprehension.

Presentation Modalities. (1) Visual–verbal; (2) auditory–verbal for instructions.

Response Modalities. (1) Simple upper-extremity movements—pressing a button; (2) timed.

Description. Numerous CPTs have been developed. In an NIMH version, 800 visual stimuli ($\frac{3}{8}''$-high digits) are sequentially presented for 100 msec on an LED display. The patient must respond when a "6" is followed by a "4" (Sostek *et al.*, 1980). Another version uses letters and requires the patient to press a button if an "X" is preceded by an "A" (Rosvold *et al.*, 1956).

The Gordon Diagnostic System (GDS) requires the patient to press a button every time a "1" is followed by a "9" in the Vigilance Task (Gordon, 1986; Gordon & Mettelman, 1988). In the Distractibility Task, irrelevant digits are flashed on either side of the target stimulus.

Localization. Impaired performance has been noted in brain-damaged patients (Rosvold *et al.*, 1956) and patients suffering from schizophrenia (Mirsky, 1988).

Norms. Adult norms are being collected for the GDS.

Source. Computerized CPTs are available from Gordon Systems Inc., PO Box 746, DeWitt, New York 13214; For Thought, Nine Trafalgar Square, Nashua, NH 03063; and Western Psychological Services.

Visual Search and Attention Test (VSAT)

Microdescription. Requires the patient to cross out symbols identical to a target.

Primary Assessment Areas. (1) Sustained attention; (2) visual scanning (Trenerry *et al.*, 1990); (3) visuomotor speed.

Secondary Assessment Areas. (1) Color vision; (2) verbal comprehension.

Presentation Modalities. (1) Visual–nonverbal; (2) visual–verbal; (3) auditory–verbal for instructions.

Response Modalities. (1) Simple upper-extremity movements—crossing out symbols; (2) timed.

Description. Color vision is first assessed by asking the patient to differentiate three colors (blue, green, and red) printed on the first page of the test booklet. The test consists of four cancellation tasks. Task 1 requires the selection of "F" from an array of ten rows of letters. Task 2 requires the selection of "]" in an array of symbols. Task 3 requires the selection of blue "H" from an array of green and red Hs and other colored letters. Task 4 requires the selection of blue "/" from an array of green and red /'s and other colored symbols. The patient is requested to cross out all the letters or symbols like the target. He or she is allowed 60 sec. Only Tasks 3 and 4 are scored. The number of targets correctly crossed out for both the left and right sides of the arrays as well as total score are calculated (Trenerry *et al.*, 1990).

Localization. The VSAT is sensitive to brain damage (Trenerry *et al.*, 1990). Cancellation tests have been used to assess visual neglect. Diller and Weinberg (1977) found that right hemisphere patients completed tasks in a normal time frame, but made errors on the left side of the page. Left hemisphere patients made fewer errors, but were slow in completing the task. Trenerry *et al.* (1990) found no relation between impaired performance on the left or right side and laterality of lesion.

Norms. Norms are provided for the age groups 18–19, 20–29, 30–39, 40–49, 50–59, and 60+ (Trenerry *et al.*, 1990). Gender and education are not significantly related to performance.

Source. Psychological Assessment Resources.

REFERENCES

Black, F. W. (1986). Digit repetition in brain-damaged adults: Clinical and theoretical implications. *Journal of Clinical Psychology, 42,* 770–782.

Brittain, J. L., La Marche, J. A., Reeder, K. P., Roth, D. L., & Boll, T. J. (1991). Effects of age and IQ on Paced Auditory Serial Addition Task (PASAT) performance. *The Clinical Neuropsychologist, 5,* 163–175.

Costa, L. D. (1975). The relation of visuospatial dysfunction to digit span performance in patients with cerebral lesions. *Cortex, 11,* 31–36.

DeRenzi, E., & Nichelli, P. (1975). Verbal and non-verbal short-term memory impairment following hemispheric damage. *Cortex, 11,* 341–354.

Diller, L., & Weinberg, J. (1977). Hemi-inattention in rehabilitation: The evolution of a rational remediation program. In E. A. Weinstein & R. P. Friedland (Eds.), *Advances in neurology,* Volume 18 (pp. 63–82). New York: Raven Press.

Egan, V. (1988). PASAT: Observed correlations with IQ. *Personality and Individual Differences, 9,* 179–180.

Folstein, M. F., Folstein, S. E., & McHugh, P. R. (1975). Mini-mental state: A practical method for grading the cognitive state of patients for the clinician. *Journal of Psychiatric Research, 12,* 189–198.

Glass, A. L., & Holyoak, K. J. (1986). *Cognition.* New York: Random House.

Golden, C. J., Purisch, A. D., & Hammeke, T. A. (1985). *Luria–Nebraska Neuropsychological Battery: Forms I and II.* Los Angeles: Western Psychological Services.

Gordon, M. (1986). Microprocessor-based assessment of attention deficit disorders. *Psychopharmacology Bulletin, 22,* 288–290.

Gordon, M., & Mettelman, B. B. (1988). The assessment of attention: Standardization and reliability of a behavior-based measure. *Journal of Clinical Psychology, 44,* 682–690.

Gregory, R. J. (1987). *Adult intellectual assessment.* Boston: Allyn and Bacon.

Gronwall, D. (1977). Paced Auditory Serial-Addition Task: A measure of recovery from concussion. *Perceptual and Motor Skills, 44,* 367–373.

Gronwall, D. (1987). Advances in the assessment of attention and information processing after head injury. In H. S. Levin, J. Grafman, & H. M. Eisenberg (Eds.), *Neurobehavioral recovery from head injury* (pp. 355–371). New York: Oxford University Press.

Gronwall, D., & Wrightson, P. (1981). Memory and information processing capacity after closed head injury. *Journal of Neurology, Neurosurgery, and Psychiatry, 44,* 889–895.

Kaplan, E., Fein, D., Morris, R., & Delis, D. C. (1991). *WAIS-R NI: Manual.* San Antonio: Psychological Corporation.

Lezak, M. D. (1983). *Neuropsychological assessment* (2nd ed.). New York: Oxford University Press.

Milner, B. (1971). Interhemispheric differences in the localization of psychological processes in man. *British Medical Bulletin, 27,* 272–277.

Mirsky, A. F. (1988). Research on schizophrenia in the NIMH Laboratory of Psychology and Psychopathology 1954–1987. *Schizophrenia Bulletin, 14,* 151–156.

Mirsky, A. F., Anthony, B. J., Duncan, C. C., Ahearn, M. B., & Kellam, S. G. (1991). Analysis of the elements of attention: A neuropsychological approach. *Neuropsychology Review, 2,* 109–145.

Morgan, S. F., & Wheelock, J. (1992). Digit Symbol and Symbol Digit Modalities Tests: Are they directly interchangeable? *Neuropsychology, 6,* 327–330.

Pyke, S., & Agnew, N. (1963). Digit Span performance as a function of noxious stimulation. *Journal of Consulting Psychology, 27,* 281.

Roman, D. D., Edwall, G. E., Buchanan, R. J., & Patton, J. H. (1991). Extended norms for the Paced Auditory Serial Addition Task. *The Clinical Neuropsychologist, 5,* 33–40.

Rosvold, H. E., Mirsky, A. F., Sarason, I., Bransome, E. D., & Beck, L. H. (1956). A continuous performance test of brain damage. *Journal of Consulting Psychology, 20,* 343–350.

Smith, A. (1967). The Serial Sevens Subtraction Test. *Archives of Neurology, 17,* 78–80.

Smith, A. (1982). *Symbol Digit Modalities Test: Manual.* Los Angeles: Western Psychological Services.

Sostek, A. J., Buchsbaum, M. S., & Rapoport, J. L. (1980). Effects of amphetamine on vigilance performance in normal and hyperactive children. *Journal of Abnormal Child Psychology, 8,* 491–500.

Spreen, O., & Strauss, E. (1991). *A compendium of neuropsychological tests: Administration, norms, and commentary.* New York: Oxford University Press.

Strub, R. L., & Black, F. W. (1985). *The mental status examination in neurology* (2nd ed.). Philadelphia: F. A. Davis.

Stuss, D. T., Stethem, L. L., & Poirier, C. A. (1987). Comparison of three tests of attention and rapid information processing across six age groups. *The Clinical Neuropsychologist, 1,* 139–152.

Stuss, D. T., Stethem, L. L., & Pelchat, G. (1988). Three tests of attention and rapid information processing: An extension. *The Clinical Neuropsychologist, 2,* 246–250.

Trenerry, M. R., Crosson, B., DeBoe, J., & Leber, W. R. (1990). *Visual Search and Attention Test: Professional Manual,* Odessa, FL: Psychological Assessment Resources.

Van Zomeren, A. H., & Brouwer, W. H. (1987). Head injury and concepts of attention. In H. S. Levin, J. Grafman, & H. M. Eisenberg (Eds.), *Neurobehavioral recovery from head injury* (pp. 398–415). New York: Oxford University Press.

Wechsler, D. (1981). *Wechsler Adult Intelligence Scale—Revised.* New York: Psychological Corporation.

Wechsler, D. (1987). *Wechsler Memory Scale—Revised.* New York: Psychological Corporation.

Weinberg, J., Diller, L., Gerstman, L., & Schulman, P. (1972). Digit span in right and left hemiplegics. *Journal of Clinical Psychology, 28,* 361.

Memory

Memory may be defined as the capacity to register, retain, and retrieve information (Ellis and Young, 1988). There are three distinct but related, psychologically and biologically validated, forms of memory: sensory memory, short-term memory, and long-term memory (Squire, 1987). *Sensory memory* holds sensory information for a second or two (Neisser, 1967). The information decays continuously, and new inputs erase residual traces of previous inputs. Sensory memory is not directly assessed clinically. *Short-term memory* is a limited-capacity store that retains information for a minute or two depending on rehearsal (Squire, 1987). *Long-term memory* is a larger, longer-lasting memory process.

Memory processes may be categorized according to sensory modality or content as, for example, verbal or visual. *Episodic memory* is memory of an individual personal experience such as remembering what you had for lunch (Baddeley, 1982). *Semantic memory* is memory of information of a general nature such as the capital of Switzerland or the chemical formula for water (Baddeley, 1982). *Declarative memory* is "memory that is directly accessible to conscious recollection" (Squire, 1987, p. 152). *Procedural memory* is "memory that is contained within learned skills or modifiable cognitive operations" (Squire, 1987, p. 152).

In clinical assessment, memory is often classified according to the procedure used to test memory: *Immediate memory* is memory for material immediately after it has been presented. *Delayed* or *recent memory* is memory for information after a delay of minutes to hours. The inclusion of a delayed-recall trial in a memory evaluation can sometimes detect a memory deficit that is otherwise equivocal (Lezak, 1983). *Remote memory* is memory for events in the distant past (Strub & Black, 1985). These clinically useful concepts of memory do not correspond in a one-to-one fashion with the psychologically validated concepts listed earlier. For example, immediate memory may not correspond directly with short-term memory. Although immediate recall of digits may provide a measure of short-term auditory memory capacity, immediate recall of a paragraph or a geometric design may require a performance lasting well beyond the 1- or 2-min duration of short-term memory (Lezak, 1983).

Free recall is recall of material without imposed structure. In *cued recall,* hints are provided. In a memory assessment, a cued-recall trial may assist in determining whether providing partial information facilitates recall (Hannay & Levin, 1985; Warrington & Weiskrantz, 1970). In *recognition,* the item to be remembered is presented either alone or with other items and must be identified or selected. A recognition trial may assist in assessing retention of information that is otherwise unavailable for retrieval (Hannay & Levin, 1985).

The following tests are categorized under verbal memory and visual memory. The LNNB Memory Scale is found at the end of the visual memory category, but assesses both verbal and visual memory. Brief reviews of memory batteries may be found at the end of this chapter. In addition to the tests reviewed here, the use of everyday memory self-report questionnaires (Gilewski & Zelinski, 1986) and assessments of remote and autobiographical memory may be appropriate (Squire, 1986).

VERBAL MEMORY

Logical Memory I and II (LM-WMS-R)

Microdescription. Requires the patient to repeat short stories from memory.

Primary Assessment Areas. (1) Immediate and (2) delayed recall of a story.

Secondary Assessment Areas. (1) Verbal comprehension; (2) speech.

Presentation Modality. Auditory–verbal.

Response Modalities. (1) Speech; (2) untimed.

Description. A story is read to the patient and the patient is asked to retell it immediately after hearing it and then after a 30-min delay. Each story contains 25 scorable memory units, and a detailed description of the scoring criteria for each unit is available in the manual (Wechsler, 1987).

Localization. Performance of patients with left hemisphere lesions may be inferior to performance of patients with right hemisphere impairment (Chelune & Bornstein, 1988).

Norms. See the WMS-R.

Source. The Psychological Corporation.

Verbal Paired Associates I and II (VP-WMS-R)

Microdescription. Assesses immediate and delayed recall of pairs of words.

Primary Assessment Areas. (1) Immediate recall; (2) learning or acquisition rate over several presentations; (3) delayed recall of verbal paired associates.

Secondary Assessment Areas. (1) Verbal comprehension; (2) speech.

Presentation Modality. Auditory–verbal.

Response Modalities. (1) Speech; (2) time-limited.

Description. A group of eight word pairs is read to the patient. The patient is then required to recall the second word of the pair when the first is read. The pairs, arranged in different orders, are read and recall is required at least three times. The process is discontinued if all eight items are answered correctly on any of the third through sixth trials. After a 30-min delay, recall is assessed a final time. Four of the word pairs are classified as "easy" and involve well-learned verbal associations (Lezak, 1983). Four are "difficult" and require learning new, unfamiliar verbal associations.

Localization. Performance of patients with left hemisphere lesions may be inferior to performance of patients with right hemisphere impairments (Chelune & Bornstein, 1988).

Norms. See the WMS-R.

Source. The Psychological Corporation.

Rey Auditory–Verbal Learning Test (RAVLT)

Microdescription. Requires the patient to learn and recall a list of words.

Primary Assessment Areas. (1) Immediate recall; (2) learning or acquisition rate over several presentations; (3) delayed recall; (4) delayed recognition of a word list.

Secondary Assessment Areas. (1) Verbal comprehension; (2) speech; (3) reading.

Presentation Modalities. (1) Auditory–verbal; (2) visual–verbal.

Response Modalities. (1) Speech; (2) untimed.

Description. A 15-word list is read at a rate of one word per second, and the patient is asked to say, in any order, as many words as he or she can remember. The list is read and recall requested five consecutive times. A different 15-word list is then read, and recall is requested. Recall is again requested for the first list. Finally, the patient is presented with a paragraph and is required to select the words from the first list. This procedure allows the examiner to construct a learning curve and to assess the effect of interpolated potentially interfering material on recall (Lezak, 1983). Geffen *et al.* (1990) require an additional recall of the first list after 20 min. Recognition is then assessed by requiring the patient to select all list words and to report whether they are from the first or the second list. The test includes 30 words from the first and second lists as well as 20 distracter words.

Localization. Performance on Trial 5 of the RAVLT has been found to distinguish patients with brain damage from controls (Powell *et al.,* 1991). Patients with left hemisphere lesions may perform more poorly than patients with right hemisphere lesions (Lezak, 1983; Miceli *et al.,* 1981).

Norms. Geffen *et al.* (1990) have provided norms for the age ranges 16–19, 20–29, 30–39, 40–49, 50–59, 60–69, and 70 and over for males and females. Ivnik *et al.* (1992a) have provided norms for adults of 56–97. Lezak (1983) has adapted the norms *Rey* based on a sample of manual laborers, professionals, students, elderly laborers (70–90 years), and elderly professionals (70–88 years).

Source. Lezak (1983) has provided test instructions and stimuli. A scoring program is available from Professor G. Geffen, School of Social Sciences, The Flinders University of South Australia, GPO Box 2100, Adelaide, SA 5001, Australia.

Selective Reminding Test (SRT)

Microdescription. Requires the patient to learn and recall a list of words.

Primary Assessment Areas. (1) Immediate recall; (2) learning or acquisition rate over several presentations; (3) cued recall; (4) recognition; (5) delayed recall of a word list.

Secondary Assessment Areas. (1) Verbal comprehension; (2) speech; (3) reading.

Presentation Modalities. (1) Auditory–verbal; (2) visual–verbal.

Response Modalities. (1) Speech; (2) untimed.

Description. The revision by Levin *et al.* (1982) of the original test devised by Buschke (1973) consists of a 12-word list that is read to the patient at the rate of a word every 2-sec. The patient is then asked to recall the words in any order. On the following trial, the patient is selectively reminded of only those items not recalled on the immediately preceding trial and recall of all the words is again requested. This procedure is repeated 12 times. After the 12th and last selective reminding trial, the first two or three letters of each word are presented on an index card, and the patient is asked to recall the list word. After all cards have been presented, cues that did not elicit a correct response are presented again. Following cued recall, a series of 12 index cards is presented for multiple-choice recognition. A delayed-recall trial is given after 30 min.

If a word is recalled on two consecutive trials, it is defined as having entered long-term storage (LTS) on the first of these trials and is scored as LTS on all subsequent trials. If an item that is in LTS is recalled, it is scored as long-term retrieval (LTR). Consistent LTR (CLTR) is scored if an item is recalled from LTS on that and all subsequent trials. Random LTR (RLTR) is scored for items recalled from LTS that are not recalled on all subsequent trials (Hannay & Levin, 1985).

Localization. The SRT appears to be sensitive to memory impairments associated with a variety of neurological disorders (Buschke & Fuld, 1974; Levin *et al.,* 1982).

Norms. Norms for the age groups 18–29, 30–39, 40–49, 50–59, 60–69, 70–79, and 80–91 may be found in Spreen and Strauss (1991). Ruff *et al.* (1989) have supplied norms for Sum of LTS and Sum of CLTR stratified by gender, age, and education. The age ranges are 16–24, 25–39, 40–54, and 55–70. In this study, the subjects repeated each word immediately after each presentation to assure initial comprehension.

Source. Levin (1986) has listed all stimulus words and cues of the four SRT forms. Instructions for administration and scoring can be found in Hannay and Levin (1985).

California Verbal Learning Test (CVLT)

Microdescription. Requires the patient to learn and recall lists of words.

Primary Assessment Areas. (1) Immediate recall; (2) learning or acquisition rate over several presentations; (3) cued recall; (4) delayed recall; (5) delayed cued recall; (6) delayed recognition of a word list.

Secondary Assessment Areas. (1) Verbal comprehension; (2) speech.

Presentation Modality. Auditory–verbal.

Response Modalities. (1) Speech; (2) untimed.

Description. This test consists of two lists of words, a "Monday List" and a "Tuesday List." The words comprising the lists are drawn from four semantic categories, four words per category. The Monday List is read to the patient, who is asked to "say back" as many words as he or she can, on five consecutive trials. The Tuesday List is then read and recall requested. Free and cued recall are then requested for the Monday List. After a 20-min delay, free and cued recall for the Monday List are again assessed, as well as recognition.

The manual describes an elaborate analysis of the patient's responses that provides information on semantic and serial learning, serial position effects, acquisition rate, recall consistency, vulnerability to proactive and retroactive interference, and learning errors in recall and recognition (Delis *et al.,* 1987, 1988). A computer program is available to assist with this analysis.

Localization. The CVLT has been used to evaluate memory and learning in patients with a variety of neurological impairments. The CVLT Manual reports data on patients with chronic alcoholism, Parkinson's disease, multiple sclerosis, Huntington's disease, and Alzheimer's disease (Delis *et al.,* 1987). Crosson *et al.* (1989) have studied head-injured patients with the CVLT.

Norms. Delis *et al.* (1987) present norms for adults stratified by age and gender. The age ranges are 17–34, 35–44, 45–54, 55–64, 65–69, 70–74, and 75–80.

Source. The Psychological Corporation.

Serial Digit Learning (SDL)

Microdescription. Assesses learning of a long series of digits.

Primary Assessment Areas. (1) Learning of a supraspan series of digits; (2) immediate recall of a supraspan series of digits.

Secondary Assessment Areas. (1) Verbal comprehension; (2) speech.

Presentation Modality. Auditory–verbal.

Response Modalities. (1) Speech; (2) untimed.

Description. The patient is presented and asked to repeat a series of numbers either 8 or 9 digits long for 12 trials or until two consecutive correct repetitions are made (Benton *et al.,* 1983).

Localization. Serial digit learning may be more sensitive to brain damage than digit span tests. It may not reliably lateralize brain lesions (Hamsher *et al.,* 1980).

Norms. Norms stratified by age and education can be found in Benton *et al.* (1983). The age ranges are 16–64 and 65–74.

Source. Oxford University Press.

Auditory Consonant Trigrams (ACT)

Microdescription. Requires the patient to recall sets of consonants after counting backward by 3s.

Primary Assessment Areas. (1) Recall of consonant trigrams with interference; (2) attention.

Secondary Assessment Areas. (1) Verbal comprehension of instructions; (2) speech.

Presentation Modalities. (1) Auditory–verbal; (2) visual–sequential–verbal (Stuss *et al.,* 1982); (3) visual–simultaneous–verbal (Samuels *et al.,* 1972; Stuss *et al.,* 1982).

Response Modalities. (1) Speech; (2) untimed.

Description. The patient is presented a series of three-consonant nonsense "words" (Brown, 1958; Peterson and Peterson, 1959; Stuss *et al.,* 1982). After the presentation of each consonant trigram and an interference-delay period, the patient is required to recall the three consonants. During the interference-delay periods of 0, 3, 9, or 18 sec, the patient is required to count backward from a random number by 3s. Stuss *et al.* (1982) presented 15 trials at each of the four delay periods. Stuss *et al.* (1987) used intervals of 9, 18, and 36 sec.

Localization. Lesions in the right and possibly the left temporal lobe may result in impaired performance on ACTs (Samuels *et al.,* 1972). Orbital–frontal lesions may impair performance (Stuss *et al.,* 1982).

Norms. Normative data are available for the age groups 16–19, 20–29, 30–39, 40–49, 50–59, and 60–69 (Stuss *et al.,* 1987, 1988). No significant gender or education differences were noted.

Source. There is no standard version of this test. Descriptions of alternative versions can be found in Brown (1958), Peterson and Peterson (1959), Samuels *et al.* (1972), and Stuss *et al.* (1982, 1987).

VISUAL MEMORY

Visual Reproduction I and II (VR-WMS-R)

Microdescription. Requires the patient to draw designs from memory.

Primary Assessment Areas. (1) Immediate and (2) delayed recall of geometric designs.

Secondary Assessment Areas. (1) Visuospatial perception; (2) visuoconstructional ability; (3) drawing; (4) upper extremity motor function; (5) verbal comprehension.

Presentation Modalities. (1) Visual–nonverbal; (2) auditory–verbal for instructions.

Response Modalities. (1) Upper extremity and hand motor functioning—drawing; (2) untimed.

Description. A black line drawing of a geometric figure is presented for 10 sec. The figure is removed and the patient is required to draw it from memory. This procedure is repeated with four different figures. After a 30-min delay, the patient is required to draw the figures from memory again (Wechsler, 1987).

Localization. Chelune and Bornstein (1988) found a within-subjects double dissociation for VR vs. LM for left vs. right hemisphere injury.

Norms. See the WMS-R.

Source. The Psychological Corporation.

Visual Paired Associates I and II (VPA-WMS-R)

Microdescription. Requires the patient to learn the color associated with each of six abstract figures.

Primary Assessment Areas. (1) Immediate recall; (2) learning, and (3) delayed recall of visual paired associates.

Secondary Assessment Areas. (1) Visuospatial perception; (2) verbal comprehension.

Presentation Modalities. (1) Visuospatial–nonverbal; (2) color; (3) auditory–verbal for instructions and feedback.

Response Modalities. (1) Simple upper extremity and hand movements—pointing; (2) time-limited.

Description. An abstract design (a black line drawing on a white background) paired with a colored square is presented for 3 sec. Six such designs paired with different colors are presented in sequence. A palette of six colors is provided, and when each of the designs is presented, the patient is required to point to the associated color. The pairs, arranged in different orders, are presented and ''recall'' is required at least three times. The process is discontinued if all six items are answered correctly on any of the third through sixth trials. After a 30-min delay, ''recall'' is assessed a final time (Wechsler, 1987).

Localization. Chelune and Bornstein (1988) found a within-subjects double dissociation for VPA vs. VP for right vs. left hemisphere injury.

Norms. See the WMS-R.

Source. The Psychological Corporation.

Figural Memory (FM-WMS-R)

Microdescription. Assesses immediate recognition memory for abstract designs.

Primary Assessment Area. Immediate visual recognition memory.

Secondary Assessment Areas. (1) Visuospatial pattern recognition; (2) verbal comprehension.

Presentation Modalities. (1) Visuospatial–nonverbal; (2) auditory–verbal for instructions.

Response Modalities. (1) simple upper extremity and hand movements—pointing; (2) time-limited.

Description. A black, gray, and white abstract design or set of three such designs is presented briefly to the patient, who is then required to identify the designs among a larger group of designs (Wechsler, 1987).

Localization. No information is available.

Norms. See the WMS-R.

Source. The Psychological Corporation.

Rey–Osterrieth Complex Figure Test: Memory (ROCFT:M)

Microdescription. Requires the patient to draw a detailed figure from memory.

Primary Assessment Areas. (1) Immediate and (2) delayed recall of a detailed figure.

Secondary Assessment Areas. (1) Visuospatial perception; (2) visuoconstructional ability; (3) drawing; (4) upper extremity motor functioning; (5) verbal comprehension.

Presentation Modalities. (1) Visual–nonverbal; (2) auditory–verbal for instructions.

Response Modalities. (1) Upper extremity and hand motor functioning—drawing; (2) untimed.

Description. The patient is required to draw a detailed line drawing from memory. This test is usually preceded by a copy trial (see ROCFT:C). The patient may be provided with different-colored drawing instruments when drawing various parts of the figure or at 1-min time intervals to obtain a record of the patient's organizational plan in drawing the figure. Several administrations (with a variety of delay intervals) and scoring systems are available (Denman, 1984; Lezak, 1983; Osterrieth, 1944; Visser, 1980). The Taylor scoring criteria may be found in Spreen and Strauss (1991).

Localization. Left-sided lesions tend to result in preserved recall of overall structure of the figure with simplification and loss of details. For right-sided lesions, there is greater impairment in recalling than in copying designs (Milner, 1975).

Norms. Norms are available for the age groups 10–12, 13–15, 16–18, 19–21, 22–29, 30–39, 40–49, 50–59, 60–69, 70–79, and 80–89 (Denman, 1987). Norms for the Taylor scoring criteria for the age groups 16–30, 31–44, 50–59, 60–69, and 70+ may be found in Spreen and Strauss (1991). Normative data for the Taylor Complex Figure have been provided by Tombaugh *et al.* (1992). Norms are also available in Lezak (1983).

Source. Examples of the figure and instructions for administration are available in several sources (Denman, 1984; Lezak, 1983; Osterrieth, 1944; Spreen & Strauss, 1991; Visser, 1980).

Benton Visual Retention Test: Memory (BVRT:A,B,D)

Microdescription. Requires the patient to draw geometric figures from memory.

Primary Assessment Areas. Immediate recall of geometric figures. Correlational studies and factor analyses have suggested that the visuospatial motor component measured by this task outweighs the memory component (Larrabee *et al.*, 1985; Silverstein, 1962).

Secondary Assessment Areas. (1) Visuospatial perception; (2) visuoconstructional ability; (3) visuoverbal conceptualization; (4) drawing; (4) upper extremity motor functioning; (5) verbal comprehension.

Presentation Modalities. (1) Visuospatial–nonverbal; (2) auditory–verbal for instructions.

Response Modalities. (1) Upper extremity and hand movements—drawing; (2) untimed.

Description. See the Benton Visual Retention Test: Copy (BVRT:C) for a description of the test materials. The following three administrations have a memory component:

Administration A: Requires the patient to draw geometric figures from memory immediately after a 10-sec exposure.

Administration B: Requires the patient to draw geometric figures from memory immediately after a 5-sec exposure.

Administration D: Requires the patient to draw geometric figures from memory 15 sec after a 10-sec exposure.

Localization. Although impaired performance may be associated with a variety of brain lesions, a greater degree of impairment may be associated with focal right hemisphere lesions (Benton, 1967, 1968).

Norms. For Administration A, Benton (1974) has provided norms for the age groups 15–44, 45–54, and 55–64 crossed with six IQ groups. Norms for Administration B are derived by subtracting 1 from the norms for Administration A. No norms are provided for

Administration D. Benton and Spreen (1961) found that individuals simulating impairment performed at a lower level and made more distortion errors and fewer omission, perseveration, and size errors than brain-damaged patients.

Source. The Psychological Corporation.

Benton Visual Retention Test: Multiple Choice-Memory (BVRT:G)

Microdescription. Requires identification of sets of geometric figures from memory.

Primary Assessment Areas. Visual recognition memory.

Secondary Assessment Areas. (1) Visuospatial perception; (2) visual–verbal conceptualization; (3) verbal comprehension.

Presentation Modalities. (1) Visuospatial–nonverbal; (2) auditory–verbal for instructions.

Response Modalities. (1) Pointing or (2) speech; (3) untimed.

Description. See the Visual Form Discrimination Test (VFDT) for a description of the materials. The administration is similar to that of the VFDT except that the stimulus card is presented alone to the patient and removed after a 10- or 15-sec exposure. The set of foils is then presented. It has been noted that the test may be successfully completed by using a systematic response strategy rather than memory (Blanton & Grouvier, 1985). It may be useful to ask patients about their response strategy.

Localization. No information is available.

Norms. There are no published norms for adults.

Source. Benton *et al.,* (1977) have described Administration F: Multiple Choice— Memory and report studies with children. Stimulus materials are available from Oxford University Press as the VFDT.

Memory for Faces (MF)

Microdescription. Requires the patient to recognize faces after presentation.

Primary Assessment Areas. Recognition memory for faces.

Presentation Modalities. (1) Visual–nonverbal; (2) auditory–verbal for instructions.

Response Modalities. (1) Speech; (2) upper extremity movements—writing or (3) pointing.

Description. In the version of the test by Denman (1984), the patient is shown a photograph with 16 peoples' faces on it for 45 sec. After 90 sec of interpolated material, the patient is required to select the 16 faces from among 48.

Localization. Patients with right temporal lobe lesions may exhibit impaired performance (Milner & Teuber, 1968). It should be noted that impaired performance can result from neglect of one side of the array of faces (Milner & Teuber, 1968).

Norms. Norms are available for the age groups 10–12, 13–15, 16–18, 19–21, 22–29, 30–39, 40–49, 50–59, 60–69, 70–79, and 80–89 (Denman, 1987).

Source. MF is available as part of the Denman Neuropsychology Memory Scale (DNMS) (Denman, 1984, 1987). The DNMS can be ordered from Sidney B. Denman, Ph.D., 1040 Fort Sumter Drive, Charleston, SC 29412.

Memory Scale (C10- and C12-LNNB)

Microdescription. Assesses various aspects of memory functioning.

Primary Assessment Areas. (1) Immediate memory (C10); (2) delayed (intermediate) memory (C12) (Golden *et al.,* 1985).

Secondary Assessment Area. Verbal comprehension.

Presentation Modalities. (1) Any–verbal instructions for all items; (2) any–verbal for items 223–225; (3) auditory–verbal for items 231–235; (4) visual–verbal for item 230; (5) auditory–nonverbal for item 228; (6) visual–nonverbal for items 226, 227, 229, and 235.

Response Modalities. (1) Any–verbal for items 223–226 and 230–235; (2) communication of "yes" or "no" for item 226; (3) any–verbal or drawing for 227; (4) hand movements for 229; (5) speech or extremity movements—tapping for 228; (6) untimed for 224 and 227–235; (7) time-limited for 223 and 225.

Description. C10- and C12-LNNB are sets of relatively heterogeneous items that assess various aspects of memory. The items of C10 generally assess immediate memory:

223–225	Learning and prediction of recall on a 7-word list
226	Recognition of a card with shapes and colors
227	Recall of geometric shapes
228	Recall of a tapped rhythm
229	Immediate recall of finger positions
230	Immediate recall of printed words
231, 232	Recall of three words after interference
233	Recall of sentences after interference
234	Immediate recall of a story
235	Immediate recall of word–picture paired associates

Two Factor Scales have been identified. Verbal Memory (ME1) is composed of items that involve recall of lists of words. Visual and Complex Memory (ME2) involves primarily visually presented nonverbal material (Golden *et al.,* 1985).

Additional items may be added to LNNB Form I to assess delayed or intermediate memory. A Complex Visual Reproduction Item requires immediate and delayed recall of a figure of moderate complexity. Items 110 R, 223 R, 227 R, 229 R, 234 R, 235 R, 223 R2, and Delayed Complex Visual Reproduction assess delayed recall or recognition for their respective previously administered items. The manual provides extremely limited norms (Golden *et al.*, 1985).

LNNB Form II contains a set of items (C12) for assessment of delayed or intermediate memory:

270 Delayed recall of hand movements from item C1-LNNB
271 Delayed recall of figures from C1-LNNB
272 Delayed recall of tactile stimuli from items 76–79
273 Delayed recall of tactile stimuli from item 82 or 84
274 Delayed recall of 7-word list
275 Delayed recall of word–picture paired associates
276, 278 Delayed recognition of pictures
277 Delayed recall of story
279 Delayed recall of song from item 56

Localization. The manual states that impaired performance on verbal items may suggest left hemisphere dysfunction, while impaired performance on nonverbal items may suggest right hemisphere dysfunction. Severe, overall impairment may suggest bilateral hemispheric dysfunction, bilateral hippocampal injury, or other subcortical dysfunction (Golden *et al.*, 1982, 1985).

Norms. See the LNNB.

Source. Western Psychological Services.

MEMORY BATTERIES

Wechsler Memory Scale—Revised (WMS-R)

The WMS-R is a substantial revision of the WMS. Its subtests are (1) Information and Orientation (O), (2) Mental Control (MC), (3) Figural Memory (FM), (4) Logical Memory (LM) I, (5) Visual Paired Associates (VPA) I, (6) Verbal Paired Associates (VP) I, (7) Visual Reproduction (VR) I, (8) Digit Span (DS), (9) Visual Memory Span (VMS), (10) LM II, (11) VPA II, (12) VP II, and (13) VR II. All these subtests are reviewed in this book. The subtest raw scores are combined and the following indexes are computed: (1) Verbal Memory Index, (2) Visual Memory Index, (3) General Memory Index, (4) Attention/Concentration Index, and (5) Delayed Recall Index. The indexes have a mean of 100 with a standard deviation of 15. Percentiles are available for DS Forward and Backward, VMS Forward and Backward, LM I and II, and VR I and II (Wechsler, 1987).

Reliability and validity information may be located in the manual (Wechsler, 1987). *The Clinical Neuropsychologist* (1988), Vol. 2, No. 2, is devoted to studies of the test.

Normative data are available in the manual for the age groups 16–17, 20–24, 35–54, 55–64, 65–69, and 70–74 (Wechsler, 1987). Norms for the age groups 18–19, 25–34, and 45–54 were "empirically derived." D'Elia *et al.* (1989) have recommended that the WMS be used for these groups until appropriate normative data are available. This recommendation has been disputed by Bowden and Bell (1992). Mittenberg *et al.* (1992) have provided normative data for 25- to 34-year-olds. Ivnik *et al.* (1992b) have provided norms for ages 56–94. A detailed appraisal of the psychometric characteristics of the WMS-R including formulae for calculation of confidence intervals may be found in Elwood (1991).

Wechsler Memory Scale (WMS)

The WMS is composed of: I—Personal and Current Information, II—Orientation, III—Mental Control, IV—Logical Memory, V—Digits Forward and Backward, VI—Visual Reproduction, and VII—Associate Learning (verbal paired associates). These subtests are similar but not identical to their respective subtests on the WMS-R, although there is no delayed recall trial. The revision of the WMS by Russell (1975) obtains delayed recall for LM (IV) and VR (VI).

Reliability and validity studies for the WMS are reviewed in Franzen (1989). Normative studies are summarized and critiqued in D'Elia *et al.* (1989).

Randt Memory Test (RMT)

The RMT (Randt & Brown, 1983) is composed of seven sections: General Information, Five Items, Repeating Numbers, Paired Words, Short Story, Picture Recognition, and Incidental Learning. General Information assesses orientation and factual information such as who is the President. In Five Items, the patient is required to learn a 5-word list. After the presentation of the words, the patient is required to serially subtract 3s before repeating the words. Acquisition is assessed over three trials using a selective reminding procedure. Repeating Numbers is a digit-span task. Paired Words is a paired-associates learning task with a procedure similar to that of Five Items except for the substitution of restricted reminding for selective reminding. Short Story assesses recall of narrative material. Picture Recognition assesses recognition and recall of line drawings of everyday objects. Incidental Learning is assessed by requesting the patient to recall the names of the six previous sections of the test. Recall is assessed for Five Items, Paired Words, Short Story, and Picture Recognition after 5-min and 24-hr delays.

Norms are presented in the manual (Randt & Brown, 1983) for ages 20–89 grouped by decade.

Memory Assessment Scales (MAS)

The MAS consist of 12 subtests: List Learning, Prose Memory, List Recall, Verbal Span, Visual Span, Visual Recognition, Visual Reproduction, Names–Faces, Delayed List Recall, Delayed Prose Memory, Delayed Visual Recognition, and Delayed Names–Faces Recall (Williams, 1991).

On the List Learning subtest, the patient is required to learn a list of 12 common words—3 from each of four semantic categories. The list is repeated until perfect recall is achieved or for a maximum of six trials. Additional scores provide measures of clustering strategies and intrusions. In Prose Memory, the patient is presented with a story and required to answer 9 questions about it. List Recall is administered after a several-minute delay. Verbal Span requires the repetition of digits forward and backward. Visual Span requires the patient to repeat the sequence in which the examiner points to a series of printed stars. The Visual Recognition subtest assesses recognition memory of designs. Visual Reproduction requires the patient to draw a geometric design after performing a distracter task. The Names–Faces subtest requires the patient to learn the names of individuals who are portrayed in photographs. Delayed memory is assessed for some of the memory tasks: Delayed List Recall, Delayed Prose Memory, Delayed Visual Recognition, and Delayed Names–Faces Recall.

Norms are presented in the manual (Williams, 1991) for ages 18–70+ by decade and for the age groups 18–49, 50–59, 60–69, and 70+ crossed with education (≤11 years, 12 years, ≥13 years).

Denman Neuropsychology Memory Scale (DNMS)

The DNMS (Denman, 1984) is administered in a 12-stage procedure. A story is presented and immediate recall is assessed. Then a list of 14 paired associates is presented and immediate recall is requested on three consecutive trials. After copying the Rey–Osterrieth Complex Figure, the patient is required to draw it from memory. A scoring system unique to the DNMS is provided. Digits Forward and Digits Backward are then assessed. In the Memory for Musical Tones and Melodies subtest, the patient is required to compare successive groups of tones. The Remotely Stored Verbal Information subtest assesses general knowledge. The patient then views a photograph with 16 different faces on it (see under *Memory for Faces* above). After a delay, the patient is asked to select the 16 faces from a photograph containing 48 faces. The Remotely Stored Non-Verbal Information subtest requires the patient to describe, draw, or demonstrate familiar objects, structures, designs, or gestures. Delayed recall of the Complex Figure, Paired Associates, and Story is then requested.

Norms are available for the age groups 10–12, 13–15, 16–18, 19–21, 22–29, 30–39, 40–49, 50–59, 60–69, 70–79, and 80–89 (Denman, 1987).

REFERENCES

Baddeley, A. (1982). *Your memory: A user's guide.* New York: Macmillan.

Benton, A. L. (1967). Constructional apraxia and the minor hemisphere. *Confinia Neurologica, 29,* 1–16.

Benton, A. L. (1968). Differential behavioral effects in frontal lobe disease. *Neuropsychologia, 6,* 53–60.

Benton, A. L. (1974). *Revised visual retention test: Clinical and experimental applications.* New York: Psychological Corporation.

Benton, A. L., & Spreen, O. (1961). Visual memory test: The simulation of mental incompetence. *Archives of General Psychiatry, 4,* 79–83.

Benton, A. L., Hamsher, K., & Stone, E. (1977). *Visual Retention Test: Multiple Choice Form (Visual Form Discrimination).* Iowa City: University of Iowa, Department of Neurology.

Benton, A. L., Hamsher, K., Varney, N. R., & Spreen, O. (1983). *Contributions to neuropsychological assessment: A clinical manual.* New York: Oxford University Press.

Blanton, P. D., & Gouvier, W. D. (1985). A systematic solution to the Benton Visual Retention Test: a caveat to examiners. *International Journal of Clinical Neuropsychology, 7,* 95–96.

Bowden, S. C., & Bell, R. C. (1992). Relative usefulness of the WMS-R: A comment on D'Elia *et al.* (1989). *Journal of Clinical and Experimental Neuropsychology, 14,* 340–346.

Brown, J. (1958). Some tests of the decay theory of immediate memory. *Quarterly Journal of Experimental Psychology, 10,* 12–21.

Buschke, H. (1973). Selective reminding for analysis of memory and learning. *Journal of Verbal Learning and Verbal Behavior, 12,* 543–550.

Buschke, H., & Fuld, P. A. (1974). Evaluating storage, retention, and retrieval in disordered memory and learning. *Neurology, 24,* 1019–1025.

Chelune, G. J., & Bornstein, R. A. (1988). WMS-R patterns among patients with unilateral brain lesions. *The Clinical Neuropsychologist, 2,* 121–132.

The Clinical Neuropsychologist. (1988). Initial validity studies of the new Wechsler Memory Scale—Revised. *The Clinical Neuropsychologist, 2,* 101–196.

Crosson, B., Novack, T. A., Trenerry, M. R., & Craig, P. L. (1989). Differentiation of verbal memory deficits in blunt head injury using the recognition trial of the California Verbal Learning Test: An exploratory study. *The Clinical Neuropsychologist, 3,* 29–44.

Delis, D. C., Kramer, J. H., Kaplan, E., & Ober, B. A. (1987). *The California Verbal Learning Test—Research edition.* San Antonio: The Psychological Corporation.

Delis, D. C., Freeland, J., Kramer, J. H., & Kaplan, E. (1988). Integrating clinical assessment with cognitive neuroscience: Construct validation of the California Verbal Learning Test. *Journal of Consulting and Clinical Psychology, 56,* 123–130.

Denman, S. B. (1984). *Denman Neuropsychology Memory Scale.* Privately published: Sidney B. Denman, Ph.D., 1040 Fort Sumter Drive, Charleston, SC 29412.

Denman, S. B. (1987). *Denman Neuropsychology Memory Scale: Norms—1987.* Charleston, SC: Privately published.

D'Elia, L., Satz, P., & Schretlen, D. (1989). Wechsler Memory Scale: A critical appraisal of the normative studies. *Journal of Clinical and Experimental Neuropsychology, 11,* 551–568.

Ellis, A. W., & Young, A. W. (1988). *Human cognitive neuropsychology.* London: Lawrence Erlbaum Associates.

Elwood, R. W. (1991). The Wechsler Memory Scale—Revised: Psychometric characteristics and clinical application. *Neuropsychology Review, 2,* 179–201.

Franzen, M. (1989). *Reliability and validity in neuropsychological assessment.* New York: Plenum Press.

Geffen, G., Moar, K. J., O'Hanlon, A. P., Clark, C. R., & Geffen, L. B. (1990). Performance measures of 16- to 86-year-old males and females on the Auditory Verbal Learning Test. *The Clinical Neuropsychologist, 4,* 45–63.

Gilewski, M. J., & Zelinski, E. M. (1986). Questionnaire assessment of memory complaints. In L. Poon (Ed.), *Clinical memory assessment of older adults* (pp. 93–107). Washington, DC: American Psychological Association.

Golden, C. J., Hammeke, T. A., Purisch, A. D., Berg, R. A., Moses, J. A., Jr., Newlin, D. B., Wilkening, G. N., & Puente, A. E. (1982). *Item interpretation of the Luria–Nebraska Neuropsychological Battery.* Lincoln: University of Nebraska Press.

Golden, C. J., Purisch, A. D., & Hammeke, T. A. (1985). *Luria–Nebraska Neuropsychological Battery: Forms I and II.* Los Angeles: Western Psychological Services.

Hamsher, K., Benton, A. L., & Digre, K. (1980). Serial digit learning: Normative and clinical aspects. *Journal of Clinical Neuropsychology, 2,* 39–50.

Hannay, H. J., & Levin, H. S. (1985). Selective reminding test: An examination of equivalent forms. *Journal of Experimental Neuropsychology, 7,* 251–263.

Ivnik, R. J., Malec, J. F., Smith, G. E., Tangalos, E. G., Petersen, R. C., Kokmen, E., & Kurland, L. T. (1992a). Mayo's older Americans normative studies: WMS-R norms for ages 56 to 94. *The Clinical Neuropsychologist, 6,* 83–104.

Ivnik, R. J., Malec, J. F., Smith, G. E., Tangalos, E. G., Petersen, R. C., Kokmen, E., & Kurland, L. T. (1992b). Mayo's older Americans normative studies: AVLT norms for ages 56 to 94. *The Clinical Neuropsychologist, 6,* 49–82.

Larrabee, G. L., Kane, R. L., Schuck, J. R., & Francis, D. J. (1985). Construct validity of various memory testing procedures. *Journal of Clinical and Experimental Neuropsychology, 7,* 239–250.

Levin, H. S. (1986). Learning and memory. In H. J. Hannay (Ed.), *Experimental techniques in human neuropsychology* (pp. 309–362). New York: Oxford University Press.

Levin, H. S., Benton, A. L., & Grossman, R. G. (1982). *Neurobehavioral consequences of closed head injury.* New York: Oxford University Press.

Lezak, M. (1983). *Neuropsychological assessment* (2nd ed.). New York: Oxford University Press.

Miceli, G., Caltagirone, C., Gainotti, G., Masullo, C., & Silveri, M. C. (1981). Neuropsychological correlates of localized cerebral lesions in nonaphasic brain-damaged patients. *Journal of Clinical Neuropsychology, 3,* 53–63.

Milner, B. (1975). Psychological aspects of focal epilepsy and its neurological management. In D. P. Purpura, J. K. Penny, & R. D. Walters (Eds.), *Advances in neurology.* (Volume 8) (pp. 291–321). New York: Raven Press.

Milner, B., & Teuber, H. L. (1968). Alteration of perception and memory in man: Reflections on methods. In L. Weiskrantz (Ed.), *Analysis of behavioral change* (pp. 268–375). New York: Harper & Row.

Mittenberg, W., Burton, D. B., Darrow, E., & Thompson, G. B. (1992). Normative data for the Wechsler Memory Scale—Revised: 25- to 34-year olds. *Psychological Assessment, 4,* 363–368.

Neisser, U. (1967). *Cognitive psychology.* New York: Appleton-Century-Crofts.

Osterrieth, P. A. (1944). Le test de copy d'une figure complexe. *Archives de Psychologie, 30,* 206–356.

Peterson, L. R., & Peterson, M. J. (1959). Short-term retention of individual verbal items. *Journal of Experimental Psychology, 58,* 193–198.

Powell, J. B., Cripe, L. I., & Dodrill, C. B. (1991). Assessment of brain impairment with the Rey Auditory Verbal Learning Test: A comparison with other neuropsychological measures. *Archives of Clinical Neuropsychology, 6,* 241–249.

Randt, C. T., & Brown, E. R. (1983). *Administration Manual: Randt Memory Test.* Bayport, NY: Life Science Associates.

Rey, A. (1964). *L'examen clinique en psychologie.* Paris: Press Universitaire de France.

Ruff, R. M., Light, R. H., & Quayhagen, M. (1989). Selective reminding tests: A normative study of verbal learning in adults. *Journal of Clinical and Experimental Neuropsychology, 11,* 539–550.

Russell, E. W. (1975). A multiple scoring method for the assessment of complex memory functions. *Journal of Consulting and Clinical Psychology, 43,* 800–809.

Samuels, I., Butters, N., & Fedio, P. (1972). Short-term memory disorders following temporal lobe removals in humans. *Cortex, 8,* 283–298.

Silverstein, A. B. (1962). Perceptual, motor, and memory functions in the Visual Retention Test. *American Journal of Mental Deficiency, 66,* 613–617.

Spreen, O., & Strauss, E. (1991). *A compendium of neuropsychological tests: Administration, norms, and commentary.* New York: Oxford University Press.

Squire, L. R. (1986). The neuropsychology of memory dysfunction and its assessment. In I. Grant & K. M. Adams (Eds.), *Neuropsychological assessment of neuropsychiatric disorders* (pp. 268–299). New York: Oxford University Press.

Squire, L. R. (1987). *Memory and brain.* New York: Oxford University Press.

Strub, R. L., & Black, F. W. (1985). *The mental status examination in neurology* (2nd ed.). Philadelphia: F. A. Davis.

Stuss, D. T., Kaplan, E. F., Benson, D. F., Weir, W. S., Chuilli, S., & Sarazin, F. F. (1982). Evidence for the involvement of orbitofrontal cortex in memory functions: An interference effect. *Journal of Comparative and Physiological Psychology, 16,* 913–925.

Stuss, D. T., Stethem, L. L., & Poirier, C. A. (1987). Comparison of three tests of attention and rapid information processing across six age groups. *The Clinical Neuropsychologist, 1,* 139–152.

Stuss, D. T., Stethem, L. L., & Pelchat, G. (1988). Three tests of attention and rapid information processing: An extension. *The Clinical Neuropsychologist, 2,* 246–250.

Tombaugh, T. N., Schmidt, J. P., & Faulkner, P. (1992). A new procedure for administering the Taylor Complex Figure: Normative data over a 60-year age span. *The Clinical Neuropsychologist, 6,* 63–79.

Visser, R. S. H. (1980). *Manual of the complex figure test CFT.* Swets Test Services, 347b Heereweg, 2161 CA LISSE, The Netherlands.

Warrington, E. K., & Weiskrantz, L. (1970). Amnestic syndrome: Consolidation or retrieval? *Nature, 228,* 628–630.

Wechsler, D. A. (1987). *Wechsler Memory Scale—Revised.* New York: The Psychological Corporation.

Williams, J. M. (1991). *Memory Assessment Scales: Professional manual.* Odessa, FL: Psychological Assessment Resources.

18

Intelligence, General Knowledge, and Social Understanding

The tests reviewed in this chapter assess an assortment of abilities and areas of knowledge: general knowledge, practical intelligence, social understanding, sequencing, and verbal arithmetic problem-solving.

INFORMATION [I-WAIS-R (NI)]

Microdescription. Assesses general verbal knowledge.

Primary Assessment Areas. (1) Knowledge of general information; (2) remote, semantic memory (Lezak, 1983).

Secondary Assessment Areas. (1) Verbal comprehension; (2) speech.

Presentation Modality. Auditory–verbal.

Response Modalities. (1) Speech; (2) untimed.

Description. The patient is asked questions that test general knowledge normally available to persons who grew up in the United States. The test consists of 29 items arranged in order of increasing difficulty. The items assess knowledge of geography, famous people, scientific facts, literature, religion, and the United States (Wechsler, 1981).

In the WAIS-R NI, administration continues unless the patient becomes discouraged or frustrated. Information Multiple Choice is a multiple-choice version of the subtest that can be read by the patient (Kaplan *et al.,* 1991). Raw, Raw Scatter, Multiple Choice, and Multiple-Choice Scatter scores are recorded. The content areas of missed items should be noted: number facts: 3, 7, 22, 23, 25, 27; directions: 5, 9; geography: 9, 11, 16, 19, 23; classic writings: 12, 18, 28, 29; history and civics: 6, 10, 13, 14, 17, 22, 27; science: 4, 15, 20, 21, 24–26; and production or comprehension of names: 6, 8, 12–14, 17, 20, 26, 29 (Kaplan *et al.,* 1991).

Localization. The subtest is among the WAIS subtests least affected by brain injury. It may therefore provide an estimate of premorbid functioning, in the absence of left hemisphere dysfunction (Golden, 1978; Lezak, 1983). Impaired performance on the I-WAIS is suggestive of left hemisphere damage (Reitan, 1955; Spreen & Benton, 1965).

Norms. See the WAIS-R.

Source. The Psychological Corporation.

COMPREHENSION [C-WAIS-R (NI)]

Microdescription. Assesses the patient's understanding of social norms and practices, practical reasoning, and understanding of proverbs.

Primary Assessment Areas. (1) Practical reasoning; (2) social understanding; (3) comprehension of proverbs (Peck *et al.,* 1987); (4) remote, semantic memory.

Secondary Assessment Areas. (1) Verbal comprehension; (2) speech.

Presentation Modality. Auditory–verbal.

Response Modalities. (1) Speech; (2) untimed.

Description. The patient is asked questions that assess knowledge of practically and socially appropriate behavior, governmental policies, and proverbs. The test consists of 14 open-ended questions, of which 3 concern proverbs, arranged in order of difficulty from easy to hard (Wechsler, 1981). The clinician should be wary of making inferences about the patient's capacity to behave appropriately in complex, multidimensional, real-life situations on the basis of performance on this subtest (Lezak, 1983).

In the WAIS-R NI administration, Items 12 and 14–15 (proverbs) are given regardless of the patient's performance on other items. Multiple-choice renditions of these items are provided. Raw and Raw Scatter scores are recorded.

Localization. The Comprehension subtest may be minimally affected by brain injury. It may therefore provide an estimate of premorbid functioning, in the absence of left-hemisphere dysfunction (Peck *et al.,* 1987). Impaired performance on the Comprehension subtest of the WAIS is suggestive of left-hemisphere damage (Lezak, 1983). However, impairment on proverbs may be suggestive of right-hemisphere pathology (Kaplan *et al.,* 1991).

Norms. See the WAIS-R.

Source. The Psychological Corporation.

PICTURE ARRANGEMENT [PA-WAIS-R (NI)]

Microdescription. Requires the patient to rearrange a set of cartoon-like pictures to tell a sensible story.

Primary Assessment Areas. (1) Visual analysis and synthesis; (2) interpretation of social situations (Lezak, 1983; Sattler, 1988); (3) capacity to anticipate and understand the consequences and antecedents of social events (Lezak, 1983; Sattler, 1988).

Secondary Assessment Areas. (1) Verbal comprehension; (2) upper extremity motor functioning.

Presentation Modalities. (1) Visual–nonverbal; (2) auditory–verbal for instructions.

Response Modalities. (1) Simple upper extremity movements—moving cards; (2) time-limited.

Description. The patient is presented with a series of pictures and is asked to arrange them in an order that tells a story that makes sense. The materials consist of 10 sets of cartoon pictures. The sets vary in length from three to six pictures (Wechsler, 1981).

The WAIS-R NI administration offers two alternatives. In one administration, the patient is requested, to tell me the story of what is happening after all the items have been administered. In the other, this request is made after the patient produces each arrangement (Kaplan *et al.,* 1991). Raw, Raw Scatter, Overtime, and Sequence scores are recorded. Sequence scores give credit for a partially correct sequencing of cards.

Sentence Arrangement provides a verbal analog to PA-WAIS-R and allows for the comparison of sequencing ability for verbal vs. visual material (Kaplan *et al.,* 1991).

Localization. Impaired performance on the PA-WAIS-R is associated with right hemisphere dysfunction (Warrington *et al.,* 1986).

Norms. See the WAIS-R.

Source. The Psychological Corporation.

INTELLECTUAL PROCESSES (C11-LNNB)

Microdescription. Assesses intellectual functions, complex reasoning, and problem-solving skills (Golden *et al.,* 1985).

Primary Assessment Areas. (1) Understanding thematic pictures and texts; (2) vocabulary, concepts, and verbal relationships; (3) verbal arithmetic problem-solving.

Secondary Assessment Areas. Verbal comprehension and communication.

Presentation Modalities. (1) Any verbal modality may be used to convey the instructions and items; (2) items 236–243 are visual–nonverbal.

Response Modalities. (1) Any verbal modality may be used; (2) untimed for items 236, 237, and 242–257; (3) evens are time-limited and odds are timed for items 238–241 and 258–269.

Description. The items may be briefly described as follows:

236, 237 Identification of relationships in a picture
238–241 Picture arrangement
242, 243 Absurdities
244 Understanding the moral of a story
245–247 Proverbs
248 Definitions
249 Similarities
250 Differences
251 Categorization
252 Member of a group
253 Part when given whole
254 Whole when given part
255 Opposites
256 Analogies
257 Identification of word that doesn't belong
258–269 Verbal arithmetic problems

Three Factor Scales have been identified: General Verbal Intelligence (I1) contains items in the general area of verbal intelligence. Complex Verbal Arithmetic (I2) contains difficult verbal arithmetic problems and Simple Verbal Arithmetic (I3) primarily contains simple arithmetic problems. C11 correlates 0.8 with Full Scale IQ.

Localization. Poor performance on C11 in the absence of poor performance on C5 and C6 scales and in the absence of significant psychiatric thought disorder has been reported to be generally associated with prefrontal dysfunction. Elevation of C11 can be associated with impairment in either hemisphere; however, an elevation combined with elevation of C2, C4, C10, and C9 may suggest right hemisphere dysfunction, while an elevation combined with elevation of C6, C8, and C7 may suggest left hemisphere dysfunction (Golden *et al.,* 1982; Golden *et al.,* 1985).

Norms. See the LNNB.

Source. Western Psychological Services.

REFERENCES

Golden, C. J. (1978). *Diagnosis and rehabilitation in clinical neuropsychology.* Springfield, IL: Charles C. Thomas.
Golden, C. J., Hammeke, T. A., Purisch, A. D., Berg, R. A., Moses, J. A., Jr., Newlin, D. B., Wilkening, G. N., & Puente, A. E. (1982). *Item interpretation of the Luria–Nebraska Neuropsychological Battery.* Lincoln: University of Nebraska Press.
Golden, C. J., Purisch, A. D., & Hammeke, T. A. (1985). *Luria–Nebraska Neuropsychological Battery: Forms I and II.* Los Angeles: Western Psychological Services.
Kaplan, E., Fine, D., Morris, R., & Delis, D. C. (1991). *WAIS-R NI: Manual.* San Antonio: The Psychological Corporation.
Kaufman, A. S. (1990). *Assessing adolescent and adult intelligence.* Boston: Allyn & Bacon.
Lezak, M. (1983). *Neuropsychological assessment* (2nd ed.). New York: Oxford University Press.
Peck, E. A., Stephens, V., & Martelli, M. F. (1987). A descriptive summary of essential neuropsychological tests. In L. C. Hartlage, M. J. Aske, & J. L. Horsby (Eds.), *Essentials of neuropsychological assessment.* New York: Springer.

Reitan, R. M. (1955). Certain differential effects of right and left cerebral lesions in human adults. *Journal of Comparative and Physiological Psychology, 48,* 474–477.

Sattler, J. M. (1988). *Assessment of children* (3rd ed.). San Diego: Jerome M. Sattler.

Spreen, O., & Benton, A. L. (1965). Comparative studies of some psychological tests for cerebral damage. *Journal of Nervous and Mental Disease, 140,* 323–333.

Warrington, E. K., James, M., & Maciejewski, C. (1986). The WAIS as a lateralising and localising diagnostic instrument: A study of 656 patients with unilateral cerebral lesions. *Neuropsychologia, 24,* 223–239.

Wechsler, D. (1981). *Wechsler Adult Intelligence Scale—Revised.* New York: Psychological Corporation.

Speech and Language

The speech/language area of cognitive functioning can be broken down into several subareas—fluency, repetition, naming, auditory comprehension, oral reading, reading comprehension, writing, and spelling. *Verbal fluency* is production of an uninterrupted, flowing series of speech sounds. *Prosody* is the rhythmic intonation or melody of speech. *Word fluency* is production of words representative of a category (e.g., animals, foods, words that begin with the letter "S"). *Repetition* is oral reproduction of patterns of speech sounds from auditory presentation. *Paraphasias* are word substitutions in speech. In a literal or phonemic paraphasia, syllables are substituted ("pell" for "bell"). In a verbal or semantic paraphasia, an unintended word is substituted (Goodglass & Kaplan, 1983). *Naming* is the ability to produce appropriate names for things. Impaired naming is termed *anomia. Auditory comprehension* is the ability to understand spoken language. *Oral reading* is the ability to read aloud. *Reading comprehension* is the ability to read and understand written material. Impaired reading comprehension is called *alexia*. Impairment in writing is termed *agraphia*. Impairments may occur in any of these areas of language functioning.

Cognitive neuropsychologists have devised elaborate cognitive models to account for these processes and their interrelationships. A review of these models is beyond the scope of this book. The reader is referred to the writings of Caramazza (1991), Ellis and Young (1988), McCarthy and Warrington (1990), and Shallice (1988).

APHASIAS

This section presents a listing of some of the aphasias and their major characteristics (Benson, 1979, 1985; A. R. Damasio, 1991; H. Damasio, 1991; Goodglass & Kaplan, 1983).

Broca's Aphasia

Speech fluency	Nonfluent, telegraphic
Paraphasias	Literal
Repetition	Impaired
Auditory comprehension	Relatively intact
Confrontation naming	Impaired

Reading
    Aloud   Impaired
    Comprehension   Sometimes impaired
Writing   Impaired

Lesions in Broca's aphasia may involve the frontal operculum (areas 44 and 45) and include the premotor and motor regions behind and above and extend into the underlying white matter and the basal ganglia as well as the insula (H. Damasio, 1991).

Wernicke's Aphasia

Speech fluency	Good
Paraphasias	Verbal and literal
Repetition	Impaired
Auditory comprehension	Impaired
Confrontation naming	Impaired
Reading	
Aloud	Impaired
Comprehension	Impaired
Writing	Impaired

Lesions occur in the posterior region of the left superior temporal gyrus (H. Damasio, 1991).

Conduction Aphasia

Speech fluency	Good
Paraphasias	Phonemic, literal
Repetition	Impaired
Auditory comprehension	Good
Confrontation naming	Impaired
Reading	
Aloud	Impaired
Comprehension	Good
Writing	Impaired

Lesions may be in the left perisylvian region and may involve primary auditory cortex (areas 41 and 42), a portion of the surrounding association cortex (area 22), and the insula and its subcortical white matter as well as the supramarginal gyrus (H. Damasio, 1991).

Anomic Aphasia

Speech fluency	Fluent
Paraphasias	Absent
Repetition	Good
Auditory comprehension	Good
Confrontation naming	Impaired

Reading
    Aloud   Sometimes impaired
    Comprehension   Sometimes impaired
Writing   Sometimes impaired

Lesions of the left anterior temporal cortices are necessary for the syndrome (H. Damasio, 1991).

Transcortical Motor Aphasia

Speech fluency	Nonfluent
Paraphasias	Absent
Repetition	Good (echolalia)
Auditory comprehension	Good
Confrontation naming	Impaired
Reading	
Aloud	Impaired
Comprehension	Usually good
Writing	Impaired

This aphasia may be caused by a lesion that disrupts connections between the supplementary motor area and structures of Broca's area and the motor area (H. Damasio, 1991). Lesions tend to be outside Broca's area, either anteriorly or superiorly, deep in the left frontal lobe or in the cortex.

Transcortical Sensory Aphasia

Speech fluency	Fluent
Paraphasias	Neologistic and semantic
Repetition	Good (echolalia)
Auditory comprehension	Impaired
Confrontation naming	Impaired
Reading	
Aloud	Impaired
Comprehension	Impaired
Writing	Impaired

Lesions occur in the posterior sector of the middle temporal gyrus (area 37) and in the angular gyrus (area 39) or in the underlying white matter (H. Damasio, 1991).

Mixed Transcortical Aphasia

Speech fluency	Nonfluent
Paraphasias	Absent
Repetition	Good (echolalia)
Auditory comprehension	Impaired
Confrontation naming	Impaired
Reading	
Aloud	Impaired
Comprehension	Impaired
Writing	Impaired

Lesions may spare the perisylvian area but involve the surrounding area or border zones (Benson, 1985).

Global Aphasia

Speech fluency	Nonfluent
Paraphasias	Sometimes present
Repetition	Impaired
Auditory comprehension	Impaired
Confrontation naming	Impaired
Reading	
Aloud	Impaired
Comprehension	Impaired
Writing	Impaired

The lesion may occur in the entire left perisylvian region (H. Damasio, 1991).

RHYTHM

Seashore Rhythm Test (SR)

Microdescription. Assesses perception of rhythm.

Primary Assessment Areas. (1) Perception of nonverbal auditory stimuli; (2) sustained attention (Reitan & Wolfson, 1993).

Secondary Assessment Area. Verbal comprehension.

Presentation Modalities. (1) auditory–verbal for instructions; (2) auditory–nonverbal for stimulus items.

Response Modalities. (1) Upper extremity movements—writing; (2) paced.

Description. A tape recording is played and the patient is required to discriminate between 30 pairs of rhythmic beats. The patient writes "S" for "same" or "D" for "different" on an answer sheet (Reitan & Wolfson, 1993).

Localization. SR is an indicator of the general adequacy of cerebral functioning and has no lateralizing significance (Reitan & Wolfson, 1993; Steinmeyer, 1984).

Norms. Heaton *et al.* (1991) have reported norms broken down by age, gender, and education.

Source. Reitan Neuropsychology Laboratory.

Rhythm Scale (C2-LNNB)

Microdescription. Assesses perception and production of pitches, rhythms, and melodies.

Primary Assessment Areas. (1) Perception and reproduction of pitch relationships and melodies; (2) perception of acoustic signals; (3) reproduction and production of rhythms (Golden *et al.,* 1982).

Secondary Assessment Area. Verbal comprehension.

Presentation Modalities. (1) auditory–verbal instructions for all items, but instructions may be varied and written, except for item 63, to ensure understanding; (2) auditory–nonverbal for items 52–55 and 57–62.

Response Modalities. (1) Any signal for items 52–54, (2) humming for items 55, 56, and 58–61; (3) speech for item 57; (4) any motor response for items 62 and 63; (5) all items are untimed.

Description. Items may be summarized as follows:

52	Identification of different pitches
53	Identification of higher pitch
54	Identification of different groups of tones
55	Repeating (humming) tones
56	Repeating (humming) a tune
57	Singing a tune
58–61	Counting beeps
62	Copy rhythm
63	Produce rhythm

All items except for the singing items are loaded on RH1 (Rhythm and Pitch Perception).

Localization. C2 is sensitive to disorders of attention and concentration (Golden *et al.,* 1985). When C2 is high and also the highest of the scales, this configuration is most often associated with right hemisphere injuries, although it may also occur with left hemisphere injuries. Very good scores are generally inconsistent with severe right hemisphere injury (Golden *et al.,* 1985). However, Steinmeyer (1984) found that C2 was not differentially sensitive to right temporal lobe lesions.

Norms. See the LNNB.

Source. Western Psychological Services.

SPEECH PERCEPTION

Speech Sounds Perception Test (SSPT)

Microdescription. Assesses auditory perception of consonants.

Primary Assessment Area. Auditory consonant perception.

Secondary Assessment Areas. (1) Attention; (2) reading of nonsense words; (3) verbal comprehension.

Presentation Modalities. (1) Auditory–verbal for instructions and presentation of nonsense word stimuli; (2) visual–verbal presentation of nonsense words.

Response Modalities. (1) Simple upper extremity and hand motor movements—pointing or underlining; (2) paced.

Description. The test assesses the patient's ability to match a spoken "nonsense word" with the correct alternative among a group of similar printed nonsense words. The test is administered with a tape recorder and consists of 60 groups of four nonsense words. All words are single syllable and have "ee" in the middle and may be discriminated by comparing the consonants at the beginning or end of each word (Reitan & Wolfson, 1993). Versions of the test with 30 items per group have been found to be equivalent to the original test (Margolis *et al.*, 1984).

Localization. The SSPT is a complex task that is sensitive to general cerebral dysfunction (Crockett *et al.*, 1982). It does not clearly lateralize (Bornstein & Leason, 1984; Sherer *et al.*, 1991). Care should be taken in inferring a central auditory processing deficit on the basis of impaired performance on the SSPT, since high-frequency hearing loss may result in impaired performance (Schear *et al.*, 1988).

Norms. Norms stratified by age, gender, and education may be found in Heaton *et al.* (1991).

Source. Reitan Neuropsychology Laboratory.

Phoneme Discrimination

Microdescription. Assesses auditory perception of vowels.

Primary Assessment Areas. (1) Auditory perception of vowels nonsense words; (2) verbal comprehension.

Presentation Modalities. (1) Auditory–verbal for instructions and presentation of nonsense-word stimuli; (2) visual–verbal presentation of nonsense words.

Response Modalities. (1) Simple vocal response or simple motor movements—pointing or nodding to indicate "same" or "different"; (2) untimed.

Description. The test consists of 30 pairs of "nonsense words" (10 pairs of one-syllable and 20 pairs of two-syllable words) administered with a tape recorder. Since the test assesses only a small subset of possible phonemic contrasts, it cannot be used to assess perception of vowels vs. consonants or of voicing contrasts vs. place contrasts (Benton *et al.*, 1983).

Localization. A subset of aphasic left-brain-damaged patients produce defective performances (Benton *et al.*, 1983). Varney and Benton (1979) found only aphasics with impaired aural comprehension to have defects in phoneme discrimination.

Norms. A score of less than 22 is classified as defective (Benton *et al.,* 1983).

Source. Oxford University Press.

COMPREHENSION

Vocabulary [V-WAIS-R (NI)]

Microdescription. Requires the patient to define words.

Primary Assessment Areas. (1) Vocabulary; (2) remote, semantic memory.

Secondary Assessment Areas. (1) Verbal comprehension; (2) speech.

Presentation Modality. Auditory–verbal.

Response Modalities. (1) Speech; (2) untimed.

Description. The patient is asked to provide the meanings of words. The test consists of 35 words presented in order of difficulty (Wechsler, 1981). Vocabulary is one of the best measures of verbal and general mental ability (Lezak, 1983).

The WAIS-R NI Stimulus Book contains the words in large print (Kaplan *et al.,* 1991). It can be used to present words singly by covering the multiple choices with a shield. A multiple-choice version of the Vocabulary subtest (Vocabulary Multiple Choice) for testing the limits of the patient's vocabulary is provided. Raw, Raw Scatter, Multiple Choice, and Multiple-Choice Scatter can be scored.

Localization. V-WAIS-R is one of the subtests least affected by bilateral or diffuse brain injury (Lezak, 1983). It may therefore provide an estimate of premorbid functioning, in the absence of left hemisphere dysfunction. Impaired performance on the V-WAIS-R is suggestive of left hemisphere damage (Parsons *et al.,* 1969).

Norms. See the WAIS-R.

Source. The Psychological Corporation.

Similarities (S-WAIS-R)

Microdescription. Requires the patient to explain what each of two members of a verbal class has in common.

Primary Assessment Areas. (1) Verbal concept formation (Lezak, 1983; Sattler, 1988); (2) remote, semantic memory.

Secondary Assessment Areas. (1) Verbal comprehension; (2) speech.

Presentation Modality. Auditory–verbal.

Response Modalities. (1) Speech; (2) untimed.

Description. The patient is required to explain what two words have in common. The test consists of 14 pairs of words arranged from least to most difficult (Wechsler, 1981).

The WAIS-R NI Stimulus Book includes a multiple-choice version (Similarities Multiple Choice) that can be used for testing limits (Kaplan *et al.,* 1991). Raw, Raw Scatter, Multiple Choice, and Multiple-Choice Scatter can be scored.

Localization. S-WAIS-R is the verbal subtest most sensitive to brain damage. Impairment on the S-WAIS-R is associated with left hemisphere lesions (McFie, 1975; Reitan, 1955; Warrington *et al.,* 1986).

Norms. See the WAIS-R.

Source. The Psychological Corporation.

Peabody Picture Vocabulary Test—Revised (PPVT-R)

Microdescription. Requires the patient to select a picture that best represents a word.

Primary Assessment Areas. (1) Receptive vocabulary (Dunn & Dunn, 1981); (2) auditory–verbal comprehension.

Secondary Assessment Areas. Object recognition.

Presentation Modalities. (1) Auditory–verbal presentation of instructions and stimulus words; (2) visual–spatial presentation of line drawings.

Response Modalities. (1) Simple upper extremity movements—pointing or (2) speech; (3) untimed.

Description. The patient is shown a page in a booklet containing four black and white drawings of objects or scenes and is asked to select the picture that depicts the word spoken by the examiner. There are 5 training items and 175 test items of increasing difficulty. Because administration involves locating basal (highest 8 consecutive correct responses) and ceiling (lowest 8 responses containing six errors) performance levels, all items are not given (Dunn & Dunn, 1981; Shea, 1989). There are two equivalent forms (L and M).

Localization. No information is available.

Norms. Norms are available for ages 2.5–40 years (Dunn & Dunn, 1981). The test has been found to be highly correlated with intelligence (Crofoot & Bennett, 1980).

Source. American Guidance Service.

Auditory Comprehension (AC-BDAE)

Microdescription. Patient demonstrates comprehension of orally presented words, commands, sentences, and paragraphs.

Primary Assessment Areas. (1) Verbal comprehension; (2) comprehension of verbal descriptions of objects, actions, letters, colors, forms, numbers, body parts, and commands (Goodglass & Kaplan, 1983); (3) comprehension of complex ideational material (Goodglass & Kaplan, 1983).

Secondary Assessment Areas. (1) Form perception; (2) color vision; (3) right–left orientation (Goodglass & Kaplan, 1983); (4) upper extremity motor functioning.

Presentation Modalities. (1) Auditory–verbal; (2) visual–verbal for Word Discrimination; (3) visual–nonverbal for Word Discrimination, Body-Part Discrimination, and Commands.

Response Modalities. (1) Upper extremity movements; (2) timed (Word Discrimination and Body-Part Discrimination); (3) untimed (Commands and Complex Ideational Material); (4) expression of agreement or disagreement via ''yes''/''no'' responses such as head nods for Complex Ideational Material.

Description. Auditory Comprehension is composed of four subtests:

Word Discrimination (WD-BDAE): The patient is presented two cards containing pictures of objects and actions, geometric shapes, colors, letters, and numbers. The patient is asked to show the examiner items on the cards, 36 items in all. Two points are scored for a correct response within 5 sec and one point for a correct response after 5 sec. One-half point is scored for an incorrect response in the correct category or a correct response after cuing to the appropriate category.

Body-Part Identification (BPI-BDAE): The patient is asked to show the examiner body parts. The identification of 18 body parts is required. Eight additional questions require identification of the left and right sides of the body. One point is scored for a correct response within 5 sec. One-half point is scored for a correct response after 5 sec. A total of 18 points may be earned from the first 18 items, and a maximum of 2 additional points may be earned from the right–left items for a maximum of 20.

Commands (C-BDAE): The patient is asked to perform five commands with one to five informational elements. A point is earned for conformance with each informational unit for a maximum of 15.

Complex Ideational Material (CIM-BDAE): The patient is required to express agreement or disagreement concerning eight simple facts. Sixteen questions test comprehension of brief paragraphs orally presented to the patient. The questions are arranged in yes/no pairs. One point is scored for each correct pair for a maximum of 12 points (Goodglass & Kaplan, 1983).

Localization. See the BDAE.

Norms. See the BDAE. CIM-BDAE norms may be found in Heaton *et al.* (1991).

Source. Lea & Febiger.

Aural Comprehension of Words and Phrases (ACWP-MAE)

Microdescription. Requires the identification of pictures corresponding to spoken words.

Primary Assessment Areas. (1) Understanding of words and simple phrases (Benton & Hamsher, 1989); (2) verbal comprehension.

Secondary Assessment Areas. (1) Visual object recognition; (2) upper extremity motor functioning.

Presentation Modalities. (1) Auditory–verbal; (2) visual–verbal.

Response Modalities. (1) Upper extremity movements—pointing; (2) time-limited.

Description. Materials consist of a six-page booklet with each page containing four pictures. The patient is instructed "Point to the picture which best shows what I say," and a word is orally presented. Eleven single words and seven short phrases are presented. One point is scored for a correct response within 20 sec for a maximum of 18 (Benton & Hamsher, 1989).

Localization. See the Multilingual Aphasia Examination (MAE).

Norms. Benton and Hamsher (1989) provide percentile norms for a group of ages 16–69 years and with 8 years or more of education. The scores for patients with 8–11 years of education are adjusted by adding 1 point.

Source. Psychological Assessment Resources.

Token Test (TT-MAE)

Microdescription. Requires the patient to manipulate tokens in response to commands.

Primary Assessment Areas. (1) Ability to comprehend and carry out simple commands (Benton & Hamsher, 1989); (2) verbal comprehension.

Secondary Assessment Areas. (1) Upper extremity motor functioning; (2) visual form recognition; (3) color vision; (4) praxis.

Presentation Modalities. (1) Auditory–verbal; (2) visual–nonverbal; (3) color.

Response Modalities. (1) Upper extremity movements; (2) time-limited.

Description. The patient is presented with an array of 20 plastic tokens: large and small, circles and squares in five colors (red, black, green, yellow, and white). The patient is asked to do things regarding the tokens (e.g., "Point to the large, red circle"). If the patient fails on the first attempt, the item is repeated. Two points are scored for success on the first attempt and one point for success on the second attempt. A total of 22 commands are made in all for a total of 44 possible points (Benton & Hamsher, 1989).

Localization. The test discriminates well between aphasic and nonaphasic adults (Sarno, 1986).

Norms. Benton and Hamsher (1989) provide percentile norms for a group of ages 16–69 years and with 8 years or more of education.

Source. Psychological Assessment Resources.

Receptive Speech Scale (C5-LNNB)

Microdescription. Assesses the patient's ability to understand spoken speech (Golden *et al.,* 1985).

Primary Assessment Areas. (1) Phoneme perception; (2) repetition; (3) comprehension of words, sentences, and complex grammatical constructions.

Presentation Modalities. Although instructions may be provided in a variety of modalities, the items are presented auditorily only, with the examiner behind or beside the patient. All items are presented in the auditory–verbal modality. In addition, items 110, 113, 116–121, and 127 are visual–nonverbal.

Response Modalities. For most items, any response modality may be used (Golden *et al.,* 1985). See the LNNB Manual (Golden *et al.,* 1985) for exceptions. Responses are untimed for items 100–120 and 123 and time-limited for items 121, 122, and 124–132.

Description. The items of the LNNB Receptive Speech Scale may be summarized as follows:

100, 102, 104	Repetition of spoken sounds
101, 103, 105	Writing spoken sounds
106	Signaling to spoken sounds
107	Identification of same or different consonants
108, 109, 111	Pointing to named body parts
110, 113	Pointing to named objects
112	Definition of similar words with different beginning consonants
114	Following simple commands
115, 116	Understanding simple sentences
117	Understanding conflicting instructions
118–120	Understanding simple inflective constructions
121–132	Understanding grammatical constructions

Four Factor Scales have been identified. Phonemic Discrimination (R1) is self-explanatory. Relational Concepts (R2) consists of items that require the patient to understand verbally expressed relationships. Concept Recognition (R3) assesses basic understanding of concepts. Verbal–Spatial Relationships (R4) involves understanding of simple prepositional relationships, performing simple actions, and visual identification of simple objects.

Localization. Elevation on C5 may be associated with left hemisphere damage (Golden *et al.,* 1985).

Norms. See the LNNB.

Source. Western Psychological Services.

READING

Reading (R-WRAT-R)

Microdescription. Requires the patient to read words aloud.

Primary Assessment Areas. (1) Oral word reading (Jastak & Wilkinson, 1984; Wilkinson, 1989); (2) word recognition (Jastak & Wikinson, 1984; Wilkinson, 1989).

Secondary Assessment Area. Speech.

Presentation Modalities. (1) Visual–verbal; (2) auditory–verbal for instructions.

Response Modalities. (1) Speech; (2) untimed.

Description. There are two versions of the WRAT-R, a Level 1 version for children 5–11 and a Level 2 version for individuals 12–75 years. In both versions, the patient is required to read a list of gradually more difficult words aloud. Under certain conditions, the patient is required to read and recognize letters in a prereading section of the test. There are 75 words on the Level 1 Reading Test and 74 words on the Level 2 Reading Test. Administration time is approximately 10 min (Jastak & Wilkinson, 1984).

Localization. Localization data are not available for this test.

Norms. Norms are provided for 28 age groups from 5 to 75 (Jastak & Wilkinson, 1984)—standard scores, percentiles, and grade equivalents. Comparisons are made with other test performances using standard scores and percentiles rather than grade equivalents.

Source. Jastak Assessment Systems.

Oral Reading (OR-BDAE)

Microdescription. Requires the patient to read words and sentences aloud.

Primary Assessment Areas. (1) Oral reading (Goodglass & Kaplan, 1983); (2) word finding.

Secondary Assessment Area. Verbal comprehension.

Presentation Modalities. (1) Visual–verbal; (2) auditory–verbal for instructions.

Response Modalities. (1) Speech; (2) timed (Word Reading); (3) untimed (Oral Sentence Reading).

Description. OR-BDAE consists of two subtests:

Word Reading (WR-BDAE): One at a time, using a card as a shield the examiner displays 10 words printed on a card. The patient is asked to read the 10 words aloud. Three points are earned for a correct response within 3 sec for each word, two points within 10 sec, one point within 30 sec, and otherwise 0.

Oral Sentence Reading (OSR-BDAE): This subtest requires the patient to read complete sentences, 10 in all (Goodglass & Kaplan, 1983). One point is scored for each correctly read sentence.

Localization. See the BDAE.

Norms. See the BDAE.

Source. Lea & Febiger.

Reading Comprehension (RC-BDAE)

Microdescription. Requires the patient to demonstrate recognition and comprehension of written material.

Primary Assessment Areas. (1) Recognition of written letters or words (SWR-BDAE, WRec-BDAE, WPM-BDAE, RSP-BDAE) (Goodglass & Kaplan, 1983); (2) understanding of written words or sentences (WPM-BDAE, RSP-BDAE); (3) visual object recognition (WPM-BDAE); (4) auditory–visual phonetic associations (WRec-BDAE) (Goodglass & Kaplan, 1983); (5) ability to respond to the connative meaning of a written word without appreciating its phonetic value (WRec-BDAE) (Goodglass & Kaplan, 1983); (6) understanding of orally spelled words (COS-BDAE) (Goodglass & Kaplan, 1983).

Presentation Modalities. (1) Visual–verbal (SWD-BDAE, WRec-BDAE, WPM-BDAE, RSP-BDAE); (2) auditory–verbal (WREc-BDAE, COS-BDAE); (3) auditory–verbal for instructions (WREc-BDAE, COS-BDAE, WPM-BDAE, RSP-BDAE); (4) visual–nonverbal (WPM-BDAE).

Response Modalities. (1) Upper extremity movements (SWD-BDAE, WRec-BDAE, WPM-BDAE, RSP-BDAE); (2) speech (COS-BDAE); (3) untimed.

Description. RC-BDAE, or Understanding Written Language, consists of five subtests:

Symbol and Word Discrimination (SWD-BDAE): A letter or brief word is presented on a card along with the same word or letter in different writing and four foils. The patient is required to match the stimuli. Ten items are presented for a maximum of ten points.

Word Recognition (WRec-BDAE): The patient is asked to select from five printed words the one spoken by the examiner. A total of eight words are presented. One point is scored for each correct selection.

Comprehension of Oral Spelling (COS-BDAE): The patient identifies words orally spelled by the examiner. One point is scored for each of eight words identified correctly.

Words Picture Matching (WPM-BDAE): The patient is required to select pictures of things corresponding to written words. One point is scored for each correct match for a maximum of ten.

Reading Sentences and Paragraphs (RSP-BDAE): The patient reads a sentence or paragraph and is required to select the word or phrase from four alternatives that will correctly complete the sentence. After two practice examples, ten items are presented for a maximum of ten points (Goodglass & Kaplan, 1983).

Localization. See the BDAE.

Norms. See the BDAE.

Source. Lea & Febiger.

Reading Comprehension of Words and Phrases (RCWP-MAE)

Microdescription. Requires the identification of pictures corresponding to read words.

Primary Assessment Areas. (1) Reading and understanding of words and simple phrases (Benton & Hamsher, 1989); (2) verbal comprehension.

Secondary Assessment Areas. (1) Visual object recognition; (2) upper extremity motor functioning.

Presentation Modalities. (1) Visual–verbal; (2) visual–nonverbal; (3) auditory–verbal for instructions.

Response Modalities. (1) Upper extremity movements—pointing; (2) time-limited.

Description. Materials consist of a six-page booklet with each page containing four pictures. The patient is presented a word or short phrase printed on a card and is instructed, "Read this word and point to the picture which best fits it." Eighteen single words or short phrases are presented. One point is scored for a correct response within 20 sec for each word or phrase (Benton & Hamsher, 1989).

Localization. See the MAE.

Norms. Benton and Hamsher (1989) provide percentile norms for a group age 16–69 years and with 8 years or more of education. The scores of patients with 8–11 years of education are adjusted by adding 1 point.   .

Source. Psychological Assessment Resources.

North American Adult Reading Test (NAART)

Microdescription. Requires the patient to read words aloud.

Primary Assessment Areas. (1) Oral reading; (2) word recognition.

Secondary Assessment Areas. Speech.

Presentation Modalities. (1) Visual–verbal; (2) auditory–verbal for instructions.

Response Modalities. (1) Speech; (2) untimed.

Description. The test consists of a list of 61 words printed in two columns on both sides of an $8\frac{1}{2}'' \times 11''$ card that is given to the patient to read aloud. The test is composed of ''irregular'' words that cannot be correctly pronounced through the use of common rules of phonetic interpretation. The error score is used to calculate premorbid IQ. The NAART is the north American version of the National Adult Reading Test (NART) designed for British patients by Nelson and O'Connell (1978). Nelson and McKenna (1975) found that although WAIS scores of a group of patients with cerebral atrophy were one standard deviation below those of a control group, there was no difference in NART scores. Hart *et al.* (1986) found that performance on the NART was a better estimator of premorbid function in demented subjects than VIQ–PIQ discrepancy or Schonell's Graded Reading Test. Blair and Spreen (1989) found the NAART to predict IQ more accurately than the Barona equations in a normal sample (Barona *et al.,* 1984). Although these results are encouraging, deterioration in reading test performance has been found in patients having moderate and severe dementia and in patients having mild dementia with linguistic deficits (Stebbins *et al.,* 1988, 1990).

Localization. No localization studies have been performed.

Norms. Equations for calculating estimated VIQ, PIQ, and FSIQ are available in Spreen and Strauss (1991).

Source. Spreen and Strauss (1991).

Reading Scale (C8-LNNB)

Microdescription. Assesses reading aloud.

Primary Assessment Areas. Reading of letters, words, sentences, and paragraphs aloud.

Presentation Modalities. (1) Except for items 188 and 189, instructions can be written (Golden *et al.,* 1985); (2) items 190 and 192–200 are visual–verbal in presentation.

Response Modalities. (1) All responses are oral speech; (2) all items except 200, which is timed, are time-limited.

Description. The items may be summarized as follows:

          188 Production of sounds
          189 Production of words from letters
     190, 194 Reading letters
          191 Recognition of letters
          192 Reading syllables
193, 195, 196 Reading words

196–198 Reading sentences
199, 200 Reading a paragraph

Two Factor Scales have been identified. Reading Complex Material (RE1) involves reading complex words and paragraphs. Reading Simple Material (RE2) involves reading letters, words with silent letters, and simple sentences.

Localization. For individuals who have achieved good reading skills earlier in life, the C8 scale yields the best estimate of the premorbid functioning of the LNNB scales. For patients with good premorbid reading ability, impairment on the C8 scale is suggestive of left hemisphere dysfunction (Golden *et al.*, 1985).

Norms. See the LNNB.

Source. Western Psychological Services.

PRAXIS

Apraxia Test, BDAE Supplementary Test (AT-BDAE)

Microdescription. Requires the patient to perform movements to command, imitation, or when cued with an object.

Primary Assessment Area. Praxis.

Secondary Assessment Areas. (1) Facial motor functioning; (2) upper extremity motor functioning; (3) entire body motor functioning; (4) visual object identification; (5) verbal comprehension.

Presentation Modalities. (1) Auditory–verbal; (2) visual–nonverbal.

Response Modalities. (1) Upper extremity movement; (2) facial movement; (3) whole-body movement.

Description. The patient is required to perform a variety of purposeful movements involving the face, upper extremities, and the whole body. If an item is failed on command, the examiner performs the movement and asks the patient to imitate. If this trial is failed, the patient is asked to perform with a real object (if appropriate for the item). The patient is also required to perform a sequences of actions (Goodglass & Kaplan, 1983).

Localization. Apraxia may result from a variety of lesions, depending on the type of intentional act and the quality of the impairment. A summary is presented in Joseph (1990).

Norms. Norms were not available when this test was published (Goodglass & Kaplan, 1983).

Source. Lea & Febiger.

ORAL EXPRESSION

Fluency (F-BDAE)

See the BDAE.

Rating of Articulation (RA-MAE)

See the MAE.

Repetition (R-BDAE)

Microdescription. Requires the patient to repeat words, phrases, and sentences.

Primary Assessment Areas. (1) Repetition; (2) speech.

Secondary Assessment Areas. Verbal comprehension.

Presentation Modality. Auditory–verbal.

Response Modalities. (1) Speech; (2) untimed.

Description. Repetition consists of two subtests:

Repetition of Words (RW-BDAE): The patient is required to repeat words. Paraphasias and articulation are noted. Ten items are presented and scored one point each.

Repeating Phrases and Sentences (RepPS-BDAE): The patient is required to repeat phrases and sentences. Paraphasias and articulation are noted. Eight "high probability" and eight "low probability" sentences are presented and scored separately. One point is scored for each correct repetition.

Localization. See the BDAE.

Norms. See the BDAE.

Source. Lea & Febiger.

Sentence Repetition (SR-MAE)

Microdescription. Requires the repetition of sentences.

Primary Assessment Area. Repetition.

Secondary Assessment Area. Verbal comprehension.

Presentation Modality. Auditory–verbal.

Response Modalities. (1) Speech; (2) untimed.

Description. The patient is required to repeat 14 sentences from 3 to 18 words in length. One point is scored for each sentence repeated without any error for a maximum of 14 points (Benton & Hamsher, 1989).

Localization. See the MAE.

Norms. Benton and Hamsher (1989) provide percentile norms for a group age 16–69 years and with 8 years or more of education. The scores of patients with less than 9 years of education are adjusted by adding 3 points; 9–11 years, +2 points; 12–15 years, +1 point. If the patient is in the age range 60–69 and has had less than 16 years of education, an additional point is added.

Source. Psychological Assessment Resources.

Expressive Speech Scale (C6-LNNB)

Microdescription. Assesses fluency and articulatory speech skills (Golden *et al.,* 1985).

Primary Assessment Areas. (1) Repetition; (2) reading aloud; (3) recitation of automatic series; (4) naming; (5) narrative speech (Golden *et al.,* 1982).

Presentation Modalities. Although instructions are usually auditory–verbal, various methods of communication of instructions may be used (Golden *et al.,* 1985). Generally, the presentation is auditory–verbal for items 133–142, 154–156, 159, and 160, visual–verbal for items 143–153, 166, and 170–174, and visual–nonverbal for items 157 and 158.

Response Modalities. All items require speech. Responses are untimed for items 133–156, time-limited for items 157–163, 170, 172, and 173, and timed for items 163–169, 171, and 174.

Description. The items of the Expressive Speech Scale may be summarized as follows:

133, 134 Repetition of speech sounds
135–142 Repetition of words
143, 144 Saying sounds that go with letters
145–153 Reading words aloud
154–156 Repeating sentences
157, 158 Confrontation naming
      159 Naming objects from description
160–163 Recitation of automatic series
164, 165 Describing a scene
166, 167 Paraphrasing a story
168, 169 Giving a speech
170–174 Forming grammatical sentences

Factor Scales are E1 (Simple Phonemic Reading), E2 (Word Repetition)—repetition of sounds, words, and phrases from auditory input, and E3 (Reading Polysyllabic Words).

Localization. Significant elevations may be associated with left hemisphere dysfunction (Golden *et al.,* 1985).

Norms. See the LNNB.

Source. Western Psychological Services.

NAMING

Boston Naming Test (BNT)

Microdescription. Requires the patient to name line drawings of objects.

Primary Assessment Areas. (1) Naming; (2) visual object recognition; (3) verbal comprehension; (4) speech.

Presentation Modalities. (1) Visual–nonverbal; (2) auditory–verbal for instructions.

Response Modalities. (1) Speech; (2) untimed.

Description. The patient is required to name 60 line drawings of objects arranged in order of increasing difficulty. One point is scored for each correct name. If the patient fails to provide the correct name, a phonemic cue is provided. The test is discontinued after six successive failures if the patient becomes frustrated (Goodglass & Kaplan, 1983). Both longer and shorter alternative forms are available (Huff *et al.,* 1986; Thompson & Heaton, 1989).

Localization. Confrontation naming is often impaired by left hemisphere lesions (Knopman *et al.,* 1984). Picture-naming deficits may have limited use in the diagnosis of different aphasia syndromes (Kohn & Goodglass, 1985).

Norms. Norms are available for males in the age groups 20–29, 30–39, 40–49, 50–59, 60–69, and 70+ (Borod *et al.,* 1980; Goodglass & Kaplan, 1983). Van Gorp *et al.,* (1986) provide norms for adults aged 59–64, 65–69, 70–74, 75–79, and 80+. LaBarge *et al.* (1986) have provided norms for ages 60–64, 65–69, 70–74, 75–79, and 80–85. Heaton *et al.* (1991) have published norms stratified by age, education, and gender.

Source. Lea & Febiger.

Naming (N-BDAE)

Microdescription. Requires the patient to provide names.

Primary Assessment Areas. (1) Naming; (2) word fluency (AN-BDAE), (3) visual object recognition (VCN-BDAE); (4) verbal comprehension; (5) speech.

Presentation Modalities. (1) Auditory–verbal; (2) auditory–verbal for instructions; (3) visual–nonverbal.

Response Modalities. (1) Speech; (2) timed.

Description. Naming consists of three subtests:

Responsive Naming (RN-BDAE): The patient provides one-word answers to simple questions. Paraphasias and articulation are noted. Three points are earned for a correct response within 3 sec for each question, 2 points within 10 sec, 1 point within 30 sec, and otherwise 0. A maximum of 30 points is possible.

Visual Confrontation Naming (VCN-BDAE): Pictures of objects, geometric forms, letters, actions, numbers, colors, and body parts are presented to the patient, who is asked to name them. Paraphasias and articulation are noted. Three points are earned for a correct response within 3 sec for each picture, 2 points within 10 sec, 1 point within 30 sec, and otherwise 0. A maximum of 30 points is possible.

Animal Naming (AN-BDAE): The patient is requested to name as many animals as he or she can. The starting word ''dog'' is provided. The patient's words are recorded in 15-sec intervals for 90 sec. The score is the number of names in the most productive consecutive 60 sec (Goodglass & Kaplan, 1983).

Localization. See the BDAE.

Norms. See the BDAE.

Source. Lea & Febiger.

Visual Naming (VN-MAE)

Microdescription. Requires the patient to name line drawings of objects and parts of objects.

Primary Assessment Areas. (1) Naming (applying semantically correct verbal labels to visually perceived stimuli) (Benton & Hamsher, 1989); (2) visual object recognition; (3) verbal comprehension; (4) speech.

Presentation Modalities. (1) Visual–nonverbal; (2) auditory–verbal.

Response Modalities. (1) Speech; (2) time-limited.

Description. Ten pictures are presented requiring 30 naming responses. The patient is presented with a picture and asked to name whole objects or parts of objects. A maximum of 10 sec (15 if the patient is trying to produce an answer) is allowed for each picture. Two points are credited for each correct response.

Localization. See the MAE.

Norms. Benton and Hamsher (1989) provide percentile norms for a group age 16–69 years and with 8 years or more of education. Adjustments are made to the raw score for level of education (6–8 years, +8; 9–11 years, +6; 12–13 years, +4, 14–15 years, +2).

Source. Psychological Assessment Resources.

SPELLING

Spelling (S-WRAT-R)

Microdescription. Requires the patient to write words from dictation.

Primary Assessment Areas. (1) Written spelling (Jastak & Wilkinson, 1984; Wilkinson, 1989); (2) auditory perception of spoken words.

Presentation Modality. Auditory–verbal.

Response Modality. Skilled upper extremity movement—writing.

Description. There are two versions of the WRAT-R, a Level 1 version for children 5–11 and a Level 2 version for individuals 12–75 years. In both versions, the patient is required to write words to dictation. Under certain conditions, the patient is asked to copy some figures and write his or her name. Administration time is approximately 10 min.

Localization. No localization studies are available for this test.

Norms. Norms are provided for 28 age groups from 5 to 75 years (Jastak & Wilkinson, 1984), including standard scores, percentiles, and grade equivalents. Comparisons are made with other test performances using standard scores and percentiles rather than grade equivalents.

Source. Jastak Assessment Systems.

Spelling Test Battery (STB-MAE)

Microdescription. Requires the patient to spell words.

Primary Assessment Area. Spelling.

Secondary Assessment Areas. (1) Speech; (2) writing; (3) letter identification.

Presentation Modalities. (1) Auditory–verbal; (2) visual–verbal (BS-MAE).

Response Modalities. (1) Speech (OS-MAE); (2) upper extremity movements—writing (WS-MAE); (3) upper extremity movements—block letter manipulation.

Description

Oral Spelling (OS-MAE): The patient is asked to spell 11 words. The examiner reads a word, uses it in a sentence, and repeats the word. The patient then attempts to spell the word orally. One point is scored for each correct response.

Written Spelling (WS-MAE): This test is the same as OS-MAE except the patient attempts to write the words on an unlined sheet of white paper.

Block Spelling (BS-MAE): This test is the same as OS-MAE except the patient attempts to spell the words with black plastic block letters (Benton & Hamsher, 1989).

Localization. See the MAE.

Norms. Benton and Hamsher (1989) provide percentile norms for a group age 16–69 years and with 8 years or more of education. Adjustments are made to the raw score for level of education and for gender. Two points are added to the raw scores of males with less than 12 years of education and one point for scores of females with less than 12 years of education.

Source. Psychological Assessment Resources.

Spelling Scale (01 LNNB)

See the C7-LNNB.

WRITING

Writing (W-BDAE)

Microdescription. The patient is required to write letters, numbers, words, sentences, and paragraphs when presented with a variety of stimuli.

Primary Assessment Area. Writing.

Secondary Assessment Areas. (1) Upper extremity motor functioning; (2) visual object recognition (WCN-BDAE, NW-BDAE); (3) verbal comprehension.

Presentation Modalities. (1) Auditory–verbal (PLD-BDAE, SD-BDAE, SenD-BDAE); (2) visual–verbal (MW-BDAE); (3) visual–nonverbal (WCN-BDAE, NW-BDAE); (4) auditory verbal for instructions (MW-BDAE, SW-BDAE, PLD-BDAE, SD-BDAE, NW-BDAE, SenD-BDAE).

Response Modalities. (1) Upper extremity movements—writing; (2) untimed.

Description

Mechanics of Writing (MW-BDAE): The patient is requested to write his or her name and address on an unlined sheet of paper. If failed, the name and address are block-printed by the examiner and the patient is asked to transcribe in his or her own writing. Failing this, the patient is asked to copy. The patient is also required to copy a sentence in his or her own handwriting. This writing and all other writing on the Writing subtests is rated on a 5-point scale: 1 = no legible letters; 2 = occasional success on single letters (block printing); 3 = block printing with some malformed letters; 4 = legible but impaired cursive writing and/or upper- and lower-case printing; and 5 = judged to be the same as premorbid printing, with allowance made for the use of the nonpreferred hand (Goodglass & Kaplan, 1983).

Serial Writing (SW-BDAE): The patient is asked to write the alphabet and the numbers 1 to 21. The score is the total number of different, correct letters and numbers for a maximum score of 47.

Primer-Level Dictation (PLD-BDAE): The patient writes numbers, letters, and simple words to dictation. One point is scored for each correct item for a maximum of 15.

Spelling to Dictation (SD-BDAE): The patient is asked to write ten words to dictation. A point is scored for each correct word.

Written Confrontation Naming (WCN-BDAE): The examiner points silently to objects, colors, and other items printed on cards. The patient is instructed, orally or in pantomine, to write their names. One point is earned for each correct response for a maximum of ten.

Narrative Writing (NW-BDAE): The patient is asked to write as much as he or she can about what is going on in a picture ("cookie theft") that shows some children taking cookies from a jar while a woman washes dishes. The patient's writing is rated on a scale from 0 to 5.

Sentences to Dictation (SenD-BDAE): The patient is required to write three sentences from dictation. The sentences are scored for correctness on a 0–4 scale and paragraphic substitutions are noted.

Localization. See the BDAE.

Norms. See the BDAE.

Source. Lea & Febiger.

Rating of Praxic Features of Writing (RPFW-MAE)

See the MAE.

Writing Scale (C7-LNNB)

Microdescription. Assesses writing and spelling.

Primary Assessment Areas. (1) Writing to dictation; (2) spontaneous writing; (3) spelling (Golden *et al.,* 1985).

Presentation Modalities. Items 175, 176, and 180–187 are auditory–verbal in instruction or presentation. Instructions but not stimulus items may be written. Stimulus items 177–179 are visual–verbal.

Response Modalities. All items except 175 and 176, which may be signaled, spoken, or written, require the patient to respond by writing. Responses are untimed for items 177 and 182–185, time-limited for items 175, 176, 178–181, and 186, and timed for item 187.

Description. Items may be summarized as follows:

175, 176 Oral spelling

177, 178 Copying letters
    179 Writing words from memory
    180 Writing name
    181 Writing letters from dictation
    182 Writing sounds from dictation
183–185 Writing words and phrases from dictation
186, 187 Writing on a topic

Derivative scales are O1 (Spelling) and O2 (Motor Writing). O1 is the same as C7 except item 187 is omitted. O2 requires the rescoring of items 177–185 and 187 for motor writing performance (Golden *et al.*, 1985).

Localization. Four major cognitive systems are involved in writing: acoustic system, sensorimotor system, visual–spatial system, and inattentional/attentional system (Golden *et al.*, 1982). Localization therefore involves the systematic elimination of possible explanations of impairment (Golden *et al.*, 1985).

Norms. See the LNNB.

Source. Western Psychological Services.

GESTURAL COMMUNICATION

Pantomime Recognition (PR)

Microdescription. Requires the patient to point to objects whose uses are pantomimed.

Primary Assessment Area. Pantomime recognition (ability to understand meaningful, nonlinguistic pantomimed actions) (Benton *et al.*, 1983).

Secondary Assessment Areas. (1) Visual object recognition; (2) verbal comprehension; (3) upper extremity motor functioning.

Presentation Modalities. (1) Visual–nonverbal; (2) auditory–verbal for instructions.

Response Modalities. (1) Upper extremity movements—pointing; (2) untimed.

Description. Materials consist of a response booklet containing line drawings of objects and a videotape of a man pretending to use common objects. The response booklet contains four practice items printed on the first page. The remaining 30 pages contain four drawings each: (1) correct choice; (2) semantic foil—an object belonging to the same class of objects as the pantomimed object; (3) neutral foil—an object whose use is pantomimed elsewhere on the test, and (4) odd foil—an object whose use is not suitable for pantomime. The patient is shown a videotaped pantomime and required to point to the object that the man was pretending to use. If the patient passes three of the four practice items, the remaining 30 items are administered. Each correct response is scored 1 point for a maximum of 30 points (Benton *et al.*, 1983).

Localization. Varney and Benton (1982) found that errors made by aphasic patients impaired on pantomime recognition were predominantly semantic in type.

Norms. Norms are provided for a group ranging in age from 38 to 60 years and in educational level from 8 to 16 years. A score of less than 26 is classed as defective (Benton *et al.,* 1983).

Source. Oxford University Press.

SPEECH/LANGUAGE BATTERIES

In the following discussion, some of the more popular aphasia batteries are briefly reviewed. Numerous batteries and tests have been developed that are not reviewed here [e.g., Communicative Abilities in Daily Living (Holland, 1980) and Porch Index of Communicative Ability (Porch, 1971)]. For a comprehensive review of aphasia tests, see Spreen and Risser (1991).

Reitan–Indiana Aphasia Screening Test (AST)

Although the AST is not a battery, it is included under this heading because it contains a highly heterogeneous set of items. It is best viewed as a screening test for specific areas of deficit such as reading, writing, naming, arithmetic, and copying (Graves, 1987; Reitan, 1984).

Microdescription. Briefly assesses a variety of abilities.

Primary Assessment Areas. (1) Copying; (2) spelling; (3) naming; (4) reading; (5) repetition; (6) writing; (7) calculation; (8) right–left body orientation; (9) praxis.

Secondary Assessment Area. Verbal comprehension.

Presentation Modalities. (1) Auditory–verbal instructions for all items; (2) visual–nonverbal for items 1–12, 26, and 28; (3) visual–verbal for items 13–16, 20, 21a, 24, and 29.

Response Modalities. See below. All items are untimed.

Description. The stimuli are administered using a small booklet of cards containing the visual stimuli. Instructions for administration may be found in Reitan (1984) and Reitan and Wolfson (1993). The items involve the following:

           1, 4, 7, 28 Copying
    2, 5, 8, 10, 12, 26 Naming
              3, 6, 9 Spelling
           11, 20, 23 Writing
        13–16, 21a, 29 Reading
           17–19, 21 Repetition
                  22 Repeating and explaining

24, 25 Calculating
27 Praxis
30, 31 Body orientation

A system for scoring the items and for obtaining Aphasia and Spatial Relations scores is available in Russell *et al.* (1970). It is important to note the quality of the patient's performance on each item as well as the summed Aphasia and summed Spatial Relations scores (Barth *et al.*, 1984). A scoring system has also been developed by Williams and Shane (1986).

Localization. Localization varies depending on the items impaired.

Norms. Norms are available, using the scoring system of Russell *et al.* (1970) in Heaton *et al.* (1991). VIQ has been found to be significantly related to the Aphasia score and PIQ significantly related to the Spatial Relations score in epileptic patients (Barth *et al.*, 1984).

Source. Reitan Neuropsychology Laboratory.

Boston Diagnostic Aphasia Examination (BDAE)

In the BDAE, a general rating of the severity of the patient's aphasia from 1 to 5 is made on the Aphasia Severity Rating Scale (Goodglass & Kaplan, 1983). The BDAE contains a Rating Scale Profile of Speech Characteristics on which conversational and expository speech is rated for Melodic Line, Phrase Length, Articulatory Agility, Grammatical Form, Paraphasia in Running Speech, Repetition, Word Writing, and Auditory Comprehension. Speech is elicited by asking the patient simple questions and by presentation of the Cookie Theft Card, which is a line drawing of a scene.

Subtests not reviewed above include Verbal and Nonverbal Agility, Automatized Sequences, Reciting, Singing, and Rhythm. In Nonverbal Agility, the patient is required to perform simple, repetitive mouth movements after they have been described and demonstrated. The movements are timed. Verbal agility is tested by having the patient repeat words rapidly. The repetitions are timed. In the Automatized Sequences subtest, patients say overlearned series. Recitation, Singing, and Rhythm require the patient to recite overlearned material, sing a familiar song, and copy tapped rhythms. Information on additional supplementary language and nonlanguage tests may be found in Goodglass and Kaplan (1983).

Areas assessed by the BDAE include: Severity Rating, Fluency, Auditory Comprehension, Naming, Oral Reading, Repetition, Paraphasia, Automatic Speech, Reading Comprehension, Writing, Music, and Spatial and Computational. The scores of subtests in each of these categories are recorded on the Subtest Summary Profile. The BDAE was standardized on a sample of aphasic patients and a sample of normals. The Subtest Summary Profile is based on the sample of aphasics and provides percentiles on each of the subtests relative to this group. Using Pattern Analysis based on the Rating Profile of Speech Characteristics and the Subtest Summary Profile, the examiner can diagnose and classify a given patient's aphasia. Examples may be found in Goodglass and Kaplan (1983) for Broca's, Wernicke's, Anomic, Conduction, and Transcortical Sensory Aphasias. General descriptions may be found for other aphasias. The BDAE has been reported to be useful as a diagnostic instrument and in measuring progress in therapy (Helm-Estabrooks & Ramsberger, 1986). Norms are available for a Spanish version of the test (Rosselli *et al.*, 1990).

Multilingual Aphasia Examination (MAE)

The MAE (Benton & Hamsher, 1989) contains the following subtests: I—Visual Naming, II—Sentence Repetition, III—Controlled Word Association, IV—Oral Spelling, V—Written Spelling, VI—Block Spelling, VII—MAE Token Test, VIII—Aural Comprehension of Words and Phrases, and IX—Reading Comprehension of Words and Phrases. These tests are described in more detail in this chapter and in Chapter 24. Two rating scales are also part of the battery: X—Rating of Articulation (from "speechless or usually unintelligible speech" to "normal speech") and XI—Rating of Praxic Features of Writing (from "illegible scrawl" to "good penmanship"). The MAE was standardized on a sample of 360 subjects aged 16–69. Distributions of adjusted scores for aphasic patients are available in the manual and may be useful for diagnosis. Equivalent tests are being developed in Chinese, French, German, Italian, Portuguese, and Spanish (Spreen & Risser, 1991).

Minnesota Test for the Differential Diagnosis of Aphasia (MTDDA)

The MTDDA (Schuell, 1973) subtests are classified under Auditory Disturbances, Visual and Reading Disturbances, Speech and Language Disturbances, Visuomotor and Writing Disturbances, and Numerical Relations and Arithmetic Processes. The numerous subtests (69 total) in each category begin at a low level of difficulty that increases as the testing progresses. Differential diagnosis involves the distinction of five aphasic syndromes: simple aphasia, aphasia with visual involvement, aphasia with sensorimotor involvement, aphasia with scattered findings compatible with generalized brain damage, and irreversible aphasic syndrome. The MTDDA has been used primarily for assessment of baseline language functioning, treatment planning, and assessment of recovery. The test has not been standardized (Kertesz, 1989).

Western Aphasia Battery (WAB)

The WAB assesses Spontaneous Speech (Information Content, Fluency), Comprehension (Yes–No Questions, Auditory Word Recognition, Sequential Commands), Repetition, and Naming (Object Naming, Word Fluency, Sentence Completion, Responsive Speech). A global measure of speech functioning (Aphasia Quotient) is calculated on the basis of these scales. Reading and Writing, Praxis, and Construction (Drawing, Block Design, Calculation, Raven's Score) are also assessed and yield a performance quotient (Kertesz, 1979, 1982). The two quotients are summed to form the Cortical Quotient. The profile of the patient's scores on Fluency, Comprehension, Repetition, and Naming is used to diagnose global, Broca's isolation, transcortical motor, Wernicke's, transcortical sensory, conduction, or anomic aphasia.

Neurosensory Center Comprehensive Examination for Aphasia (NCCEA)

The NCCEA (Spreen & Benton, 1977; Spreen & Strauss, 1991) assesses name finding, immediate verbal memory, verbal production and fluency, receptive ability, reading, writing, and articulation. There are 20 subtests and 4 control subtests. Tests include visual naming, description of use, tactile naming with the right and left hands, repetition and reversal of digits, sentence construction, identification by name, oral reading of names and sentences, reading of names and sentences for meaning, visual–graphic naming, writing of names and writing to dictation, writing from copy, and articulation. Four control tests may also be administered: tactile–visual matching for the right and left hands, visual–visual matching, and form perception. A variety of stimuli are used, including four trays of objects and tape-recorded stimuli.

The test is standardized using reference groups of aphasic patients, brain-damaged patients, and normals (Spreen & Strauss, 1991). Corrections are available for education and age when necessary. The resulting scores can then be entered on profile sheets corresponding to the three reference groups.

REFERENCES

Barona, A., Reynolds, C. R., & Chastain, R. (1984). A demographically based index of premorbid intelligence for the WAIS-R. *Journal of Consulting and Clinical Psychology, 52,* 885–887.

Barth, J. T., Macciocchi, S. N., Giordani, B., Berent, S., & Boll, T. J. (1984). Interrater reliability and prediction of verbal and spatial functioning with a modified scoring system for the Reitan–Indiana Aphasia Screening Examination. *International Journal of Clinical Neuropsychology, 6,* 135–138.

Benson, D. F. (1979). *Aphasia, alexia, and agraphia.* New York: Churchill Livingston.

Benson, D. F. (1985). Aphasia. In K. M. Heilman & E. Valenstein (Eds.), *Clinical neuropsychology* (2nd ed.) (pp. 17–47). New York: Oxford University Press.

Benton, A. L., & Hamsher, K. (1989). *Multilingual aphasia examination* (2nd ed.). Iowa City: AJA Associates.

Benton, A. L., Hamsher, K., Varney, N., & Spreen, O. (1983). *Contributions to neuropsychological assessment: A clinical manual.* New York: Oxford University Press.

Blair, J. R., & Spreen, O. (1989). Predicting premorbid IQ: A revision of the National Adult Reading Test. *Clinical Neuropsychologist, 3,* 129–136.

Bornstein, R. A., & Leason, M. (1984). Item analysis of Halstead's Speech-Sounds Perception Test: Quantitative and qualitative analysis of errors. *Journal of Clinical Neuropsychology, 6,* 205–214.

Borod, J., Goodglass, H., & Kaplan, E. (1980). Normative data on the Boston Diagnostic Aphasia Examination, Parietal Lobe Battery, and Boston Naming Test. *Journal of Clinical Neuropsychology, 2,* 209–216.

Caramazza, A. (1991). *Issues in reading, writing, and speaking: A neuropsychological perspective.* Dordrecht: Kluwer Academic Publishers.

Crockett, D., Campbell, C., Labreche, T., Lacoste, D., & Klonoff, H. (1982). Shortening of the speech sounds perception test. *Journal of Clinical Neuropsychology, 4,* 167–171.

Crofoot, M. J., & Bennett, T. S. (1980). A comparison of three screening tests and the WISC-R in special education evaluations. *Psychology in the Schools, 17,* 474–478.

Damasio, A. R. (1991). Signs of aphasia. In M. T. Sarno (Ed.), *Acquired aphasia* (2nd ed.) (pp. 27–43). San Diego: Academic Press.

Damasio, H. (1991). Neuroanatomical correlates of the aphasia. In M. T. Sarno (Ed.), *Acquired aphasia* (2nd ed.) (pp. 45–71). San Diego: Academic Press.

Dunn, L. M., & Dunn, L. M. (1981). *Peabody Picture Vocabulary Test—Revised: Manual for forms L and M.* Circle Pines, MN: American Guidance Service.

Ellis, A. W., & Young, A. W. (1988). *Human cognitive neuropsychology.* London: Laurence Erlbaum Associates.

Golden, C. J., Hammeke, T. A., Purisch, A. D., Berg, R. A., Moses, J. A., Jr., Newlin, D. B., Wilkening, G. N., & Puente, A. E. (1982). *Item interpretation of the Luria–Nebraska Neuropsychological Battery.* Lincoln: University of Nebraska Press.

Golden, C. J., Purisch, A. D., & Hammeke, T. A. (1985). *Luria–Nebraska Neuropsychological Battery: Forms I and II.* Los Angeles: Western Psychological Services.

Goodglass, H., & Kaplan, E. (1983). *The assessment of aphasia and related disorders* (2nd ed.). Philadelphia: Lea & Fibiger.

Graves, R. E. (1987). Test review: Aphasia and sensory–perceptual deficits in adults. *Journal of Clinical and Experimental Neuropsychology, 9,* 461–466.

Hart, S., Smith, C. M., & Swash, M. (1986). Assessing intellectual deterioration. *British Journal of Clinical Psychology, 25,* 119–124.

Heaton, R. K., Grant, I., & Matthews, C. G. (1991). *Comprehensive norms for an expanded Halstead–Reitan Battery: Demographic corrections, research findings, and clinical applications.* Odessa, FL: Psychological Assessment Resources.

Helm-Estabrooks, N., & Ramsberger, G. (1986). Treatment of agrammatism in long-term Broca's aphasia. *British Journal of Disorders of Communication, 21,* 39–45.

Holland, A. L. (1980). *Communicative Abilities in Daily Living: Manual.* Baltimore: University Park Press.

Huff, F. J., Collins, C., Corkin, S., & Rosen, T. J. (1986). Equivalent forms of the Boston Naming Test. *Journal of Clinical and Experimental Neuropsychology, 8,* 556–562.

Jastak, S., & Wilkinson, G. (1984). *Wide Range Achievement Test—Revised.* Wilmington, DE: Jastak Associates.

Joseph, R. (1990). *Neuropsychology, neuropsychiatry, and behavioral neurology.* New York: Plenum Press.

Kaplan, E., Fein, D., Morris, R., & Delis, D. C. (1991). *WAIS-R NI: Manual.* San Antonio: The Psychological Corporation.

Kertesz, A. (1979). *Aphasia and associated disorders: Taxonomy, localization, and recovery.* New York: Grune & Stratton.

Kertesz, A. (1982). *Western Aphasia Battery: Test Manual.* San Antonio: The Psychological Corporation.

Kertesz, A. (1989). Assessing aphasic disorders. In E. Perecman (Ed.), *Integrating theory and practice in clinical neuropsychology* (pp. 245–264). Hillsdale, NJ: Lawrence Erlbaum Associates.

Knopman, D. S., Selnes, O. A., Niccum, N., & Rubens, A. (1984). Recovery of naming in aphasia: Relationship to fluency, comprehension and CT findings. *Neurology, 34,* 1461–1470.

Kohn, S. E., & Goodglass, H. (1985). Picture-naming in aphasia. *Brain and Language, 24,* 266–283.

LaBarge, E., Edwards, D., & Knesevich, J. W. (1986). Performance of normal elderly on the Boston Naming Test. *Brain and Language, 27,* 380–384.

Lezak, M. (1983). *Neuropsychological assessment* (2nd ed.). New York: Oxford University Press.

Margolis, R. B., Taylor, J. M., & Dunn, E. J. (1984). An abbreviated Speech Sounds Perception Test with a geriatric population. *International Journal of Clinical Neuropsychology, 7,* 167–169.

McCarthy, R. A., & Warrington, E. K. (1990). *Cognitive neuropsychology: A clinical introduction.* San Diego: Academic Press.

McFie, J. (1975). *Assessment of organic intellectual impairment.* London: Academic Press.

Nelson, H. E., & McKenna, P. (1975). The use of reading ability in the assessment of dementia. *British Journal of Clinical Psychology, 25,* 157–158.

Nelson, H. E., & O'Connell, A. (1978). Dementia: The estimation of pre-morbid intelligence levels using the new adult reading test. *Cortex, 14,* 234–244.

Parsons, O. A., Vega, A., & Burn, J. (1969). Differential psychological effects of lateralized brain damage. *Journal of Consulting and Clinical Psychology, 33,* 551–557.

Porch, B. E. (1971). *Porch Index of Communicative Ability: Administration, scoring, and interpretation.* Palo Alto, CA: Consulting Psychologists Press.

Reitan, R. M. (1955). Certain differential effects of right and left cerebral lesions in human adults. *Journal of Comparative and Physiological Psychology, 48,* 474–477.

Reitan, R. M. (1984). *Aphasia and sensory–perceptual deficits in adults.* Tucson: Ralph M. Reitan, Ph.D.

Reitan, R. M., & Wolfson, D. (1993). *The Halstead–Reitan Neuropsychological Test Battery: Theory and clinical interpretation* (2nd ed.). Tucson: Neuropsychology Press.

Rosselli, M., Ardila, A., Florez, A., & Castro, C. (1990). Normative data on the Boston Diagnostic Aphasia Examination in a Spanish-speaking population. *Journal of Clinical and Experimental Neuropsychology, 12,* 313–322.

Russell, E. W., Neuringer, C., & Goldstein, G. (1970). *Assessment of brain damage: A neuropsychology key approach.* New York: Wiley-Interscience.

Sarno, M. T. (1986). Verbal impairment in head injury. *Archives of Physical and Medical Rehabilitation, 67,* 399–404.

Sattler, J. M. (1988). *Assessment of children* (3rd. ed.). San Diego: Jerome M. Sattler.

Schear, J. M., Skenes, L. L., & Larson, V. D. (1988). Effect of simulated hearing loss on speech sounds perception. *Journal of Clinical and Experimental Neuropsychology, 10,* 597–602.

Schuell, H. (1973). *Differential diagnosis of aphasia with the Minnesota test* (2nd ed.). Minneapolis: University of Minnesota Press.

Shallice, T. (1988). *From neuropsychology to mental structure.* Cambridge, England: Cambridge University Press.

Shea, V. (1989). Peabody Picture Vocabulary Test—Revised. In Newmark, C. S. (Ed.), *Major psychological assessment instruments,* Volume II (pp. 271–283). Boston: Allyn & Bacon.

Sherer, M., Parsons, O. A., Nixon, S. J., & Adams, R. L. (1991). Clinical validity of the speech-sounds perception test and the seashore rhythm test. *Journal of Clinical and Experimental Neuropsychology, 13,* 741–751.

Spreen, O., & Benton, A. L. (1977). *Neurosensory Center Comprehensive Examination for Aphasia.* Victoria, BC: University of Victoria.

Spreen, O., & Risser, A. (1991). Assessment of aphasia. In M. T. Sarno (Ed.), *Acquired aphasia* (2nd ed.) (pp. 73–150). San Diego: Academic Press.

Spreen, O., & Strauss, E. (1991). *A compendium of neuropsychological tests: Administration, norms, and commentary.* New York: Oxford University Press.

Stebbins, G. T., Wilson, R. S., Gilley, D. W., Bernard, B. A., & Fox, J. H. (1988). Estimation of premorbid intelligence in dementia. *Journal of Clinical and Experimental Neuropsychology, 10,* 63–64.

Stebbins, G. T., Gilley, D. W., Wilson, R. S., Bernard, B. A., & Fox, J. H. (1990). Effects of language disturbances on premorbid estimates of IQ in mild dementia. *The Clinical Neuropsychologist, 4,* 64–68.

Steinmeyer, C. H. (1984). Are the rhythm tests of the Halstead–Reitan and Luria–Nebraska Batteries differentially sensitive to right temporal lobe lesions? *Journal of Clinical Psychology, 40,* 1464–1466.

Thompson, L. L., & Heaton, R. K. (1989). Comparison of different versions of the Boston Naming Test. *The Clinical Neuropsychologist, 3,* 184–192.

Van Gorp, W. G., Satz, P., Kiersch, M. E., & Henry, R. (1986). Normative data on the Boston Naming Test for a group of normal older adults. *Journal of Clinical and Experimental Neuropsychology, 8,* 702–705.

Varney, N. R., & Benton, A. L. (1979). Phonemic discrimination and aural comprehension among aphasic patients. *Journal of Clinical Neuropsychology, 1,* 65–73.

Varney, N. R., & Benton, A. L. (1982). Qualitative aspects of pantomine recognition in aphasia. *Brain and Cognition, 1,* 132–139.

Warrington, E. K., James, M., & Maciejewski, C. (1986). The WAIS as a lateralising and localising diagnostic instrument: A study of 656 patients with unilateral cerebral lesions. *Neuropsychologia, 24,* 223–239.

Wechsler, D. (1981). *Wechsler Adult Intelligence Scale—Revised.* New York: Psychological Corporation.

Wilkinson, G. S. (1989). Wide Range Achievement Test—Revised. In Newmark, C. S. (Ed.), *Major psychological assessment instruments,* Volume II (pp. 233–250). Boston: Allyn & Bacon.

Williams, J. M., & Shane, B. (1986). The Reitan–Indiana Aphasia Screening Test: Scoring and factor analysis. *Journal of Clinical Psychology, 42,* 156–160.

Arithmetic

Calculation is a complicated process and can require a variety of cognitive, motor, and sensory abilities. Impaired calculation (*acalculia*) has been grossly classified as: (1) *alexic or agraphic acalculia*—impairment in calculation due to impaired reading or writing of numbers; (2) *spatial acalculia*—impairment in calculation due to spatial disorganization of written calculations; and (3) *anarithmetria* or *primary acalculia*—impairment in calculation per se excluding the previous two causes. Cognitive models have been developed by Grafman (1988), McCarthy and Warrington (1990), and others on the basis of studies isolating specific cognitive subprocesses in very selectively impaired individuals.

Alexia or agraphic acalculia or both are commonly associated with left temporal–parietal lesions, spatial acalculia with left or right pathology, and anarithmetria with left–posterior lesions (Grafman, 1988).

In addition to the standardized tests reviewed below, a neuropsychological evaluation of calculation may benefit from the inclusion of items assessing specific impairments in calculation. Kahn and Konewko [(1986) cited in Kahn, 1988] have developed an acalculia exam that assesses: "1) magnitude judgment of digits in written and oral and lexical representation; 2) ordering numbers sequentially; 3) counting numbers; 4) identifying, copying, reading, and writing to oral dictation; 5) transcoding in both directions (lexical to digit and digit to lexical representation); 6) addition, subtraction and multiplication problems in production and multiple choice tasks (written and auditory presentation)" (Kahn, 1988, p. 33). Benton [(1963), cited in Levin & Spiers, 1985] has developed a detailed examination of calculation.

An assessment of the patient's ability to use a simple electronic calculator may assist the examiner in determining the effect the patient's impairment might have on everyday functioning.

Arithmetic (A-WRAT-R)

Microdescription. Requires the patient to solve written arithmetic problems.

Primary Assessment Area. Written arithmetic (Jastak & Wilkinson, 1984; Wilkinson, 1989).

Presentation Modality. Visual–verbal.

Response Modalities. (1) Skilled upper extremity movement—writing; (2) timed.

Description. There are two versions of the A-WRAT-R, a Level 1 version for children 5–11 and a Level 2 version for individuals 12–75 years. In both versions, the patient is required to perform written computations. Under certain conditions described in the manual, the patient is asked to count, read numbers, and solve simple verbally presented arithmetic problems. The patient is given 10 min to complete the test.

Localization. No localization data are available for this test.

Norms. Norms are provided for 28 age groups from 5 to 75 (Jastak & Wilkinson, 1984). (Standard scores, percentiles, and grade equivalents.) Comparisons are made with other test performances using standard scores and percentiles rather than grade equivalents.

Source. Jastak Assessment Systems.

Arithmetic [A-WAIS-R (NI)]

Microdescription. Requires the patient to solve verbally posed arithmetic problems.

Primary Assessment Areas. (1) Mental calculation; (2) attention (Kaufman, 1990); (3) memory (Kaplan *et al.*, 1991); (4) mental manipulation of information (Kaplan *et al.*, 1991); (5) "conversion of the verbal problems to the correct operations" (Kaplan *et al.*, 1991, p. 39).

Secondary Assessment Areas. (1) Verbal comprehension; (2) speech.

Presentation Modality. Auditory–verbal for all items.

Response Modalities. (1) Speech; (2) time-limited for items 1–9 and (3) timed for items 10–14.

Description. There are 14 items. In 13 of the items, the patient is required to solve verbally posed arithmetic problems without writing them. Administration begins with the third item. If this simple addition is failed, the patient is presented with seven of the Block Design blocks, red side up in groups of three and four, and asked how many there are. The specific protocol may be found in the *WAIS-R Manual* (Wechsler, 1981). An easy verbal arithmetic problem, item 2, is also posed before continuing with the remainder of the test.

In the A-WAIS-R NI administration, the items are first presented as in the A-WAIS-R, except that the patient is allowed to work past the time limit and the standard discontinue rule is not necessarily observed (Kaplan *et al.*, 1991). For failed items, the patient is asked to read the problem aloud from the WAIS-R Stimulus Booklet. Reading may be assisted. If the item is again failed, the Stimulus Booklet is left open in front of the patient and paper and pencil are allowed. Items that continue to be failed are presented as written numerical problems in the WAIS-R NI Response Booklet. Time, Raw, Raw Scatter, Overtime, score after presentation of Stimulus Booklet, score after use of paper and pencil, and score using Response Booklet are recorded (Kaplan *et al.*, 1991).

Localization. Impairment on the A-WAIS has been associated primarily with left hemisphere dysfunction (McFie, 1975; Warrington *et al.*, 1986).

Norms. See the WAIS-R.

Source. The Psychological Corporation.

Arithmetic Scale (C9-LNNB)

Microdescription. Assesses number identification and calculational–mathematical ability.

Primary Assessment Areas. (1) Mathematical ability; (2) writing and reading numbers.

Secondary Assessment Areas. (1) Verbal comprehension; (2) attention.

Presentation Modalities. (1) Auditory–verbal instructions for all items; (2) auditory presentation of numbers for items 201–205, 210, 212–215, 221, and 222; (3) visual presentation of numbers for items 204–209, 211, and 216–220.

Response Modalities. (1) Writing (items 201–205); (2) speech (items 206–210 and 216–222); (3) writing or speech (items 212–215); (4) pointing (item 211); (5) all items are time-limited.

Description. The (Arithmetic) C9-LNNB Scale is a set of relatively heterogeneous items that assess either mathematical ability or number identification. Brief descriptions of the items are as follows:

201, 203, 204, 205	Writing numbers
202	Writing Roman numerals
206, 208, 209	Reading numbers
207	Reading Roman numerals and two-digit numbers
210, 211	Determining the larger of two numbers
212, 213, 214, 215, 216, 217, 220	Arithmetic
218, 219	Equations
221, 222	Subtracting serial 7s and 13s

Factors Scales include A1 (Arithmetic Calculations) and A2 (Number Reading). A1 items involve identification of Roman numerals and arithmetic calculations. A2 items assess writing and reading numbers and include a simple calculation item (Golden *et al.,* 1985).

Localization. C9 is sensitive to educational deficits. In patients with an average education, it may be in the severely pathological range even when there is no brain damage. C9 may be sensitive to lesions anywhere in the brain and therefore may not be useful for localizing brain injury. Although A2 may be spuriously elevated by single errors, elevations can be correlated with lesions in the left cerebral hemisphere (Golden & Berg, 1983; Golden *et al.,* 1985).

Norms. See the LNNB.

Source. Western Psychological Services.

REFERENCES

Golden, C. J., & Berg, R. A. (1983). Interpretation of the Luria–Nebraska Neuropsychological Battery by item intercorrelation: The Arithmetic scale. *Clinical Neuropsychology, 5,* 122–127.

Golden, C. J., Purisch, A. D., & Hammeke, T. A. (1985). *Luria–Nebraska Neuropsychological Battery: Forms I and II.* Los Angeles: Western Psychological Services.

Grafman, J. (1988). Acalculia. In F. Boller & J. Grafman (Eds.), *Handbook of neuropsychology,* Volume 1 (pp. 415–431). Dordrecht: Elsevier Science Publishers.

Jastak, S., & Wilkinson, G. (1984). *Wide Range Achievement Test—Revised.* Wilmington, DE: Jastak Associates.

Kahn, H. J. (1988). Acalculia: Multiplication fact retrieval in normal and impaired subjects. In J. M. Williams & C. J. Long (Eds.), *Cognitive approaches to neuropsychology* (pp. 27–43). New York: Plenum Press.

Kaplan, E., Fein, D., Morris, R., & Delis, D. C. (1991). *WAIS-R NI: Manual.* San Antonio: The Psychological Corporation.

Kaufman, A. S. (1990). *Assessing adolescent and adult intelligence.* Boston: Allyn & Bacon.

Levin, H. S., & Spiers, P. A. (1985). Acalculia. In K. M. Heilman & E. Valenstein (Eds.), *Clinical neuropsychology* (2nd ed.). New York: Oxford University Press.

McCarthy, R. A., & Warrington, E. K. (1990). *Cognitive neuropsychology: A clinical introduction.* San Diego: Academic Press.

McFie, J. (1975). *Assessment of organic intellectual impairment.* London: Academic Press.

Warrington, E. K., James, M., & Maciejewski, C. (1986). The WAIS as a lateralising and localising diagnostic instrument: A study of 656 patients with unilateral cerebral lesions. *Neuropsychologia, 24,* 223–239.

Wechsler, D. (1981). *Wechsler Adult Intelligence Scale—Revised.* New York: Psychological Corporation.

Wilkinson, G. S. (1989). Wide Range Achievement Test—Revised. In Newmark, C. S. (Ed.), *Major psychological assessment instruments:* Volume II (pp. 233–250). Boston: Allyn & Bacon.

Visual–Spatial Functioning

Visual–spatial functioning, as used in this book, is a general term referring to visuoperceptual, visuospatial, or visuoconstructive abilities. The visual system may be divided into a number of areas of functioning and anatomically separate subsystems. *Visual object perception* or *pattern recognition* involves the identification of spatial collections of visual qualities. Impairment is termed *visual agnosia.* The neuroanatomical substrate of object recognition appears to involve the posterior temporal or inferotemporal cortex (Benton, 1985; Ungerleider & Mishkin, 1982). Other forms of recognition include recognition of familiar faces (impairment is termed *prosopagnosia*) and recognition of unfamiliar faces. A review of the different varieties of visual agnosia may be found in *Visual Agnosia* (Farah, 1990). *Visual synthesis* is the ability to grasp the relationships between simultaneously presented stimuli and integrate them into a meaningful whole (Benton, 1985). *Visuospatial abilities* involve the localization of objects or the self in space. The neuroanatomical substrate of the ability to localize objects appears to involve the posterior parietal cortex (Benton, 1985; Ungerleider & Mishkin, 1982). Subcategories of visuospatial abilities include the ability to localize points in space and to judge direction, distance, and depth. Topographical orientation is the ability to find one's way around in or to describe various environments, e.g., home, neighborhood, or city. *Visuo-constructive ability* or *constructional praxis* is the ability to put parts together to form a single object (Benton, 1985). Successful performance of this activity requires accurate perception of the parts and their spatial relationships and unimpaired organization and performance of the motor activities necessary to construct the object (Benton, 1985).

The tests in this chapter are reviewed under the subheadings of copying, construction, spatial perception and reasoning, neglect, and other.

COPYING

Benton Visual Retention Test (BVRT:C)

Microdescription. Requires the patient to copy geometric figures.

Primary Assessment Areas. (1) Visuospatial perception; (2) visual–constructional ability; (3) drawing.

Secondary Assessment Areas. (1) Upper extremity motor functioning; (2) verbal comprehension.

Presentation Modalities. (1) Visuospatial–nonverbal; (2) auditory–verbal for instructions.

Response Modalities. (1) Upper extremity and hand motor movements—drawing; (2) untimed.

Description. The patient is required to copy 10 line drawings. The first 2 drawings are single figure designs. The remaining 8 contain three figures—two major figures and one peripheral figure usually appearing on either the right or the left. Both the number of correct designs and the number of errors are scored. Errors are classified as omissions, distortions, perseverations, rotations, and relative misplacements of figures (Benton, 1974).

There are three different forms of the test. Form D may be a bit more difficult than Form C or E.

Localization. Impaired performance is more likely to be associated with right hemisphere damage than left (Benton, 1968), although this may not always be the case (Arena & Gainotti, 1978). Visual–spatial inattention, which may be associated with impairment in the hemisphere contralateral to the field of inattention, may be suggested by a consistent absence of figures on one side of the patient's drawings (Lezak, 1983).

Norms. Error score norms with no age or intelligence corrections are available for adults (Benton, 1974).

Source. The Psychological Corporation.

Rey–Osterrieth Complex Figure Test: Copy (ROCFT:C)

Microdescription. Assesses copying of a detailed figure.

Primary Assessment Areas. (1) Visuospatial perception; (2) constructional ability; (3) drawing.

Secondary Assessment Areas. (1) Upper extremity motor functioning; (2) verbal comprehension.

Presentation Modalities. (1) Verbal instructions; (2) visuospatial–nonverbal.

Response Modalities. (1) Upper extremity and hand motor functioning—drawing; (2) untimed.

Description. The patient is required to copy a detailed line drawing. The patient may be provided with different-colored drawing instruments when drawing various parts of the figure or at 1-min time intervals to obtain a record of the patient's organizational plan in drawing the figure. Immediate and delayed recall reproductions may also be required. Several scoring systems are available (Denman, 1984; Lezak, 1983; Osterrieth, 1944; Visser, 1980).

Localization. Copies made by patients with right hemisphere dysfunction tend to lack representation of the overall configuration of the design. Copies made by patients with left hemisphere dysfunction tend to retain overall configuration but lack details (Binder, 1982).

Norms. Norms may be found in Lezak (1983) and Spreen and Strauss (1991).

Source. Examples of the figure and instructions for administration are available in several sources (Denman, 1984; Lezak, 1983; Osterrieth, 1944; Visser, 1980).

Bender Visual Motor Gestalt Test (BVMGT)

Microdescription. Requires the patient to copy drawings.

Primary Assessment Areas. (1) Visuospatial perception; (2) constructional ability; (3) drawing.

Secondary Assessment Areas. (1) Upper extremity motor functioning; (2) verbal comprehension.

Presentation Modalities. (1) Verbal instructions; (2) visuospatial–nonverbal.

Response Modalities. (1) Upper extremity and hand motor functioning—drawing; (2) untimed.

Description. The test materials consist of black figures drawn on nine white cards. Figure A is used as an introductory figure and Figures 1–8 are given in sequence. According to the original instructions of Bender (1938), the patient is given a sheet of unlined white paper $8\frac{1}{2}''\times 11''$ and a pencil with an eraser. The cards are presented one at a time and laid at the top of the sheet of paper. The patient is told, "Here are some figures (or designs) for you to copy; just copy them the way you see them" (Bender, 1938, p. 6). Numerous variations on this procedure have been developed (Lezak, 1983), and even more numerous methods have been developed for scoring the BVMGT (Franzen, 1989; Lezak, 1983). Scoring systems in use include those of Hutt (1969) and Marley (1982).

Canter (1966, 1976) devised a Background Interference Procedure for use with the BVMGT. The patient first draws the designs using the standard administration. He or she is then asked to reproduce the designs on sheets of paper covered with black, wavy lines. Scoring involves a comparison of both administrations.

Localization. Studies suggest that the BVMGT may be sensitive to some forms of brain damage (Lacks, 1984). Impaired performance has been associated with parietal lesions (Garron & Cheifetz, 1965). The Canter Procedure has been reported to increase the sensitivity of the BVMGT to brain damage (Lezak, 1983). Because patients with severe brain damage may exhibit no impairment on this test, Bigler and Ehrfurth (1980) have cautioned against using the BVMGT as a lone screening instrument for brain damage. Delaney (1982) found patients with epilepsy to be indistinguishable from controls using the BVMGT with the Background Interference Procedure.

Norms. Normative data using the Hutt scoring method are available for patients 17–80+ years of age (Lacks, 1984; Lacks & Storandt, 1982). The cutoff for organicity is 5 errors.

Source. The original BVMGT is available in Bender (1938), which may be purchased from Psychological Assessment Resources. The Canter Background Interference Procedure is available in Canter (1976).

CONSTRUCTION

Block Design [BD-WAIS-R (NI)]

Microdescription. Requires the patient to copy designs using colored blocks.

Primary Assessment Areas. (1) Visuoconstructive ability; (2) visuospatial perception; (3) visual analysis and synthesis (Sattler, 1988).

Secondary Assessment Areas. (1) Upper extremity motor functioning; (2) verbal comprehension.

Presentation Modalities. (1) Visual–nonverbal; (2) auditory–verbal for instructions.

Response Modalities. (1) Upper extremity motor movements; (2) timed.

Description. The materials consist of 9 cubes colored red on two sides, white on two sides, and red/white on two sides. On the first trial, the examiner makes a design using four blocks and provides the patient with four blocks to make a duplicate. For the second trial, the patient is shown a two-dimensional red and white design in a booklet, and the examiner demonstrates construction using the patient's blocks. The patient is then asked to construct the design. The patient is required to construct the remaining seven designs without a demonstration. Designs 6–9 require nine blocks. More points are scored for faster correct constructions. No points are scored for incorrect designs (Wechsler, 1981).

The WAIS-R NI administration of Block Design differs significantly from that of the WAIS-R (Kaplan *et al.,* 1991) and a scaled score cannot be obtained: (1) Blocks beyond those needed to complete the design are provided to the patient; (2) for each item, the patient is allowed to work beyond the standard time limit; (3) the patient is asked to judge the correctness of his or her solution; and (4) if any of the designs are failed, they are presented in a grid. The Record Form contains a series of blank grids for each design. Using the Block Design Notation System, the examiner can code the patient's progress in attempting to copy the design. Scores recorded include Raw, Raw Scatter, Overtime, Number of Blocks Correctly Placed—[Timed (Left, Right), Overtime (Left, Right), Grid (Left, Right)], Broken Configurations—(En Route, Final), Rotations—(Block, Design). Percentages of Blocks Correctly Placed and percentages of Broken Configurations can be calculated.

Localization. Impaired performance on BD tends to be associated with right hemisphere lesions (Black & Strub, 1976; Warrington *et al.,* 1986), although the performance of patients with left parietal injuries also may be impaired (McFie, 1975).

The more extensive administration and scoring of the WAIS-R NI may provide information on laterality of lesion. Right-hemisphere-damaged patients may tend to break the configuration and distort the pattern. Left-hemisphere-damaged patients may tend to misalign internal details of the design, especially on the right side. "The percentage of broken configurations relative to the number of items administered is the single best Block Design index reflecting right-hemisphere or bilateral involvement" (Kaplan *et al.,* 1991, p. 88). Akshoomoff-Haist *et al.* (1989) found the mean percentage of broken configurations for patients with right hemisphere damage to be 40.0%; left hemisphere damage, 9.7%; and normals, 10.9%. Kaplan *et al.* (1991, p. 88) provided the following clinical rules of thumb: "Whereas a broken configuration score lower than 25% does not rule out right-hemisphere damage, a score higher than 25% lends support for the hypothesis of at least right-hemisphere, and possibly bilateral involvement."

Norms. See the WAIS-R.

Source. The Psychological Corporation.

Object Assembly [OA-WAIS-R (NI)]

Microdescription. Requires the patient to put together the pieces of a cut-up object.

Primary Assessment Areas. (1) Object recognition (Sattler, 1988); (2) visual analysis and synthesis (Sattler, 1988); (3) visuoconstructive ability (Peck *et al.,* 1987); (4) visual–motor coordination (Sattler, 1988).

Secondary Assessment Areas. (1) Upper extremity motor functioning; (2) remote memory; (3) verbal comprehension.

Presentation Modalities. (1) Visual–nonverbal; (2) auditory–verbal for instructions.

Response Modalities. (1) Upper extremity motor movements; (2) timed.

Description. The patient is required to assemble cut-up cardboard figures of familiar objects. The test consists of four figures presented in order of increasing difficulty. More points are scored for faster correct assemblies. Points may be scored for partially correct assemblies (Wechsler, 1981).

The WAIS-R NI contains an Object Assembly Layout Shield that stands on its own while the examiner places the pieces for each puzzle (Kaplan *et al.*, 1991). It also adds three Object Assembly puzzles—Car, Circle, and Cow puzzles. The WAIS-R NI allows for two administrations of Object Assembly. It is administered as in the WAIS-R except that the solution status is noted at the usual time limit and the patient is allowed to keep working. Also, the three additional puzzles are administered. In the second way of administering Object Assembly, the patient is instructed to tell the examiner when he or she first sees what the puzzle is. This provides information relevant to determining the strategy used in solving the puzzle. If the Manikin is failed, the correct solution is demonstrated. The remainder of the items are then administered.

The order and time of each correct juncture are recorded. Strategies are noted for each puzzle. These strategies include Trial and Error, Edge Alignment, and Internal-Detail Matching. Raw and Overtime scores are recorded.

Localization. Impaired performance on OA tends to be associated with right hemisphere and posterior lesions (Black & Strub, 1976). Overreliance on internal-detail matching is common in right hemisphere damage (Kaplan *et al.*, 1991). Matching of details may result in an incorrect construction of the Car. The Circle and Cow may be difficult for the patient, especially if the lesions are posterior. Patients with left hemisphere lesions complete the

Circle, which can be solved by an edge-alignment strategy, more rapidly than the Cow, which cannot. Patients with right anterior lesions may do better with the Cow than with the Circle (Kaplan *et al.*, 1991).

Norms. See the WAIS-R.

Source. The Psychological Corporation.

Three-Dimensional Block Construction (TDBC)

Microdescription. Requires the patient to copy three-dimensional block constructions.

Primary Assessment Areas. (1) Visuoconstructive ability; (2) visuospatial perception.

Secondary Assessment Areas. (1) Upper extremity motor functioning; (2) verbal comprehension.

Presentation Modalities. (1) Visual–nonverbal; (2) auditory–verbal for instructions.

Response Modalities. (1) Upper extremity motor movements; (2) timed.

Description. The test materials consist of three block constructions or photographs of the constructions that the patient attempts to re-create using a set of 29 blocks laid out in a predetermined arrangement. The models are (1) a pyramid composed of 6 cubes; (2) an 8-block, four-level construction; and (3) a 15-block, four-level construction. One point is scored for each correctly placed block. If the total time to complete the constructions exceeds 380 sec, two points are subtracted from the total score. Errors, classed as (1) omissions, (2) additions, (3) substitutions, and (4) displacements, are also scored. There are two forms available.

Localization. Failure tends to be more frequent and more severe in right hemisphere injuries than in left hemisphere injuries (Benton & Fogel, 1962; Benton *et al.*, 1983). In patients with left hemisphere injuries, aphasics with receptive language deficits exhibited a high frequency of constructional disability.

Norms. Benton *et al.* (1983) have provided normative observations for a group aged 16–63. The variables of education and age may affect performance.

Source. Oxford University Press.

SPATIAL PERCEPTION AND REASONING

Picture Completion (PC-WAIS-R)

Microdescription. Requires the patient to identify missing parts in pictures.

Primary Assessment Areas. (1) Ability to identify missing details in pictures (Lezak,

1983); (2) object recognition (Peck *et al.,* 1987; Sattler, 1988); (3) visual analysis and synthesis; (4) judgment of practical and conceptual relevancy (Saunders, 1960).

Secondary Assessment Areas. (1) Remote memory (Lezak, 1983); (2) verbal comprehension.

Presentation Modalities. (1) Visual–nonverbal; (2) auditory–verbal for instructions.

Response Modalities. (1) Speech; (2) pointing; (3) time-limited.

Description. The patient is required to describe or point to the place where an important detail is missing in a picture. Twenty seconds are allowed for a response. The test consists of 20 pictures arranged in order of increasing difficulty (Wechsler, 1981).
   WAIS-R NI administration is similar to that of the WAIS-R except that overtime is allowed (Kaplan *et al.,* 1991). Time, Raw, Raw Scatter, and Overtime are recorded. Kaplan *et al.* (1991) suggest that the examiner should note where missed details are located in the picture—right, left, up, or down. These notes may provide information about impairment in the visual system. Items may classified as involving: (1) accurate long-term memory of a missing part and identification of it (1, 5, 7, 8, 15, 18, 19); (2) appreciation of a violation of symmetry (9, 12, 13, 17); and (3) higher-level cognitive inferences (2, 4, 6, 10, 11, 14, 20).

Localization. The PC subtest tends to be resilient to brain damage and may provide an estimate of premorbid functioning (Lezak, 1983).

Norms. See the WAIS-R.

Source. The Psychological Corporation.

Facial Recognition Test (FR)

Microdescription. Requires the patient to discriminate unfamiliar faces.

Primary Assessment Area. Identification and discrimination of photographs of unfamiliar human faces (Benton *et al.,* 1983).

Secondary Assessment Area. Verbal comprehension.

Presentation Modalities. (1) Visual–nonverbal; (2) auditory–verbal for instructions.

Response Modalities. (1) Simple upper extremity motor movements—pointing or (2) speech; (3) untimed.

Description. The stimulus materials consist of a spiral-bound book with stimulus photographs and response photographs printed on facing pages. The test is composed of three parts. In the first part, the patient is required to match identical front-view photographs. The second part requires the patient to match front-view photographs of individuals with three-quarter view photographs of those same individuals. Finally, matching is required between front-view photographs of individuals and photographs under different lighting conditions of those same individuals. A point is scored for each correct response. Both a Short Form (27 items) and a Long Form (54 items) are available. A table is provided to convert Short Form scores to Long Form scores (Benton *et al.,* 1983).

Localization. For nonaphasic patients with unilateral brain disease, impaired performance appears to be associated with lesions in the right hemisphere (Benton *et al.,* 1983). FR may have some utility for distinguishing neurological from psychiatric impairment (Kronfol *et al.,* 1978; Levin & Benton, 1977). Levin *et al.* (1977) have reported that head-injured patients, especially those who have been comatose for at least 24 hr, may perform defectively on FR.

Norms. Norms are provided for the age groups 16–54, 55–64, and 65–74. Since age and education were found to affect performance, corrections are available for both these factors (Benton *et al.,* 1983).

Source. Oxford University Press.

Hooper Visual Organization Test (HVOT)

Microdescription. Requires the patient to identify cut-up objects.

Primary Assessment Areas. (1) Object recognition; (2) visual synthesis; (3) naming (Western Psychological Services, 1983).

Secondary Assessment Area. Verbal comprehension.

Presentation Modalities. (1) Visual–nonverbal; (2) auditory–verbal for instructions.

Response Modalities. (1) Writing or (2) speech; (3) untimed.

Description. The test consists of 30 line drawings of simple objects that have been cut into pieces. The pieces are separated and may be rotated. The patient is asked to identify what each object would be if the pieces were put together correctly (Western Psychological Services, 1983). Scores of 1 point, $\frac{1}{2}$ point, or 0 may be obtained on each item according to a scoring key. Errors have been categorized as (1) isolate responses—only one part of the picture is used to formulate a response, (2) perseverative responses, (3) bizarre responses that lack direct relationship to the test item, and (4) neologistic responses (Hooper, 1958; Walker, 1956, 1957).

Localization. The HVOT is sensitive to brain damage (Boyd, 1981; Wang, 1977). Fitz *et al.* (1992) found HVOT scores to be lower in patients with right parietal lobe lesions.

Norms. Mason and Ganzler (1964) have derived multiple regression equations to correct for age (25–69 years) and education (6–16+ years) with and without the Shipley Institute of Living Vocabulary score (Shipley, 1967):

HVOT (predicted) = 23.990 + 0.224 Vocabulary + 0.075 Education − 0.125 Age

HVOT (predicted) = 25.708 + 0.368 Education − 0.092 Age

Corrected Raw Scores are obtained as follows:

$$HVOT \text{ (corrected)} = HVOT \text{ (obtained)} - HVOT \text{ (predicted)}/4.779$$

The corrected scores may be classified according to probability of impairment in the areas of functioning assessed by the HVOT: (1) 24–30 = Very Low; (2) 21–23 = Low; (3) 19–20 = Moderate; (4) 16–18 = High; and (5) <16 = Very High (Western Psychological Services, 1983). T scores may also be calculated and are available in the manual.

Source. Western Psychological Services.

Judgment of Line Orientation (JLO)

Microdescription. Requires the patient to match the orientation of lines.

Primary Assessment Areas. (1) Perception and judgment of line orientation; (2) visuospatial perception.

Secondary Assessment Areas. (1) Verbal comprehension; (2) speech or (3) upper extremity motor functioning.

Presentation Modalities. (1) Visual–nonverbal; (2) auditory–verbal for instructions.

Response Modalities. (1) Speech or (2) simple upper extremity motor movements—pointing; (3) untimed.

Description. The test is administered using a spiral-bound booklet containing 35 stimuli and multiple-choice response diagrams on facing pages. Each of the multiple-choice response diagrams consists of a set of lines that diverge from an origin at 18° intervals. The 3.8-cm lines are labeled "1" through "11." Five practice stimuli, each consisting of two full-length lines, are presented first. A correct response requires the patient to identify the orientation of both lines by pointing to or calling out the numbers of the lines having an identical orientation on the response diagram. If the patient is unable to respond correctly to at least two of the stimuli, the test is discontinued. Each of the 30 test items contains partial lines. Two forms of the test are available (Benton *et al.*, 1983).

Localization. Impaired performance is more likely to be associated with right than with left hemisphere lesions (Benton *et al.*, 1975, 1978, 1983).

Norms. Norms are available for the age groups 16–49, 50–64, and 65–74. Scores of 19–20 are borderline, 17–18 are moderately defective, and below 17 are severely defective. Corrections are available for age and gender: Add 1 point for 50–64 years, 3 points for 65–74 years, and 2 points for females (Benton *et al.*, 1983).

Source. Oxford University Press.

Raven's Progressive Matrices (RPM)

Microdescription. Requires the patient to solve visual pattern matching or analogy problems.

Primary Assessment Areas. (1) Visual reasoning and conceptualization; (2) conceptualization of spatial, design, and numerical relationships (Lezak, 1983); (3) visual–spatial perception.

Secondary Assessment Area. Verbal comprehension.

Presentation Modalities. (1) Visual–nonverbal; (2) auditory–verbal for instructions.

Response Modalities. (1) Writing numbers; (2) saying numbers or (3) pointing; (4) untimed.

Description. The patient is presented with a grid of abstract designs in which the lower-right-hand design is missing. In the Standard Progressive Matrices, the patient must choose from among eight alternatives offered as possible completions of the grid. There are four groups of progressive matrices. The Standard Progressive Matrices contain 60 items in five sets of 12 (Raven *et al.,* 1983). The Coloured Progressive Matrices have a colored background to attract and hold attention (Raven *et al.,* 1986; Sattler, 1988). They include the first two sets of the Standard Progressive Matrices and a set of intermediate difficulty—36 items in all. Advanced Progressive Matrices I and II contain 12 and 36 items, respectively. The groups of progressive matrices may have different factor structures (Sattler, 1988) and may differ in their emphasis on visuospatial vs. verbal functioning (Lezak, 1983).

Localization. Although the RPM have been found to have some sensitivity to brain impairment (Zimet & Fishman, 1970; Brooks & Aughton, 1979), they do not appear to lateralize brain damage (Costa & Vaughan, 1962; DeRenzi & Faglioni, 1965; Gainotti *et al.,* 1986). Patients with unilateral lesions and visual neglect may tend to produce impaired performances (Campbell & Oxbury, 1976; Colombo *et al.,* 1976).

Norms. Norms for the Standard Progressive Matrices are available for United States children aged 6–17 (Raven & Summers, 1986). Norms for the Coloured Progressive Matrices are available for United States children aged 5–12 (Raven & Summers, 1986). Norms for a group of United States college students on the Advanced Progressive Matrices may be found in Paul (1985). Orme (1966) has provided norms for adults 65–85 years of age on Raven's Coloured Progressive Matrices.

Source. RPM is available from The Psychological Corporation. It is published by H. K. Lewis & Co.

Visual Form Discrimination Test (VFDT)

Microdescription. Requires the patient to identify sets of geometric figures.

Primary Assessment Areas. (1) Complex visual form discrimination (Benton *et al.,* 1983); (2) visual–spatial attention; (3) visuospatial perception.

Secondary Assessment Areas. (1) Visual–verbal conceptualization; (2) verbal comprehension.

Presentation Modalities. (1) Visuospatial–nonverbal; (2) auditory–verbal for instructions.

Response Modalities. (1) Pointing or (2) speech; (3) untimed.

Description. The test consists of 16 items. The patient is presented a black line drawing of three geometric figures. Four drawings are displayed beneath this stimulus drawing: one correct foil—2 points; a foil with a displacement or rotation of a small, peripheral figure—1 point; (3) a foil with a distortion of a major figure—0 points; and (4) a foil with a distortion of a major figure—0 points. The peripheral figure is presented eight times on both the right and the left. The patient is asked to find the stimulus design among the four foils. A 2-1-0 scoring method is used for adults. Absence of a response is scored 0 points.

Localization. The test appears to be sensitive to a variety of impairments of brain function (Benton *et al.*, 1983). Posterior right hemisphere lesions appear to be associated with the highest frequency of failure (Varney, 1981).

Norms. Norms are available for adults aged 16–54 and 55–75 crossed with gender (Benton *et al.*, 1983).

Source. Oxford University Press.

Right–Left Orientation (RLO)

Microdescription. Assesses right–left orientation toward one's own body and a confronting person.

Primary Assessment Area. Right–left orientation.

Secondary Assessment Areas. (1) Verbal comprehension; (2) upper extremity motor functioning.

Presentation Modality. Auditory–verbal.

Response Modalities. (1) Simple right and left upper extremity motor movements; (2) untimed.

Description. The patient is instructed to perform actions, which increase in difficulty, with either his or her right or left hand. The actions include (1) pointing to lateral parts of his or her own body; (2) performing double uncrossed commands (e.g., left hand to left ear); (3) performing double crossed commands (e.g., right hand to left ear); (4) pointing to lateral parts of the examiner's body; and (5) placing left or right hand on a specific lateral body part of the examiner. There are two 20-item forms of this test. One point is scored for each correct performance. Although the patient may receive credit by self-correcting his or her performance, no partial credit is given for a partially correct performance. The test's demands on motor skill are minimal (Benton *et al.*, 1983).

Localization. Right–left disorientation with respect to one's own body is not common in brain-injured patients who are not aphasic or demented (Benton *et al.*, 1983).

Norms. Benton *et al.* (1983) have provided norms for an age range of 16–64.

Source. Oxford University Press.

NEGLECT

Line Bisection Test (LBT)

Microdescription. Requires the patient to divide lines into two equal parts.

Primary Assessment Areas. (1) Visual–spatial inattention; (2) visual–spatial functioning; (3) visual–spatial perception.

Secondary Assessment Areas. (1) Upper extremity motor functioning; (2) verbal comprehension.

Presentation Modalities. (1) Visual–nonverbal; (2) auditory–verbal for instructions.

Response Modality. Simple upper extremity motor movements—drawing lines.

Description. The patient is presented with a sheet of white paper (21.5 × 28 cm) containing 20 lines of a variety of lengths (100, 120, 140, 150, 160, 180, and 200 mm) and positions (right, left, and center) drawn parallel to the long axis of the sheet. The patient is asked to cut each line in half with a small pencil mark. He or she is asked to make only one mark on each and every line. The number and position of the unmarked lines and the deviation of the marks from true center are recorded. Percentage deviations are calculated using the following formula:

$$\text{Percentage deviation} = (\text{measured left half} - \text{true half})/\text{true half} \times 100$$

Average deviation scores are computed for sets of lines at each position and for all lines (Schenkenberg *et al.*, 1980).

Localization. In the study performed by Schenkenberget *et al.* (1980), leaving more than two lines unmarked identified patients with right-sided brain damage. Percentage deviation of the attempted bisection from true center for left-positioned lines of right-handed individuals using their right hands was also associated with right brain damage (Schenkenberg *et al.*, 1980).

Norms. Norms are from a small control group ($N = 20$) and lesion comparison groups (Schenkenberg *et al.*, 1980).

Source. Schenkenberg *et al.* (1980) describe a standardized set of lines.

Test of Visual Neglect (TVN)

Microdescription. Requires the patient to cross out lines distributed across a sheet of paper.

Primary Assessment Areas. (1) Visual–spatial inattention; (2) visual–spatial perception; (3) visual–spatial functioning.

Secondary Assessment Areas. (1) Upper extremity motor functioning; (2) verbal or gestural comprehension.

Presentation Modalities. (1) Visual–nonverbal; (2) auditory–verbal for instructions.

Response Modality. Simple upper extremity motor movements—drawing lines.

Description. The patient is presented with a 20 × 26 cm sheet of paper containing 40 2.5-cm lines. Although the lines appear to be randomly distributed, there is one row of four lines in the center with three rows of six lines on each side. The examiner then traces over each line with a red pencil. The examiner asks the patient to cross out all the lines on the page and demonstrates by drawing a line through a line in the center. The number and position of lines left uncrossed are scored (Albert, 1973).

Localization. Severity of neglect was greater for right hemisphere lesions than for left hemisphere lesions (Albert, 1973).

Norms. Albert (1973) has provided means for different lesion groups. Control subjects made no errors.

Source. Albert (1973) has described and has provided an example of the test materials.

OTHER

Trail Making Test A (TMTA)

Microdescription. Requires the patient to draw a line connecting a sequence of numbers.

Primary Assessment Areas. (1) Number recognition (Corrigan & Hinkeldey, 1987); (2) visual scanning (Corrigan & Hinkeldey, 1987); (3) visual–spatial functioning; (4) upper extremity motor functioning (Corrigan & Hinkeldey, 1987); (5) visuomotor coordination.

Secondary Assessment Area. Verbal comprehension.

Presentation Modalities. (1) Visual–nonverbal; (2) auditory–verbal for instructions.

Response Modalities. (1) Upper extremity motor movements—drawing lines; (2) timed.

Description. After a practice trial, the patient is presented with a sheet of paper containing 25 randomly distributed, circled numbers. The patient must draw a line connecting the circled numbers, in order, without lifting the pencil from the paper. If the patient makes an error, the examiner points out the error and the patient is required to draw the line correctly. The score is the time required to complete the test (Reitan & Wolfson, 1993).

Localization. The test is generally sensitive to brain damage (Reitan, 1958; Reitan &

Wolfson, 1993), but is not useful for lateralizing brain lesions (Corrigan & Hinkeldey, 1987). It is not effective in differentiating brain-injured from psychiatric patients (Heaton *et al.*, 1978).

Norms. Fromm-Auch and Yeudall (1983) have provided norms for the age groups 15–17, 18–23, 24–32, 33–40, and 41–64. Bornstein (1985) has provided norms for the age groups 20–39, 40–59, and 60–69 crossed with gender. Davies (1968) has provided percentiles for the age groups 20–39, 40–49, 50–59, 60–69, and 70–79. Stuss *et al.* (1987) have provided norms for the age groups 16–19, 20–29, 30–39, 40–49, 50–59, and 60–69. This paper also summarizes norms from seven other studies. Reitan and Wolfson (1993) have provided cutoff scores. Performance on the test is affected by intelligence (Boll & Reitan, 1973; Kennedy, 1981) and, to a lesser degree, by education (Kennedy, 1981). Extensive norms stratified by age, education, and gender have been developed by Heaton *et al.* (1991).

Source. Reitan Neuropsychology Laboratory.

Visual Functions (C4-LNNB)

Microdescription. Assesses visual abilities.

Primary Assessment Areas. (1) Object perception; (2) visual–spatial functioning; (3) spatial orientation; (4) visual analysis and synthesis; (5) ability to tell time; (6) naming.

Secondary Assessment Areas. (1) Verbal comprehension; (2) speech, writing, or pointing.

Presentation Modalities. (1) Visual–nonverbal for items 86–99; (2) visual–verbal for items 94 and 95; (3) auditory–verbal or visual–verbal for instructions for items 86–99.

Response Modalities. (1) Speech or writing for items 86–91, 94, 97, and 98; (2) speech, writing, or pointing for items 92, 93, 96, and 99; (3) drawing for item 95; (4) time-limited for items 86–92, 94–97, and 99; (5) timed for items 93 and 98.

Description. Items may be described as:

86 Object naming
87 Object naming from pictures
88, 89 Object naming from degraded pictures
90, 91 Naming of overlapping objects
92, 93 Ravens-like matrices
94 Telling time
95 Drawing hands on clocks
96 Reading a compass
97, 98 Counting blocks in a picture of a 3-D stack
99 Matching spatially rotated geometric designs

Two Factors have been identified: Visual Acuity and Naming (V1) involves the identification of difficult-to-recognize objects and the spatial rotation item. Visual–Spatial Organization (V2) contains items that assess complex visual spatial skills.

Localization. "Profiles in which the C4 scale is the highest, in combination with any secondary scale, generally reflect impairment in the right hemisphere or the occipital areas of the left hemisphere" (Golden *et al.*, 1985).

Norms. See the LNNB.

Source. Western Psychological Services.

REFERENCES

Akshoomoff-Haist, N. A., Delis, D. C., & Kiefner, M. G. (1989). Block constructions of alcoholic and unilateral brain damaged patients: A test of the right hemisphere vulnerability hypothesis of alcoholism. *Archives of Clinical Neuropsychology, 4,* 275–281.

Albert, M. L. (1973). A simple test of visual neglect. *Neurology, 23,* 658–664.

Arena, R., & Gainotti, G. (1978). Constructional apraxia and visuoperceptive disabilities in relation to laterality of cerebral lesions. *Cortex, 14,* 463–473.

Bender, L. (1938). *Instructions for the use of Visual Motor Gestalt Test.* New York: American Orthopsychiatric Association.

Benton, A. L. (1968). Differential behavioral effects in frontal lobe disease. *Neuropsychologia, 6,* 53–60.

Benton, A. L. (1974). *Revised Visual Retention Test* (4th ed.). New York: The Psychological Corporation.

Benton, A. L. (1985). Perceptual and spatial disorders. In K. Heilman & E. Valenstein (Eds.), *Clinical neuropsychology* (2nd ed.) (pp. 151–185). New York: Oxford University Press.

Benton, A. L., & Fogel, M. L. (1962). Three-dimensional constructional praxis: A clinical test. *Archives of Neurology, 7,* 347.

Benton, A. L., Hannay, H. J., & Varney, N. R. (1975). Visual perception of line direction in patients with unilateral brain disease. *Neurology, 25,* 907–910.

Benton, A. L., Varney, N. R., & Hamsher, K. (1978). Visuospatial judgment: A clinical test. *Archives of Neurology, 35,* 364–367.

Benton, A. L., Hamsher, K., Varney, N. R., & Spreen, O. (1983). *Contributions to neuropsychological assessment: A clinical manual.* New York: Oxford University Press.

Bigler, E. D., & Ehrfurth, J. W. (1980). Critical limitations of the Bender Gestalt Test in clinical neuropsychology: Response to Lacks. *Clinical Neuropsychology, 2,* 88–90.

Binder, L. M. (1982). Constructional strategies on complex figure drawings after unilateral brain damage. *Journal of Clinical Neuropsychology, 4,* 51–58.

Black, F. W., & Strub, R. L. (1976). Constructional apraxia in patients with discrete missile wounds of the brain. *Cortex, 12,* 212–220.

Boll, T. J., & Reitan, R. M. (1973). Effect of age on performance of the Trail Making Test. *Perceptual and Motor Skills, 36,* 691–694.

Bornstein, R. A. (1985). Normative data on selected neuropsychological measures from a nonclinical sample. *Journal of Clinical Psychology, 41,* 651–659.

Boyd, J. L. (1981). A validity study of the Hooper Visual Organization Test. *Journal of Consulting and Clinical Psychology, 49,* 15–19.

Brooks, D. N., & Aughton, M. E. (1979). Psychological consequences of blunt head injury. *International Rehabilitation Medicine, 1,* 160–165.

Campbell, D. C., & Oxbury, J. M. (1976). Recovery from unilateral spatial neglect? *Cortex, 12,* 303–312.

Canter, A. (1966). A background interference procedure to increase sensitivity of the Bender-Gestalt test to organic brain disorders. *Journal of Consulting Psychology, 30,* 91–97.

Canter, A. (1976). *The Canter Interference Procedure for the Bender-Gestalt Test: Manual for administration, scoring, and interpretation.* Nashville: Counselor Recordings and Tests.

Colombo, A., DeRenzi, E., & Faglioni, P. (1976). The occurrence of visual neglect in patients with unilateral cerebral disease. *Cortex, 12,* 221–231.

Corrigan, J. D., & Hinkeldey, N. S. (1987). Relationships between parts A and B of the Trail Making Test. *Journal of Clinical Psychology, 43,* 402–409.

Costa, L. D., & Vaughan, H. G. (1962). Performance of patients with lateralized cerebral lesions. 1. Verbal and perceptual tests. *Journal of Nervous and Mental Disease, 132,* 162–168.

Davies, A. (1968). The influence of age on Trail Making Test performance. *Journal of Clinical Psychology,* *24,* 96–98.

Delaney, R. C. (1982). Screening for organicity: The problem of subtle neuropsychological deficit and diagnosis. *Journal of Clinical Psychology, 38,* 843–846.

Denman, S. B. (1984). *Denman Neuropsychology Memory Scale.* Privately published: Sidney B. Denman, Ph.D., 1040 Fort Sumter Drive, Charleston, SC 29412.

DeRenzi, E., & Faglioni, P. (1965). The comparative efficiency of intelligence and vigilance tests in detecting hemispheric cerebral damage. *Cortex, 1,* 410–433.

Farah, M. J. (1990). *Visual agnosia: Disorders of object recognition and what they tell us about normal vision.* Cambridge, MA: MIT Press.

Fitz, A. G., Conrad, P. M., Hom, D. L., Sarff, P. L., & Majovski, L. V. (1992). Hooper Visual Organization Test performance in lateralized brain injury. *Archives of Clinical Neuropsychology, 7,* 243–250.

Franzen, M. (1989). *Reliability and validity in neuropsychological assessment.* New York: Plenum Press.

Fromm-Auch, D., & Yeudall, L. T. (1983). Normative data for the Halstead–Reitan tests. *Journal of Clinical Psychology, 5,* 221–238.

Gainotti, G., D'Erme, P., Villa, G., & Caltagirone, C. (1986). Focal brain lesions and intelligence: A study of a new version of Raven's Coloured Matrices. *Journal of Clinical and Experimental Neuropsychology, 8,* 37–50.

Garron, D. C., & Cheifetz, D. I. (1965). Comment on "Bender Gestalt discernment of organic pathology." *Psychological Bulletin, 63,* 197–200.

Golden, C. J., Purisch, A. D., & Hammeke, T. A. (1985). *Luria–Nebraska Neuropsychological Battery: Forms I and II.* Los Angeles: Western Psychological Services.

Heaton, R. K., Baade, L. E., & Johnson, K. L. (1978). Neuropsychological test results associated with psychiatric disorders in adults. *Psychological Bulletin, 85,* 141–162.

Heaton, R. K., Grant, I., & Matthews, C. G. (1991). *Comprehensive norms for an expanded Halstead–Reitan Battery: Demographic corrections, research findings, and clinical applications.* Odessa, FL: Psychological Assessment Resources.

Hooper, H. E. (1958). *The Hooper Visual Organization Test manual.* Los Angeles: Western Psychological Services.

Hutt, M. L. (1969). *The Hutt adaptation of the Bender-Gestalt Test* (2nd ed.). New York: Grune & Stratton.

Kaplan, E., Deborah, F., Morris, R., & Delis, D. C. (1991). *WAIS-R NI: Manual.* San Antonio: The Psychological Corporation.

Kennedy, K. J. (1981). Age effects on Trail Making Test performance. *Perceptual and Motor Skills, 52,* 671–675.

Kronfol, Z., Hamsher, K., Digre, K., & Waziri, R. (1978). Depression and hemispheric functions: Changes associated with unilateral ECT. *British Journal of Psychiatry, 132,* 560–567.

Lacks, P. (1984). *Bender Gestalt screening for brain dysfunction.* New York: Wiley.

Lacks, P., & Storandt, M. (1982). Bender Gestalt performance of normal older adults. *Journal of Clinical Psychology, 38,* 624–627.

Levin, H. S., & Benton, A. L. (1977). Facial recognition in "pseudoneurological" patients. *Journal of Nervous and Mental Disease, 164,* 135–138.

Levin, H. S., Grossman, R. G., & Kelly, P. J. (1977). Impairment of facial recognition after closed head injuries of varying severity. *Cortex, 13,* 119–130.

Lezak, M. (1983). *Neuropsychological assessment* (2nd ed.). New York: Oxford University Press.

Marley, L. M. (1982). *Organic brain pathology and the Bender-Gestalt Test: A differential diagnostic scoring system.* New York: Grune & Stratton.

Mason, C. F., & Ganzler, H. (1964). Adult norms for the Shipley Institute of Living Scale and Hooper Visual Organization Test based on age and education. *Journal of Gerontology, 19,* 419–424.

McFie, J. (1975). *Assessment of organic intellectual impairment.* London: Academic Press.

Orme, J. E. (1966). Hypothetically true norms for the Progressive Matrices Test. *Human Development, 9,* 222–230.

Osterrieth, P. A. (1944). Le test de copy d'une figure complexe. *Archives de Psychologie, 30,* 206–356.

Paul, S. M. (1985). The Advanced Progressive Matrices: Normative data for an American university population and an examination of the relationship with Spearman's g. *Journal of Experimental Education, 54,* 95–100.

Peck, E. A., Stephens, V., & Martelli, M. F. (1987). A descriptive summary of essential neuropsychological tests. In L. C. Hartlage, M. J. Asken, & J. L. Hornsby (Eds.), *Essentials of neuropsychological assessment* (pp. 213–228). New York: Springer.

Raven, J. C., & Summers, B. (1986). *Manual for Raven's Progressive Matrices and Vocabulary Scales (Research Supplement No. 3)*. London: H. K. Lewis.

Raven, J. C., Court, J. H., & Raven, J. (1983). *Manual for Raven's Progressive Matrices and Vocabulary Scales (Section 3)—Standard Progressive Matrices* (1983 edition). London: H. K. Lewis.

Raven, J. C., Court, J. H., & Raven, J. (1986). *Manual for Raven's Progressive Matrices and Vocabulary Scales (Section 2)—Coloured Progressive Matrices* (1986 edition, with U.S. norms). London: H. K. Lewis.

Reitan, R. M. (1958). Validity of the Trail Making Test as an indicator of organic brain damage. *Perceptual and Motor Skills, 8,* 271–276.

Reitan, R. M., & Wolfson, D. (1993). *The Halstead–Reitan Neuropsychological Test Battery: Theory and clinical interpretation* (2nd ed.). Tucson: Neuropsychology Press.

Sattler, J. M. (1988). *Assessment of children* (3rd ed.). San Diego: Jerome M. Sattler.

Saunders, D. R. (1960). A factor analysis of the Picture Completion items of the WAIS. *Journal of Clinical Psychology, 16,* 146–149.

Schenkenberg, T., Bradford, D. C., & Ajax, E. T. (1980). Line bisection and unilateral visual neglect in patients with neurologic impairment. *Neurology, 30,* 509–517.

Shipley, W. C. (1967). *Shipley Institute of Living Scale.* Los Angeles: Western Psychological Services.

Spreen, O., & Strauss, E. (1991). *A compendium of neuropsychological tests: Administration, norms, and commentary.* New York: Oxford University Press.

Stuss, D. T., Stethem, L. L., & Poirier, C. A. (1987). Comparison of three tests of attention and rapid information processing across six age groups. *The Clinical Neuropsychologist, 1,* 139–152.

Ungerleider, L. G., & Mishkin, M. (1982). Two cortical visual systems. In D. J. Ingle, M. A. Goodale, & R. J. W. Mansfield (Eds.), *Analysis of visual behavior* (pp. 549–586). Cambridge, MA: MIT Press.

Varney, N. R. (1981). Letter recognition and visual form discrimination in aphasic alexia. *Neuropsychologia, 19,* 795–800.

Visser, R. S. H. (1980). *Manual of the complex figure test CFT.* SWETS Test Services, 347b Heereweg, 2161 Ca Lisse, The Netherlands.

Walker, R. G. (1956). The Revised Hooper Visual Organization Test as a measure of brain damage. *Journal of Clinical Psychology, 12,* 387–388.

Walker, R. G. (1957). Schizophrenia and cortical involvement. *Journal of Nervous and Mental Disease, 125,* 226–228.

Wang, P. L. (1977). Visual organization ability in brain-damaged adults. *Perceptual and Motor Skills, 45,* 723–728.

Warrington, E. K., James, M., & Maciejewski, C. (1986). The WAIS as a lateralising and localising diagnostic instrument: A study of 656 patients with unilateral cerebral lesions. *Neuropsychologia, 24,* 223–239.

Wechsler, D. (1981). *Wechsler Adult Intelligence Scale—Revised.* New York: Psychological Corporation.

Western Psychological Services (1983). *Hooper Visual Organization Test (VOT): Manual.* Los Angeles: Western Psychological Services.

Zimet, C. N., & Fishman, D. B. (1970). Psychological deficit in schizophrenia and brain damage. *Annual Review of Psychology, 21,* 113–154.

Tactile Functioning

According to Adams and Victor (1989), sensory testing is one of the most difficult parts of the neurological examination. Test procedures tend to be crude and inadequate. Although paresthesias may indicate dysfunction, no sensory impairment may be found. A sensory deficit may be noted when there are no complaints of sensory symptoms. Since evaluation is dependent on the patient's interpretation of sensory stimuli, extraneous, confounding factors may be introduced. Although several sensory systems might be evaluated (e.g., touch, pain, pressure, temperature, proprioception, and vibration), neuropsychological evaluations generally assess these phenomena: two-point discrimination [Spreen & Strauss, 1991 (contains procedure and norms)], identification of numbers or letters written on the skin (graphesthesia), identification of body parts, such as fingers, by touch (finger gnosis), identification of objects by touch (stereognosis), and awareness of the position and movement of limbs (proprioception). Testing is done symmetrically for each half of the body, and if impairments are not the result of peripheral damage, inferences may be made regarding the integrity of the brain hemispheres contralateral and ipsilateral to the area being tested.

Reitan–Klove Sensory–Perceptual Examination (RKSPE)

Microdescription. Assesses visual fields, sensory suppressions, finger gnosis, graphesthesia, and stereognosis.

Primary Assessment Areas. (1) Visual fields; (2) visual, auditory, and tactile inattention or sensory suppressions; (3) finger gnosis; (4) graphesthesia; (5) stereognosis.

Secondary Assessment Areas. (1) Verbal comprehension; (2) speech or simple gestures or both.

Presentation Modalities. (1) Auditory–verbal for instructions; (2) visual–nonverbal; (3) auditory–nonverbal; (4) tactile–nonverbal.

Response Modalities. (1) Speech; (2) pointing; (3) untimed for all subtests with the exception of Tactile Form Recognition, which is timed.

Description. The RKSPE is a collection of tests that assess sensory functioning, especially tactile functioning. The Sensory Imperception test assesses visual fields and sensory suppressions in the visual, auditory, and tactile modalities. Visual fields are evaluated by having the patient focus on the examiner's nose while the examiner wiggles the fingers of his or her partially outstretched hand. Sensory imperception, sensory suppression, or unilateral inattention is tested by wiggling the fingers of one hand or the other and then of both hands simultaneously and noting whether the patient perceives both. If the patient reports only "right" or "left," an error is recorded. Similar testing is performed by touching the patient's hands, then the hand and face, then stimulating the ears by lightly rubbing the fingers and thumbs together near the patient's ears. Tactile Finger Recognition assesses the patient's ability to identify fingers when they are touched. Finger-Tip Number Writing assesses the ability to discriminate between numbers written on the hand (graphesthesia). Tactile Coin Recognition and Tactile Form Recognition assess the patient's ability to recognize shape in the tactile modality (stereognosis) (Reitan, 1984; Reitan & Wolfson, 1993).

Localization. (1) Visual-field defects suggest a variety of lesions in the visual system. (2) Visual suppressions suggest impairment in the contralateral visual system. (3) Auditory suppressions suggest impairment in the contralateral temporal lobe. (4) Tactile suppressions suggest impairment in the contralateral parietal lobe. (5) Unilateral finger agnosia, impaired graphesthesia, or impaired stereognosis suggests dysfunction in the contralateral hemisphere, probably including the parietal area (assuming that peripheral dysfunction has been ruled out) (Bigler, 1988).

Norms. Norms for the Sensory Perceptual Errors Right, Left, and Total calculated according to the procedure of Russell *et al.* (1970) and norms for Tactile Form Recognition Time may be found in Heaton *et al.* (1991).

Source. Reitan Neuropsychology Laboratory.

Tactile Form Perception (TFP)

Microdescription. Requires tactile identification of figures.

Primary Assessment Areas. (1) Tactile–spatial perception; (2) visual–spatial perception.

Secondary Assessment Areas. (1) Upper extremity movements—object manipulation and pointing; (2) verbal comprehension.

Presentation Modalities. (1) Tactile–nonverbal; (2) visual–nonverbal; (3) auditory–verbal for instructions.

Response Modalities. (1) Upper extremity movements—pointing; (2) time-limited.

Description. The materials consist of two sets of 10 cards. Each card contains a geometric figure made of fine-grade sandpaper. On presentation to the patient, the sandpaper figures are concealed from the patient in a box. The patient is asked to feel the figure with his or her hand and to visually identify it, by pointing to the appropriate one of 12 line drawings on a multiple-choice card. If possible, the patient is to point with the other hand from the one with which he or she felt the figure. A maximum of 30 sec is allowed for exploration of the figure, and the patient must respond in 45 sec. A different set of 10 cards is presented to each hand. A point is scored for each correct response. Scores for right, left, and both hands are calculated (Benton *et al.,* 1983).

Localization. Impaired test performance may suggest a high-level, contralateral somesthetic defect, or an ipsilateral or bilateral impairment in spatial processing, or both (Benton *et al.,* 1983; Dee & Benton, 1970). Right hemisphere lesions are associated with a higher frequency of defective performance than non-aphasia-producing left hemisphere lesions (Benton *et al.,* 1983).

Norms. Benton *et al.* (1983) have provided norms for the age groups 15–50, 51–60, and 61–70. For single-hand performance, a score of 7 is classified as a borderline performance, and 6 or less is classified as a defective performance. For both hands, a score of 15 is classified as borderline and 14 or less as defective. A decline of 1 point for each hand may be expected with increasing age (71–80 years).

Source. Oxford University Press.

Finger Localization (FL)

Microdescription. Requires the patient to identify fingers when touched.

Primary Assessment Area. Finger gnosis.

Secondary Assessment Areas. (1) Verbal comprehension; (2) verbal expression or (3) upper extremity motor functioning.

Presentation Modalities. (1) Tactile; (2) auditory–verbal for instructions.

Response Modalities. (1) Speech; (2) upper extremity motor movement—pointing; (3) untimed.

Description. The test is administered in three parts. In part A, single fingers of the patient's hand are touched with the pointed end of a pencil (10 touches on each hand) with the hand in sight. The procedure in part B is the same as that for part A except that the hand is hidden. In part C, with the hand hidden, the patient is simultaneously touched on pairs of fingers. The patient may identify the fingers touched by naming the fingers, calling out their numbers, or pointing to them on an outline drawing of the hand. Scores for left, right, and both hands are computed (Benton *et al.,* 1983).

Localization. Bilateral impairment in finger localization may be associated with aphasic disorder or general mental impairment or both (Gainotti *et al.,* 1972; Poeck & Orgass, 1969). In cases of unilateral impairment, contralateral impairment may be seen with a significantly higher frequency in patients with right hemisphere lesions.

Norms. Norms for a group of patients aged 16–65 are available (Benton *et al.,* 1983). Neither age nor education was reported to influence the performance of the normative group.

Source. Oxford University Press.

Tactual Performance Test (TPT)

Microdescription. Requires the patient to place geometrically shaped blocks in corresponding holes in a formboard while blindfolded.

Primary Assessment Areas. (1) Tactual–spatial perception; (2) stereognosis; (3) kinesthesis; (4) tactual–spatial memory.

Secondary Assessment Areas. (1) Upper extremity, hand and arm, motor functioning; (2) verbal comprehension.

Presentation Modalities. (1) Tactual–spatial; (2) auditory–verbal for instructions.

Response Modalities. (1) Upper extremity, hand and arm, motor functioning; (2) timed.

Description. The patient is blindfolded and required to place 10 geometrically shaped blocks into their corresponding holes in a formboard (Reitan & Wolfson, 1993). The patient never sees the blocks or the formboard. He or she is required to place the blocks first with the dominant hand, second with the nondominant hand, and finally with both hands. The patient is then asked, without prior warning, to draw the board with the blocks in their correct places. The six measures obtained are: (1) dominant hand time, (2) nondominant hand time, (3) both-hands time, (4) total time, (5) number of shapes correctly recalled (Memory), and (6) number of correctly recalled shapes that also are correctly located in the patient's drawing (Location).

The TPT has been criticized as being too lengthy and stressful for some patients and as not being time-efficient (Lezak, 1983). The use of the children's version of the TPT with a 6-hole formboard with adults has been studied (Clark & Klonoff, 1988; Russell, 1985). The 6-hole TPT may require only one third the time of the 10-hold test and yet not differ significantly in reliability and validity (Clark & Klonoff, 1988). Adult norms have not been developed for the six-hole test.

Localization. Left-hand time tends to be slower for patients with right hemisphere impairment and right-hand time tends to be slower for patients with left hemisphere impairment (Dodrill, 1978; Reitan, 1964). Reitan and Wolfson (1993) state that the dominant hand is expected to perform one third faster than the nondominant and that deviations from this ratio may suggest lateralizing significance. The TPT has been found to be sensitive to brain dysfunction in multiple sclerosis (Ivnik, 1978), chronic obstructive pulmonary disease (Prigatano *et al.,* 1983), Parkinson's disease (Reitan & Boll, 1971), and Huntington's chorea (Boll *et al.,* 1974).

Norms. Norms stratified by age, gender, and education may be found in Heaton *et al.* (1991).

Source. The original test materials are available from the Reitan Neuropsychology Laboratory. The Reitan Neuropsychology Laboratory catalog cautions that norms and studies utilizing the original materials may not be generalizable to other materials. A portable version is available from Psychological Assessment Resources.

Tactile Functions Scale (C3-LNNB)

Microdescription. Assesses touch, kinesthesis, and stereognosis.

Primary Assessment Areas. (1) Cutaneous sensation; (2) kinesthesis; (3) stereognosis (Golden *et al.,* 1985).

Secondary Assessment Area. Verbal comprehension.

Presentation Modalities. Any verbal modality may be used for instructions, but the patient must have a blindfold on during stimulation. The presentation is tactile–nonverbal or proprioceptive–nonverbal for all items.

Response Modalities. Any verbal modality may be used for all items except 80 and 81, which require arm movements. All items are untimed except 82 and 84, which are time-limited, and 83 and 85, which are timed.

Description. The scale items may be summarized as follows:

64, 65   Localization of a tactile stimulus
66, 67   Discriminating sharp and dull
68, 69   Discriminating hard and soft pressure
70, 71   Two-point discrimination
72, 73   Discrimination of direction of movement
74–79   Recognition of symbols and shapes drawn on the skin
80, 81   Proprioception
82–85   Tactile recognition of objects

Factor Scales are T1 (Simple Tactile Sensation), which contains tactile items, and T2 (Stereognosis), which contains the two-point discrimination and stereognosis items (Golden *et al.,* 1985).

Localization. The C3 scale is the most sensitive of the LNNB scales to the anterior parietal lobe of either hemisphere (Golden *et al.,* 1985). The items on the C3 scale in combination with the first 20 items on the C1 scale make up the lateralization scales, S2 and S3. S2 is affected by right sensorimotor performance and relates to left hemisphere function. The opposite is true for S3.

Norms. See the LNNB.

Source. Western Psychological Association.

REFERENCES

Adams, R. D., & Victor, M. (1989). *Principles of neurology* (4th ed.). New York: McGraw-Hill.
Benton, A. L., Hamsher, K., Varney, N. R., & Spreen, O. (1983). *Contributions to neuropsychological assessment: A clinical manual.* New York: Oxford University Press.
Bigler, E. D. (1988). *Diagnostic clinical neuropsychology.* Austin: University of Texas Press.
Boll, T. J., Heaton, R. K., & Reitan, R. M. (1974). Neuropsychological and emotional correlates of Huntington's chorea. *Journal of Nervous and Mental Disease, 158,* 61–68.

Clark, C., & Klonoff, H. (1988). Reliability and construct validity of the six-block Tactual Performance Test in an adult sample. *Journal of Clinical and Experimental Neuropsychology, 10,* 175–184.

Dee, H. L., & Benton, A. L. (1970). A cross-modal investigation of spatial performances in patients with unilateral cerebral disease. *Cortex, 6,* 261–272.

Dodrill, C. B. (1978). A neuropsychological battery for epilepsy. *Epilepsia, 19,* 611–623.

Gainotti, G., Cianchetti, C., & Tiacci, C. (1972). The influence of hemispheric side of lesion on non-verbal tasks of finger localization. *Cortex, 8,* 364–381.

Golden, C. J., Purisch, A. D., & Hammeke, T. A. (1985). *Luria–Nebraska Neuropsychological Battery: Forms I and II.* Los Angeles: Western Psychological Services.

Heaton, R. K., Grant, I., & Matthews, C. G. (1991). *Comprehensive norms for an expanded Halstead–Reitan Battery: Demographic corrections, research findings, and clinical applications.* Odessa, FL: Psychological Assessment Resources.

Ivnik, R. J. (1978). Neuropsychological test performance as a function of the duration of MS-related symptomatology. *Journal of Clinical Psychiatry, 39,* 304–312.

Lezak, M. D. (1983). *Neuropsychological assessment* (2nd ed.). New York: Oxford University Press.

Poeck, K., & Orgass, B. (1969). An experimental investigation of finger agnosia. *Neurology, 19,* 801–807.

Prigatano, G. P., Parsons, O. A., Wright, E., Levin, D. C., & Hawryluk, G. (1983). Neuropsychological test performance in mildly hypoxemic patients with chronic obstructive pulmonary disease. *Journal of Consulting and Clinical Psychology, 51,* 108–116.

Reitan, R. M. (1964). Psychological deficits resulting from cerebral lesions in man. In J. M. Warren & K. Akert (Eds.), *The frontal granular cortex and behavior.* New York: McGraw-Hill.

Reitan, R. M. (1984). *Aphasia and sensory–perceptual deficits in adults.* Tucson: Neuropsychology Press.

Reitan, R. M., & Boll, T. J. (1971). Intellectual and cognitive functions in Parkinson's disease. *Journal of Consulting and Clinical Psychology, 37,* 364–369.

Reitan, R. M., & Wolfson, D. (1993). *The Halstead–Reitan Neuropsychological Test Battery* (2nd ed.). Tucson: Neuropsychology Press.

Russell, E. W. (1985). Comparison of the TPT 10- and 6-hole form board. *Journal of Clinical Psychology, 41,* 68–81.

Russell, E. W., Neuringer, C., & Goldstein, G. (1970). *Assessment of brain damage: A neuropsychological key approach.* New York: Wiley-Interscience.

Spreen, O., & Strauss, E. (1991). *A compendium of neuropsychological tests: Administration, norms, and commentary.* New York: Oxford University Press.

Motor Functioning

A detailed assessment of motor functioning, as is performed in a neurological evaluation, is generally not included in a neuropsychological evaluation. Nevertheless, understanding of the complexities of movement disorders is useful. Adams and Victor (1989) devote a substantial section of *Principles of Neurology* to disorders of motility.

The neuropsychological evaluation generally contains several measures of upper extremity motor functioning—dexterity and strength. Although performance of the preferred hand generally exceeds that of the nonpreferred hand, deviations occur in the normal population, and inferences to impaired cortical functioning on the basis of one discrepancy should be avoided (Bornstein, 1986). Discrepancies consistent across several performances are rare and are more suggestive of dysfunction of the contralateral hemisphere (Thompson *et al.,* 1987). Although measures of lower extremity functioning may provide additional information (Peters, 1990), they are rarely used.

Finger Tapping Test (FTT)

Microdescription. Measures the tapping speed of the index finger of each hand.

Primary Assessment Areas. (1) Maximal finger tapping speed (Reitan & Wolfson, 1993); (2) upper extremity motor functioning.

Secondary Assessment Area. Verbal comprehension for instructions.

Presentation Modality. Auditory–verbal for instructions.

Response Modality. Upper extremity motor functioning—finger tapping.

Description. The materials consist of a tapping key and a device for recording the number of taps. Five 10-sec trials, separated by brief rest periods, are administered for each hand. The score for each hand is the average for the five trials (Reitan & Wolfson, 1993).

Localization. Lesions of either hemisphere result in greater deficits for the contralateral hand (Finlayson & Reitan, 1980). It should be noted that the tapping speed of the dominant hand can be less than that of the nondominant hand without the existence of brain pathology. Bornstein (1986) found this to be the case for approximately 30% of males and 20% of females in a group of nonclinical subjects. Time-sequential histograms of tapping intervals have been used to distinguish patients with motor dysfunctions of cerebellar, basal ganglia, and cerebral origins from each other and from normal individuals (Shimoyama *et al.,* 1990).

Norms. Norms may be found in Reitan and Wolfson (1993). Fromm-Auch and Yeudall (1983) provide norms for ages 15–17, 18–23, 24–32, 33–40, and 41–64 crossed with gender. Bornstein (1985) has provided norms for the age groups 20–39, 40–59, and 60–69 crossed with gender and education. Variables that affect tapping speed include gender (tapping speed for women is slower) (Dodrill, 1979) and age (Bak & Green, 1980; Heaton *et al.,* 1986). Norms are also presented in Heaton *et al.* (1991).

Source. Reitan Neuropsychology Laboratory.

Grip Strength Test (GS)

Microdescription. Measures strength of grip.

Primary Assessment Areas. (1) Grip strength; (2) upper extremity–hand strength.

Secondary Assessment Area. Verbal comprehension.

Presentation Modality. Auditory–verbal for instructions.

Response Modality. Upper extremity functioning—hand.

Description. A Smedley Hand Dynamometer consists of a grip and a scale that measures the force produced when the grip is squeezed. The dynamometer is adjusted to the patient's grip. The patient then points the dynamometer toward the floor and squeezes. Two trials are given, beginning with the preferred hand and alternating with the nonpreferred hand. The score for each hand is the average of the trials with that hand (Reitan & Wolfson, 1993).

Localization. Lesions of either hemisphere result in greater deficits for the contralateral hand (Dodrill, 1978; Jarvis & Barth, 1984). It should be noted that the grip strength of the dominant hand can be less than that of the nondominant hand without the existence of brain pathology (Bornstein, 1986). A procedure has been developed for detecting malingering on the GS (Niebuhr & Marion, 1987; Stokes, 1983).

Norms. Norms may be found in Reitan and Wolfson (1993). Fromm-Auch and Yeudall (1983) provide norms for ages 15–17, 18–23, 24–32, 33–40, and 41–64 crossed with gender. Bornstein (1985) provides norms for the age groups 20–39, 40–59, and 60–69 crossed with gender and education. Norms are also to be found in Heaton *et al.* (1991).

Source. Reitan Neuropsychology Laboratory.

Grooved Pegboard Test (GP)

Microdescription. Requires the patient to fit keyed pegs into holes.

Primary Assessment Areas. (1) Visual–motor coordination; (2) finger dexterity; (3) upper extremity motor functioning.

Secondary Assessment Area. Verbal comprehension.

Presentation Modalities. (1) Visual–nonverbal; (2) auditory–verbal for instructions.

Response Modality. Upper extremity motor movements—hand and arm.

Description. The pegboard contains a 5×5 matrix of holes with randomly positioned slots. The pegs, which have a ridge on one side, must be rotated to match the hole before they can be inserted. The time for the patient to insert all 25 pegs with the dominant hand is recorded. Next, the time for the nondominant hand is recorded (Lafayette Instrument Company, 1987).

Localization. Localization data are not available.

Norms. Norms are presented in Heaton *et al.* (1991).

Source. Lafayette Instrument Company.

Purdue Pegboard Test (PPT)

Microdescription. Requires the rapid placement of pegs and construction of simple assemblies.

Primary Assessment Areas. (1) Manual or finger dexterity (Fleishman & Ellison, 1962; Lezak, 1983); (2) visual–motor coordination; (3) upper extremity motor functioning.

Secondary Assessment Area. Verbal comprehension.

Presentation Modalities. (1) Visual–nonverbal; (2) auditory verbal for instructions.

Response Modality. Upper extremity movements—hand and arm.

Description. Materials consist of a board containing two parallel rows of 25 holes each. Pegs, collars, and washers are supplied in cups at the top of the board. The patient first inserts as many pegs as possible in 30 sec with the preferred hand. The score is the number of pegs inserted. The same is then done with the nonpreferred hand and then with both hands (score = number of pairs of pegs placed). The final task requires the patient to construct as many assemblies—consisting of a peg, a washer, a collar, and a washer—as possible in 1 min. The score is the number of parts used in making assemblies.

Localization. Right–left differences on the peg placement portion of the PPT may have lateralizing significance (Costa *et al.*, 1963; Vaughan & Costa, 1962).

Norms. Yeudall *et al.* (1986) have provided norms for the age groups 15–20, 21–25, 26–30, and 31–40 crossed with gender. Spreen and Strauss (1991) have provided norms for the age groups 50–59, 60–69, and 70+ crossed with gender.

Source. Lafayette Instrument Company.

Motor Impersistence (MI)

Microdescription. Requires the patient to sustain a movement.

Primary Assessment Area. Motor impersistence.

Secondary Assessment Area. Verbal comprehension.

Presentation Modalities. (1) Auditory–verbal for instructions; (2) visual–nonverbal for demonstration of movements.

Response Modalities. (1) Facial and head motor movements; (2) untimed.

Description. The patient is required to perform and sustain the following movements: (1) Keep eyes closed, (2) protrude tongue while blindfolded, (3) protrude tongue with eyes open, (4) fix gaze in lateral visual fields, (5) keep mouth open, (6) fix eyes centrally, (7) turn head, and (8) say "Ah" (Benton *et al.*, 1983).

Localization. MI is associated with right central and frontal lesions more than with posterior or left-sided lesions (Kertesz *et al.*, 1985). It is associated with general mental impairment (Benton *et al.*, 1983; Levin, 1973). MI may be associated with increased probability of poor outcome of rehabilitation (Ben-Yishay *et al.*, 1968).

Norms. Failure on two or three subtests indicates "moderate impersistence," while failure on four or more subtests indicates "marked impersistence" (Benton *et al.*, 1983). MI is more common in older patients (Joynt *et al.*, 1962; Levin, 1973).

Source. Oxford University Press.

Motor Sequencing Tasks (MST)

Microdescription. Requires the patient to sequence motor acts.

Primary Assessment Areas. (1) Motor sequencing; (2) upper extremity motor functioning; (3) motor learning.

Secondary Assessment Areas. (1) Verbal comprehension; (2) drawing (for some tasks); (3) writing (for some tasks).

Presentation Modalities. (1) Auditory–verbal for instructions; (2) visual–nonverbal for demonstration.

Response Modalities. (1) Upper extremity movements; (2) untimed.

Description. The patient is told to alternately clench and extend the fingers of the right and left hands (LNNB Item 21). First one hand is extended and the other clenched and then the positions are reversed (Christensen, 1975; Golden *et al.,* 1985). The patient is requested to successively place his or her hand in three different positions—fist, edge, and palm—and to do this repeatedly (Christensen, 1975). The patient is required to write a series of alternating "m"'s and "n"'s (Lezak, 1983). In LNNB Item 24, the patient is required to copy a design composed of two alternating components (Christensen, 1975; Golden *et al.,* 1985).

Localization. Lesion sites may be identified on the basis of the quality of the patient's performance (Christensen, 1975).

Norms. Normal subjects have no difficulty with these tasks. Motor sequences are learned after one or two trials.

Source. Luria (1966) and Christensen (1975) describe MST. Several items in the LNNB require motor sequencing (Golden *et al.,* 1985). Descriptions of MST are also presented in Lezak (1983).

Motor Scale (C1-LNNB)

Microdescription. "Assesses the ability to organize, control, and carry out motor acts with the upper extremities and oral motor area" (Golden *et al.,* 1982, p. 4).

Primary Assessment Areas. (1) Hand, arm, and oral movement; (2) kinesthesis; (3) body orientation; (4) praxis; (5) drawing; (6) copying; (7) ability to produce and inhibit movement.

Secondary Assessment Area. Verbal comprehension.

Presentation Modalities. (1) Any modality for items 1–4; (2) kinesthetic for items 5–8; (3) any verbal for instructions; (4) visual–nonverbal for items 9–18, 21–24, 32, 42–47, and 51; (5) any verbal for items 19, 20, 25–31, 34–41, and 48–50.

Response Modalities. All responses are either upper extremity or oral motor responses. Responses are untimed for items 5–20, 25–32, 34, 35, and 48–51; time-limited for items 24 and evens 36–46; and timed for items 1–4, 21–23, 33, and odds 37–47.

Description. The items may be summarized as follows:

    1–4 Rapid simple hand movements
    5–8 Kinesthetically guided hand movements
    9–18 Reproduction of modeled hand and arm movements
    19, 20 Pointing to right or left body part on command
    21–23 Rapid bilateral hand movements
       24 Copying a repetitive asymmetrical drawing
    25–27 Complex motor praxis
    28, 29 Simple oral movements
    30, 31 Kinesthetically guided oral movements
    32, 33 Rapid complex oral movements
    34, 35 Oral praxis
    36–41 Drawing simple geometric figures

42–47 Copying simple geometric figures
48–51 Conditional discrimination

Five Factors have been identified. Kinesthesis-Based Movement (M1) contains items that require motor responses on the basis of kinesthesis and verbal commands. Drawing Speed (M2) and Fine Motor Speed (M3) are self-explanatory. Spatial-Based Movement (M4) contains items based on miming. Oral Motor Skills (M5) contains the oral movement items.

Localization. If C1 is greatly elevated over C3, and S2 (Left Hemisphere) or S3 (Right Hemisphere) is elevated, there is the suggestion of an anterior lesion in the hemisphere suggested by the higher of the S2 and S3 scales. If C1, C3, and one of the hemisphere scales are elevated, especially if the difference is 20 points or greater between S2 and S3, there is a strong involvement of the sensorimotor area in the brain (around the central sulcus) or its related subcortical areas.

Norms. See the LNNB.

Source. Western Psychology Services.

REFERENCES

Adams, R. D., & Victor, M. (1989). *Principles of neurology* (4th ed.). New York: McGraw-Hill.

Bak, J. S., & Greene, R. L. (1980). Changes in neuropsychological functioning in an aging population. *Journal of Consulting and Clinical Psychology, 48,* 395–399.

Benton, A. L., Hamsher, K., Varney, N. R., & Spreen, O. (1983). *Contributions to neuropsychological assessment: A clinical manual.* New York: Oxford University Press.

Ben-Yishay, Y., Diller, L., Gerstman, L., & Haas, A. (1968). The relationship between impersistence, intellectual function and outcome of rehabilitation in patients with left hemiplegia. *Neurology, 18,* 852–861.

Bornstein, R. A. (1985). Normative data on selected neuropsychological measures from a nonclinical sample. *Journal of Clinical Psychology, 41,* 651–659.

Bornstein, R. A. (1986). Consistency of intermanual discrepancies in normal and unilateral brain lesion patients. *Journal of Consulting and Clinical Psychology, 54,* 719–723.

Christensen, A. L. (1975). *Luria's neuropsychological investigation.* New York: Spectrum.

Costa, L. D., Vaughan, H. G., Levita, E., & Farber, N. (1963). Purdue Pegboard as a predictor of the presence and laterality of cerebral lesions. *Journal of Consulting Psychology, 27,* 133–137.

Dodrill, C. B. (1978). The Hand Dynamometer as a neuropsychological measure. *Journal of Consulting and Clinical Psychology, 46,* 1432–1435.

Dodrill, C. B. (1979). Sex differences on the Halstead–Reitan Neuropsychological Test Battery and on other neuropsychological measures. *Journal of Clinical Psychology, 35,* 236–241.

Finlayson, M. A. J., & Reitan, R. M. (1980). Effect of lateralized lesions on ipsilateral and contralateral motor functioning. *Journal of Clinical Neuropsychology, 2,* 237–243.

Fleishman, E. A., & Ellison, G. D. (1962). A factor analysis of fine manipulative tests. *Journal of Applied Psychology, 46,* 96–105.

Fromm-Auch, D., & Yeudall, L. T. (1983). Normative data for the Halstead–Reitan tests. *Journal of Clinical Psychology, 5,* 221–238.

Golden, C. J., Hammeke, T. A., Purisch, A. D., Berg, R. A., Moses, J. A., Jr., Newlin, D. B., Wilkening, G. N., & Puente, A. E. (1982). *Item interpretation of the Luria–Nebraska Neuropsychological Battery.* Lincoln: University of Nebraska Press.

Golden, C. J., Purisch, A. D., & Hammeke, T. A. (1985). *Luria–Nebraska Neuropsychological Battery: Forms I and II.* Los Angeles: Western Psychological Services.

Heaton, R. K., Grant, I., & Matthews, C. G. (1986). Differences in neuropsychological test performance associated with age, education, and sex. In I. Grant & K. M. Adams (Eds.), *Neuropsychological assessment of neuropsychiatric disorders* (pp. 100–120). New York: Oxford University Press.

Heaton, R. K., Grant, I., & Matthews, C. G. (1991). *Comprehensive norms for an expanded Halstead–Reitan Battery: Demographic corrections, research findings, and clinical applications.* Odessa, FL: Psychological Assessment Resources.

Jarvis, P. E., & Barth, J. T. (1984). *Halstead–Reitan Test Battery: An interpretive guide.* Odessa, FL: Psychological Assessment Resources.

Joynt, R. J., Benton, A. L., & Fogel, M. L. (1962). Behavioral and pathological correlates of motor impersistence. *Neurology, 12,* 876–881.

Kertesz, A., Nicholson, I., Cancelliere, A., Kassa, K., & Black, S. E. (1985). Motor impersistence: A right-hemisphere syndrome. *Neurology, 35,* 662–666.

Lafayette Instrument Company (1987). *Instructions for the Grooved Pegboard.* Lafayette, IN: Lafayette Instrument Co.

Levin, H. (1973). Motor impersistence in patients with unilateral cerebral disease: A cross validation study. *Journal of Clinical and Consulting Psychology, 41,* 287–290.

Lezak, M. D. (1983). *Neuropsychological assessment* (2nd. ed). New York: Oxford University Press.

Luria, A. R. (1966). *Higher cortical functions in man.* New York: Basic Books.

Niebuhr, B. R., & Marion, R. (1987). Detecting sincerity of effort when measuring grip strength. *American Journal of Physical Medicine, 66,* 16–24.

Peters, M. (1990). Neuropsychological identification of motor problems: Can we learn something from the feet and legs that hands and arms will not tell us? *Neuropsychology Review, 1,* 165–183.

Reitan, R. M., & Wolfson, D. (1993). *The Halstead–Reitan Neuropsychological Test Battery* (2nd ed.). Tucson: Neuropsychology Press.

Shimoyama, I., Ninchoji, T., & Uemura, K. (1990). The Finger-Tapping Test: A qualitative analysis. *Archives of Neurology, 47,* 681–684.

Spreen, O., & Strauss, E. (1991). *A compendium of neuropsychological tests: Administration, norms, and commentary.* New York: Oxford University Press.

Stokes, H. M. (1983). The seriously uninjured hand: Weakness of grip. *Journal of Occupational Medicine, 25,* 683–684.

Thompson, L. L., Heaton, R. K., Matthews, C. G., & Grant, I. (1987). Comparison of preferred and nonpreferred hand performance on neuropsychological motor tasks. *The Clinical Neuropsychologist, 1,* 324–334.

Vaughan, H. G., & Costa, L. D. (1962). Performance of patients with lateralized cerebral lesions. II. Sensory and motor tests. *Journal of Nervous and Mental Disease, 134,* 237–243.

Yeudall, L. T., Fromm, D., Reddon, J. R., & Stefanyk, W. O. (1986). Normative data stratified by age and sex for 12 neuropsychological tests. *Journal of Clinical Psychology, 42,* 918–946.

Executive Functioning

This chapter describes a variety of tests loosely categorized as tests of executive functioning. The frontal lobes and especially the prefrontal areas of the brain have been interpreted as serving an executive function (Pribram, 1973) and as a supervisory system (Shallice, 1988). Generally, the tests reviewed in this chapter assess some aspect of executive functioning. Some tests have been included in this chapter because they have been associated with frontal lobe functioning even if they don't appear to assess higher-level executive functioning.

Impaired frontal lobe functioning can result in impairments in many of the brain's functional systems (Stuss & Benson, 1984, 1986). Impairments may be noted in attention, memory, language, visual–spatial functioning, and personality functioning. Massive frontal lobe damage or damage to the prefrontal convexity may result in ainitia and in slow, apathetic responding (Luria, 1973). Orbital damage may result in hyperkinesis, restlessness, and impulsivity (Stuss & Benson, 1984). Prefrontal damage may result in impaired attention, increased distractibility, an inability to utilize internal cueing, and an inability to appropriately process contextual cues (R. M. Anderson *et al.,* 1976; Pribram, 1987; Pribram *et al.,* 1977). Memory may be impaired due to attentional impairment (Hecaen & Albert, 1978), an increased sensitivity to interference (Stuss *et al.,* 1982), and impaired motivation and organization. Language impairment may be noted, especially in verbal fluency (Benton, 1968) and syntax (Goodglass & Berko, 1960). Visual–spatial–constructional abilities may be impaired due to impaired organizational abilities. This impairment may be noted on Block Design (Walsh, 1977). Prefrontal damage may interfere with the programming of behavior and action and the ability to inhibit behavior (Luria, 1966; Pribram, 1971). Although behavioral perseveration is not pathognomonic for frontal lobe dysfunction (Hecean & Albert, 1978), it is commonly associated with frontal lobe damage (Luria, 1966, 1973).

Since impairment of executive and frontal lobe functioning can affect a wide range of cognitive abilities, assessment of executive function involves an appraisal of performance on a wide variety of cognitive tasks not specifically designed to assess executive functioning. In addition, one may administer tests specifically designed or presumed to measure executive or frontal lobe functioning or both. This chapter is divided according to several areas of functioning associated with the frontal lobes: shifting cognitive set, maintaining cognitive set, impulse control, and cognitive productivity. Tests presumed to assess these areas of functioning are reviewed.

SHIFTING COGNITIVE SET

Trail Making Test B (TMTB)

Microdescription. Requires the patient to draw a line alternating between sequences of numbers and letters.

Primary Assessment Areas. (1) Number and letter recognition (Reitan & Wolfson, 1993; Corrigan & Hinkeldey, 1987); (2) visual scanning (Corrigan & Hinkeldey, 1987); (3) cognitive flexibility (Reitan & Wolfson, 1993); (4) visual–spatial functioning; (5) upper extremity motor functioning (Corrigan & Hinkeldey, 1987); (6) visuomotor coordination.

Secondary Assessment Area. Verbal comprehension.

Presentation Modalities. (1) Visual–nonverbal; (2) auditory–verbal for instructions.

Response Modalities. (1) Upper extremity motor movements—drawing lines; (2) timed.

Description. After a practice trial, the patient is presented with a sheet of paper containing 25 randomly distributed, circles. The circles contain the numbers 1–13 and the letters A–L. The patient must draw a line connecting the circles, in order, alternating between numbers and letters, without lifting the pencil from the paper. If the patient makes an error, the examiner points out the error and requires the patient to draw the line correctly. The score is the time required to complete the test (Reitan & Wolfson, 1993).

Localization. The test is generally sensitive to brain damage (Reitan, 1958; Reitan & Wolfson, 1993; Spreen & Benton, 1965), but is not useful for lateralizing brain lesions (Corrigan & Hinkeldey, 1987; Heilbronner *et al.,* 1991). It is not effective in differentiating brain-injured from psychiatric patients (Heaton *et al.,* 1978; Spreen & Benton, 1965).

Norms. Fromm-Auch and Yeudall (1983) have provided norms for the age groups 15–17, 18–23, 24–32, 33–40, and 41–64. Bornstein (1985) has provided norms for the age groups 20–39, 40–59, and 60–69 crossed with gender. Davies (1968) has provided percentiles for the age groups 20–39, 40–49, 50–59, 60–69, and 70–79. Stuss *et al.* (1987) have provided norms for the age groups 16–19, 20–29, 30–39, 40–49, 50–59, and 60–69. This paper also summarizes norms from seven other studies. Reitan and Wolfson (1993) have provided cutoff scores. The test is affected by intelligence (Boll & Reitan, 1973; Kennedy, 1981) and, to a lesser degree, by education (Gordon, 1972; Kennedy, 1981).

Source. Reitan Neuropsychology Laboratory.

Wisconsin Card Sorting Test (WCST)

Microdescription. Assesses the patient's ability to shift cognitive set in response to performance feedback.

Primary Assessment Areas. (1) Cognitive flexibility (Lezak, 1983); (2) simple concept formation (Lezak, 1983); (3) maintenance of cognitive set; (4) learning; (5) simple reasoning.

Secondary Assessment Areas. (1) Verbal comprehension; (2) memory.

Presentation Modalities. (1) Auditory–verbal for instructions and feedback; (2) visuo-spatial–nonverbal; (3) color.

Response Modalities. (1) Simple upper extremity and hand movements—placing cards; (2) untimed.

Description. The materials include two decks of 64 cards on each of which are printed one, two, three, or four of the symbols triangle, star, cross, and circle in one of the colors red, green, yellow, and blue. In each deck of 64 cards, no two cards are identical. The patient is asked to place the cards, one after another, under one of four stimulus cards (one red triangle, two green stars, three yellow crosses, and four blue circles) according to a principle that must be deduced from the examiner's responses ("right" or "wrong") to the patient's placements. The first sorting principle is color. After 10 consecutive correct sorts, the principle changes to form, then to number, then again to color, form, and number through six sorting principles or until the 128 cards are sorted. Scoring includes total errors, total correct, and categories completed. A perseverative response is defined as one that would have been correct according to the previous principle. Two exceptions to this definition are proposed in the WCST Manual (Heaton, 1981). Since there has been some confusion about how perseverative responses should be scored, Flashman *et al.* (1991) have developed definitions and scoring rules to operationalize this task. Failure to maintain set is scored when the patient makes 5 correct responses in a row but fails to get the 10 required to complete the category.

Several short forms of the WCST have been developed (Nelson, 1976; L. J. Robinson *et al.*, 1991; Axelrod *et al.*, 1992).

Localization. The perseverative responses category is the best WCST measure of brain damage. Patients with focal frontal lobe lesions tend to make more perseverative errors than patients with nonfrontal focal lesions. However, patients with diffuse damage do not tend to differ significantly in number of perseverative errors from patients with focal frontal lesions (Drewe, 1974; Heaton, 1981; A. L. Robinson *et al.*, 1980). In contrast to previous studies, S. W. Anderson *et al.* (1991) found no significant differences in WCST performance between subjects with frontal vs. nonfrontal brain damage. They concluded that their findings "indicate that performance on the WCST cannot be interpreted in isolation as an index of frontal lobe damage" (S. W. Anderson *et al.*, 1991, p. 909). In reviewing the WCST, Mountain and Snow (1993, p. 108) concluded that "the evidence that frontal patients perform more poorly than nonfrontal patients is weak."

Norms. In the study by Heaton (1981), a cutoff score of >18 = brain-damaged classified 74% of brain-damaged patients and 72% of normal controls correctly. Heaton recommended raising the cutoff score to around 35 for individuals 60 years old or older. More recent norms stratified by age, education, and gender may be found in Heaton *et al.* (1991).

Source. Psychological Assessment Resources.

Halstead Category Test (CT)

Microdescription. Requires the patient to discover the concept or principle that governs the relationship between sets of geometric forms.

Primary Assessment Areas. (1) Abstract concept formation (Pendleton & Heaton, 1982; Reitan & Wolfson, 1993); (2) visuospatial ability (Lansdell & Donnelly, 1977); (3) ability to respond selectively to one aspect of a stimulus (Pendleton & Heaton, 1982); (4) ability to profit from feedback regarding correctness of a response (Pendleton & Heaton, 1982); (5) cognitive flexibility or ability to shift response sets (Pendleton & Heaton, 1982); (6) memory.

Secondary Assessment Areas. (1) Verbal comprehension; (2) color vision.

Presentation Modalities. (1) Visual–nonverbal; (2) auditory–verbal for instructions; (3) auditory–nonverbal for feedback (HRNB); (4) color.

Response Modalities. (1) Upper extremity movements—depressing a lever or pointing; (2) untimed.

Description. A projection apparatus is used to present the patient with a series of 208 stimulus figures on a screen. The patient responds by pressing a lever on a panel of levers numbered 1–4. Depressing a lever causes either a bell to ring (correct response) or a buzzer to sound (incorrect response). Only one response is allowed per stimulus item. The items are grouped into seven subtests. The first subtest requires the patient to match presented Roman numerals to the Arabic numerals over the answer levers. One to four designs are presented in the second subtest. In the third subtest, the patient must press a lever that corresponds to the figure that differs the most from the others. The fourth subtest requires the association of different quadrants of a figure with the numbers 1–4. The fifth and sixth subtests associate numbers with the proportion of a figure that is solid rather than dotted. The final subtest consists of items from previous subtests, the patient being required to recall the correct responses. Errors on all subtests are added to obtain total errors score (Reitan & Wolfson, 1993). Administration time may be 20–60 min (Finlayson *et al.*, 1986). In a booklet version of the test, DeFilippis *et al.* (1979) place a piece of cardboard with the numbers 1–4 running left to right. The patient is asked to respond by pointing to a number. Feedback is given by telling the patient "correct" or "incorrect."

Localization. The Halstead CT has been found to be the most sensitive single test in the HRNB for distinguishing brain-damaged from control populations (Klove, 1974; Wheeler *et al.*, 1963). It is sensitive to diffuse brain injury and cerebral lesions regardless of their locations (Bornstein, 1986) and is therefore not useful in localizing brain impairment.

Norms. Reitan and Wolfson (1993) suggest a cutoff score of 50 or more errors. This score does not take age into account. Norms are available in Fromm-Auch and Yeudall (1983) for ages 15–17, 18–23, 24–32, 33–40, and 41–64. Age appears to affect Halstead CT performance (Corrigan *et al.*, 1987; Prigatano & Parsons, 1976).

Source. The original slide version of the CT is available from the Reitan Neuropsychology Laboratory. A booklet version authored by DeFilippis and McCampbell (1991) is available from Psychological Assessment Resources. The *Short Category Test—Booklet Format* is available from Western Psychological Services (Wetzel & Boll, 1987).

MAINTAINING COGNITIVE SET

Stroop Color–Word Test (SCWT)

Microdescription. Requires the patient to inhibit a dominant set to read a word in favor of a nondominant set to report the color of ink in which a word is printed.

Primary Assessment Areas. (1) Ability to suppress an automatic word-reading response and produce a color-naming response (Golden, 1978); (2) ability to separate word- and color-naming stimuli (Golden, 1978); (3) ability to shift perceptual set to conform to changing demands (Lezak, 1983); (4) attention (Minsky, 1989).

Secondary Assessment Areas. (1) Reading; (2) color-naming; (3) verbal comprehension.

Presentation Modalities. (1) Visual–verbal; (2) visual–nonverbal (colors); (3) auditory–verbal for instructions.

Response Modalities. (1) Speech; (2) timed.

Description. Numerous forms are available. The form used by Golden (1978) consists of three sheets of 8″ × 11″ paper. The first sheet contains five columns of color names ("blue," "green," and "red") printed in black ink. The patient is asked to read aloud down the columns and is asked to correct incorrect responses. The second sheet contains five columns of blue, green, and red X's. The patient is asked to name the colors. The third sheet contains the same words as the first sheet printed in blue, green, or red ink. The ink of each word is different from the color named. The patient is asked to name the color of the ink in which each word is printed. The score for each task is the number of correct responses in 45 sec. Administration time is approximately 10 min. A gross assessment of color-naming should be performed before administering the Stroop.

The Stroop Neuropsychological Screening Test (SNST) (Trenerry *et al.,* 1989) consists of two forms. Form C contains four columns of 28 color names ("red," "green," "blue," and "tan") printed in red, green, blue, and tan, with no name printed in its named color. The patient is asked to read the color words as quickly as he or she can. The Color Score is the number of correct responses in the time limit of 120 sec. Form C-W is the same as Form C except for the order of the color names. The patient is asked to name the color of the ink in which the word is printed. The Color–Word Score is the number of correct responses in the time limit of 120 sec.

The Victoria version of the Stroop (Spreen & Strauss, 1991) uses three 21.4 cm × 14 cm cards with each containing six rows of four items. In part D, the patient must name as quickly as possible, scanning from left to right, the color of 24 dots printed in blue, green, red, or yellow. In Part W, the dots are replaced by the words "when," "hard," "and," and "over." The patient is asked to name the colors of the words. In Part C, the colored stimuli are the color names "blue," "green," "red," and "yellow." The patient is asked to name the colors in which the words are printed. Time and errors are scored.

Localization. Golden (1976) has reported that the Stroop correctly distinguished normal and psychiatric patients from brain-injured patients with 87% accuracy. Guidelines for interpreting scores may be located in the *Stroop Color and Word Test: A Manual for Clinical and Experimental Use* (Golden, 1978). Trenerry *et al.* (1989) found that patients with left hemisphere CVAs performed at the lowest level of brain-damaged patients. Closed head injury patients performed at the highest level. Optimal cutoff scores on the Color–Word Task correctly classified 79% of the 18–49 age group (cutoff < 98 for brain damage) and 92% of the 50+ age group (cutoff < 61 for brain damage). For the Victoria version of the Stroop, the interference effect of Part C (relative to Part W) has been reported to be greater for patients with left frontal damage than for other groups (Perret, 1974).

Norms. Golden (1978) has provided age corrections for the age groups 16–44, 45–64, and 65–80. Trenerry *et al.* (1989) have provided norms for the age groups 18–49 and 50+.

Spreen and Strauss (1991) have provided norms for the age groups 20–35, 50–59, 60–69, 70–79, and 80+.

Source. The form used by Golden (1978) is available from Stoelting Company. The SNST is available from Psychological Assessment Resources. The Victoria version of the Stroop is available from the Neuropsychology Laboratory, University of Victoria.

IMPULSE CONTROL

Incompatible Conditional Discrimination Tasks (ICDT)

Microdescription. Requires a response incompatible with the meaning of a stimulus.

Primary Assessment Areas. (1) Production and inhibition of responses; (2) upper extremity motor functioning.

Secondary Assessment Area. Verbal comprehension.

Presentation Modalities. (1) Auditory–verbal for instructions; (2) visual–nonverbal for demonstration.

Response Modalities. (1) Upper extremity movements; (2) untimed.

Description. The patient is required to show his or her finger when the examiner shows his fist and vice versa (Christensen, 1975). The patient is asked to knock gently when the examiner knocks hard and vice versa (Christensen, 1975; Golden *et al.,* 1985). The patient is asked to knock once when the examiner knocks twice and vice versa (Golden *et al.,* 1985).

Localization. Drewe (1975a) found that patients with frontal lesions made more errors on an ICDT than patients with other cortical lesions. Drewe (1975a) found patients with frontal lesions also to be impaired on a compatible conditional discrimination task.

Norms. Drewe (1975a) has provided data for frontal and nonfrontal groups.

Source. Luria (1966) and Christensen (1975) have described incompatible conditional discrimination tasks. An ICDT is included in the LNNB Motor Scale Items 48 and 51 (Golden *et al.,* 1985). Drewe (1975a) describes apparatus and procedures for incompatible conditional discrimination tasks.

Go–NoGo Tasks (GNGT)

Microdescription. Requires the patient to respond or to refrain from responding to cues.

Primary Assessment Areas. (1) Production and inhibition of responses; (2) upper extremity motor functioning.

Secondary Assessment Area. Verbal comprehension.

Presentation Modalities. (1) Auditory–verbal for instructions; (2) visual–nonverbal for demonstration.

Response Modalities. (1) Simple upper extremity movements; (2) untimed.

Description. The patient may be asked to squeeze the examiner's hand at the word "red" and to do nothing at the word "green" (Christensen, 1975; Golden *et al.*, 1985). On a performance version of a GNGT, Drewe (1975a) had subjects rapidly press a key to a red light and refrain from pressing to a blue light. Sixty randomized trials, 30 red light and 30 blue light, were presented. On a learning version of a GNGT, Drewe (1975b) told subjects that there was a problem to solve and that pressing the key would not always switch the light off. The subject was asked to press the key when he or she thought the light would go off immediately and to refrain from pressing when he or she thought it would not. Seventy randomized trials, 35 red light ("Go," the light switches off) and 35 blue light ("NoGo," the light doesn't switch off), were presented.

Localization. Drewe (1975a,b) found that patients with frontal lesions took longer to learn a GNGT and made more false "Go" responses than patients with other cortical lesions. Luria (1966) related impaired Go–NoGo performance to a dissociation of verbal and motor reactions and to impaired frontal lobe functioning.

Norms. Drewe (1975a,b) has provided data for left and right frontal and left and right nonfrontal groups.

Source. Luria (1966) and Christensen (1975) have described Go–NoGo tasks. A Go–NoGo task is included in the LNNB Motor Scale Item 49 (Golden *et al.*, 1985). Drewe (1975a,b) has described apparatus and procedures for performance and learning versions of Go–NoGo tasks.

Porteus Maze Test (PMT)

Microdescription. Requires the patient to trace mazes of increasing complexity.

Primary Assessment Areas. (1) Planning; (2) inhibition of impulsive behavior; (3) ability to change set (Franzen, 1989; Porteus, 1965).

Secondary Assessment Areas. (1) Verbal comprehension; (2) visual–motor coordination.

Presentation Modalities. (1) Visual–nonverbal; (2) auditory–verbal for instructions.

Response Modalities. (1) Upper extremity movements—tracing; (2) untimed (Vineland Revision).

Description. The patient is required to trace a series of mazes of increasing difficulty without going into blind alleys or crossing lines to avoid drawing around to reach an opening (Porteus, 1965).

Localization. Schizophrenic patients who have had frontal lobectomies have been found to be impaired on PMT relative to schizophrenic patients who did not have surgery (Porteus,

1965; Smith, 1960; Smith & Kinder, 1959). Thalamotomy may also effect performance (Meier & Story, 1967).

Norms. The mazes may be administered to age groups 3–12, 14, and adult.

Source. The Psychological Corporation.

COGNITIVE PRODUCTIVITY

Controlled Oral Word Association Test (COWAT-MAE)

Microdescription. Requires the oral production of words beginning with a designated letter.

Primary Assessment Areas. (1) Word fluency (Benton & Hamsher, 1989); (2) speech.

Secondary Assessment Area. (1) Verbal comprehension.

Presentation Modality. Auditory–verbal for instructions.

Response Modalities. (1) Speech; (2) timed.

Description. The patient is asked to quickly say all the words that he or she can think of beginning with a given letter. No proper names or repetitions of a word with a different ending (e.g., eat, eating) are allowed. The letter "S" is used as an example. The patient is then given 60 sec to think of and say words beginning with "C." This test is repeated with "F" and then "L." The raw score is the total number of acceptable responses for the three letters. The alternate Form B, using the letters "P," "R," and "W," is available (Benton & Hamsher, 1989).

Localization. The performance of patients with left frontal lesions or bilateral frontal lesions tends to be more impaired on oral word fluency than that of patients with lesions in other areas of the cortex (Benton, 1968; Bornstein, 1986; Parks *et al.,* 1988). In a study of the "F," "A," "S" verbal fluency test, Crowe (1992) found a greater number of errors for subjects with suspected orbital–frontal impairment.

Norms. Norms include adjustments for the age groups 25–54, 55–59, and 60–69 crossed with education < 9, 9–11, 12–15, and 16+ years (Benton & Hamsher, 1989).

Source. Psychological Assessment Resources.

Thurstone Word Fluency Test (TWFT)

Microdescription. Requires the written production of words beginning with a certain letter.

Primary Assessment Areas. (1) Word fluency; (2) upper extremity motor functioning— writing.

Secondary Assessment Area. Verbal comprehension.

Presentation Modality. Auditory–verbal for instructions.

Response Modalities. (1) Writing; (2) timed.

Description. The patient is asked to write as many words beginning with the letter "S" as he or she can in 5 min and then as many four-letter words beginning with the letter "C" as he or she can in 4 min (Thurstone, 1938).

Localization. Performance on the TWFT is sensitive to cerebral damage generally. It is more impaired by frontal than nonfrontal, left than right, and left frontal than right frontal lesions (Pendleton *et al.,* 1982). The "S" (high association) subtask may be more sensitive to cortical impairment than the "C," four-letter subtask (Bolter *et al.,* 1983). Pendleton *et al.* (1982) found that a cutoff score of <41 classified 74% of their brain-damaged group and 75% of their normals correctly. A cutoff of <36 classified 61.8% of the frontal, 63.6% of the frontal plus nonfrontal, and 61.5% of the nonfrontal groups.

Norms. Norms are available for ages 5–9, 10–15, 16–30, 31–44, and 45–60 (Kolb & Whishaw, 1985).

Source. The test may be found in Thurstone (1938).

Ruff Figural Fluency Test (RFFT)

Microdescription. Requires the patient to draw series of different designs.

Primary Assessment Areas. (1) Figural fluency; (2) initiation; (3) planning; (4) cognitive productivity; (5) cognitive flexibility (Neuropsychological Resources, 1988).

Secondary Assessment Areas. (1) Upper extremity motor functioning; (2) visual–spatial functioning; (3) verbal comprehension.

Presentation Modalities. (1) Visuospatial–nonverbal; (2) auditory–verbal for instructions.

Response Modalities. (1) Upper extremity movements—drawing; (2) timed.

Description. In each of the five parts of the test, the patient is presented with a white sheet of paper printed with stimulus items. The stimulus items are configurations of five black dots. The front of each sheet contains three identical stimulus items for practice. The back contains 35 items in a 5 × 7 array. The patient is asked to draw as many designs as possible connecting at least two dots. Sixty seconds is allowed for each part. The Part I stimulus is an arrangement of five dots. Parts II and III have the same arrangement of dots with interfering designs. Parts IV and V have different arrangements of five dots. The total number of unique designs and the total number of perseverations are scored. Calculation of an error ratio by dividing total perseverations by total unique designs provides an index of planning efficiency. The error ratio may be independent of motor functioning. Vik and Ruff

(1988) found that patients generally use rotational or enumerative strategies to produce designs. Administration time is less than 10 min (Neuropsychological Resources, 1988).

Localization. Jones-Gotman and Milner (1977) found that patients with right frontal lesions were impaired on a design fluency test. No localization studies have been performed on the RFFT.

Norms. Norms are available for the age groups 16–24, 25–39, 40–54, and 55–70 (Neuropsychological Resources, 1988). Gender does not affect performance. A correction factor adjusts for education (Ruff *et al.,* 1987).

Source. Neuropsychological Resources, 2206 Hyde Street, San Francisco, CA 94109.

TinkerToy Test (TTT)

Microdescription. Requires the patient to make a construction using a set of Tinkertoy pieces.

Primary Assessment Area. Independent initiation, planning, and structuring of a potentially complex activity (Lezak, 1983).

Secondary Assessment Areas. (1) Visuospatial constructive ability; (2) upper extremity motor functioning.

Presentation Modalities. (1) Visual–nonverbal; (2) auditory–verbal for instructions.

Response Modalities. (1) Skilled upper extremity movement; (2) untimed.

Description. The patient is provided with a set of 50 Tinkertoy pieces—24 dowels, 10 knobs, 4 wheels, 4 connectors, 4 caps, and 4 points. He or she is then told, "Make whatever you want with these. You will have at least five minutes and as much more time as you wish to make something" (Lezak, 1983, p. 514).

After a construction is produced, the patient is asked, "What is it?" The patient's construction is scored on eight dimensions: (1) production of a construction ($mc = 1, 0$); (2) number of pieces used ($np = 1$ if $n \leq 20$, $np = 2$ if $n \leq 30$, $np = 3$ if $n \leq 40$, and $np = 4$ if $n \leq 50$, where n is the total number of pieces used); (3) appropriate name (*name* $= 1, 0$); (4) mobility and moving parts (*mov* = mobility $= 1, 0$ + moving parts $= 1, 0$); (5) symmetry (*sym* times $2 = 1$, times $4 = 2$); (6) three-dimensionality (*3d* $= 1, 0$); (7) freestanding (*stand* $= 1, 0$); and (8) commission of errors such as improperly fitting pieces and not picking up dropped pieces (*error* $= -1, 0$). Two composite scores are calculated: (1) complexity or *comp* $= mc + np + name + sym + mov + 3d + stand + error;$ (2) modified complexity or *mcomp* $= comp - np$. *Comp* can vary from -1 to 12. In the modification by Bayless *et al.* (1989) of Lezak's scoring procedure, only 1 point is available for *sym*. The *name* is scored 3 points for an appropriate name, 2 points for a vague or inappropriate name, and 1 point for post hoc descriptions, for a maximum possible *comp* score of 13.

Lezak (1982, 1983) found that controls, independent brain-injured, and dependent brain-injured patients performed differently on the test. Employed head-injured and unemployed head-injured patients may perform differently (Bayless *et al.,* 1989).

Localization. Localization has not been established.

Norms. Lezak (1982, 1983) provides data for groups of controls, independent brain-injured, and dependent brain-injured patients. Bayless *et al.* (1989) provide data for controls, employed head-injured, and unemployed head-injured patients.

Source. Lezak (1983).

REFERENCES

Anderson, R. M., Hunt, S. C., Vander Stoep, A., & Pribram, K. H. (1976). Object permanency and delayed response as spatial context in monkeys with frontal lesions. *Neuropsychologia, 14,* 481–490.

Anderson, S. W., Damasio, H., Jones, R. D., & Tranel, D. (1991). Wisconsin Card Sorting Test performance as a measure of frontal lobe damage. *Journal of Clinical and Experimental Neuropsychology, 13,* 909–922.

Axelrod, B. N., Henry, R. R., & Woodward, J. L. (1992). Analysis of abbreviated form of the Wisconsin Card Sorting Test. *The Clinical Neuropsychologist, 6,* 27–31.

Bayless, J. D., Varney, N. R., & Roberts, R. J. (1989). Tinker Toy Test performance and vocational outcome in patients with closed-head injuries. *Journal of Clinical and Experimental Neuropsychology, 11,* 913–917.

Benton, A. L. (1968). Differential behavioral effects in frontal lobe disease. *Neuropsychologia, 6,* 53–60.

Benton, A. L., & Hamsher, K. (1989). *Multilingual aphasia examination* (2nd ed.). Iowa City: AJA Associates.

Boll, T. J., & Reitan, R. M. (1973). Effect of age on performance of the Trail Making Test. *Perceptual and Motor Skills, 36,* 691–694.

Bolter, J. F., Long, C. J., & Wagner, M. (1983). The utility of the Thurstone Word Fluency Test in identifying cortical damage. *Clinical Neuropsychology, 5,* 77–82.

Bornstein, R. A. (1985). Normative data on selected neuropsychological measures from a nonclinical sample. *Journal of Clinical Psychology, 41,* 651–659.

Bornstein, R. A. (1986). Contribution of various neuropsychological measures to the detection of frontal lobe impairment. *International Journal of Clinical Neuropsychology, 8,* 18–22.

Christensen, A. L. (1975). *Luria's neuropsychological investigation.* New York: Spectrum.

Corrigan, J. D., & Hinkeldey, N. S. (1987). Relationships between parts A and B of the Trail Making Test. *Journal of Clinical Psychology, 43,* 402–409.

Corrigan, J. D., Agresti, A. A., & Hinkeldey, N. S. (1987). Psychometric characteristics of the Category Test: Replication and extension. *Journal of Clinical Psychology, 43,* 368–376.

Crowe, S. F. (1992). Dissociation of two frontal lobe syndromes by a test of verbal fluency. *Journal of Clinical and Experimental Neuropsychology, 14,* 327–339.

Davies, A. (1968). The influence of age on Trail Making Test performance. *Journal of Clinical Psychology, 24,* 96–98.

DeFilippis, N. A., & McCampbell, E. (1991). *The Booklet Category Test: Manual.* Odessa, FL: Psychological Assessment Resources.

DeFilippis, N. A., McCampbell, E., & Rogers, P. (1979). Development of the booklet form of the Category Test: Normative and validity data. *Journal of Clinical Neuropsychology, 1,* 339–342.

Drewe, E. A. (1974). The effect of type and area of brain lesion on Wisconsin Card Sorting Test performance. *Cortex, 10,* 158–170.

Drewe, E. A. (1975a). An experimental investigation of Luria's theory on the effects of frontal lobe lesions in man. *Neuropsychologia, 13,* 421–429.

Drewe, E. A. (1975b). Go–No Go learning after frontal lobe lesions in humans. *Cortex, 11,* 8–16.

Finlayson, M. A. J., Sullivan, J. F., & Alfano, D. P. (1986). Halstead's Category Test: Withstanding the test of time. *Journal of Clinical and Experimental Neuropsychology, 8,* 706–709.

Flashman, L. A., Horner, M. D., & Freides, D. (1991). Note on scoring perseveration on the Wisconsin Card Sorting Test. *The Clinical Neuropsychologist, 5,* 190–194.

Franzen, M. (1989). *Reliability and validity in neuropsychological assessment.* New York: Plenum Press.

Fromm-Auch, D., & Yeudall, L. T. (1983). Normative data for the Halstead–Reitan tests. *Journal of Clinical Psychology, 5,* 221–238.

Golden, C. J. (1976). The diagnosis of brain damage by the Stroop Test. *Journal of Clinical Psychology, 32,* 652–658.

Golden, C. J. (1978). *Stroop Color and Word Test: A manual for clinical and experimental use.* Chicago: Stoelting.

Golden, C. J., Purisch, A. D., & Hammeke, T. A. (1985). *Luria–Nebraska Neuropsychological Battery: Forms I and II.* Los Angeles: Western Psychological Services.

Goodglass, H., & Berko, J. (1960). Agrammatism and inflectional morphology in English. *Journal of Speech and Hearing Research, 3,* 257–267.

Gordon, N. G. (1972). The Trail Making Test in neuropsychological diagnosis. *Journal of Clinical Psychology, 28,* 167–169.

Heaton, R. K. (1981). *A manual for the card sorting test.* Odessa, FL: Psychological Assessment Resources.

Heaton, R. K., Baade, L. E., & Johnson, K. L. (1978). Neuropsychological test results associated with psychiatric disorders in adults. *Psychological Bulletin, 85,* 141–162.

Heaton, R. K., Grant, I., & Matthews, C. G. (1991). *Comprehensive norms for an expanded Halstead–Reitan Battery: Demographic corrections, research findings, and clinical applications.* Odessa, FL: Psychological Assessment Resources.

Hecaen, H., & Albert, M. L. (1978). *Human neuropsychology.* New York: Wiley.

Heilbronner, R. L., Henry, G. K., Buck, P., Adams, R. L., & Fogle, T. (1991). Lateralized brain damage and performance on Trail Making A and B, Digit Span Forward and Backward, and TPT Memory and Location. *Archives of Clinical Neuropsychology, 6,* 251–258.

Jones-Gotman, M., & Milner, B. (1977). Design fluency: The invention of nonsense drawings after focal cortical lesions. *Neuropsychologia, 15,* 653–674.

Kennedy, K. J. (1981). Age effects on Trail Making Test performance. *Perceptual and Motor Skills, 52,* 671–675.

Klove, H. (1974). Validation studies in adult clinical neuropsychology. In R. M. Reitan & L. A. Davison (Eds.), *Clinical neuropsychology: Current status and applications* (pp. 211–235). Washington, DC: V. H. Winston & Sons.

Kolb, B., & Whishaw, I. Q. (1985). *Fundamentals of human neuropsychology* (2nd ed.). New York: W. H. Freeman.

Lansdell, H., & Donnelly, E. (1977). Factor analysis of the Wechsler Adult Intelligence scale subtests and the Halstead–Reitan Category and Tapping Tests. *Journal of Consulting and Clinical Psychology, 45,* 412–416.

Lezak, M. D. (1982). The problem of assessing executive functions. *International Journal of Psychology, 17,* 281–297.

Lezak, M. D. (1983). *Neuropsychological assessment* (2nd. ed). New York: Oxford University Press.

Luria, A. R. (1966). *Higher cortical functions in man.* New York: Basic Books.

Luria, A. R. (1973). *The working brain.* New York: Basic Books.

Meier, M. J., & Story, J. L. (1967). Selective impairment of Porteus Maze performance after right subthalamotomy. *Neuropsychologia, 5,* 181–189.

Minsky, A. F. (1989). The neuropsychology of attention: Elements of a complex behavior. In E. Perceman (Ed.), *Integrating theory and practice in clinical neuropsychology* (pp. 75–91). Hillsdale, NJ: Laurence Erlbaum Associates.

Mountain, M. A., & Snow, W. G. (1993). Wisconsin Card Sorting Test as a measure of frontal pathology: A review. *The Clinical Neuropsychologist, 7,* 108–118.

Nelson, H. E. (1976). A modified card sorting test sensitive to frontal deficits. *Cortex, 12,* 313–324.

Neuropsychological Resources (1988). *Ruff Figural Fluency Test: Administration Manual.* San Diego: Neuropsychological Resources.

Parks, R. W., Loewenstein, D. A., Dodrill, K. L., Barker, W. W., Yoshii, F., Chang, J. Y., Emran, A., Apicella, A., Sheramata, W. A., & Duara, R. (1988). Cerebral metabolic effects of a verbal fluency test: A PET scan study. *Journal of Clinical and Experimental Neuropsychology, 10,* 565–575.

Pendleton, M. G., & Heaton, R. (1982). A comparison of the Wisconsin Card Sorting Test and the Category Test. *Journal of Clinical Psychology, 38,* 392–396.

Pendleton, M. G., Heaton, R. K., Lehman, R. A. W., & Hulihan, D. (1982). Diagnostic utility of the Thurstone Word Fluency Test in neuropsychological evaluations. *Journal of Clinical Neuropsychology, 4,* 307–317.

Perret, E. (1974). The left frontal lobe of man and the suppression of habitual responses in verbal categorical behavior. *Neuropsychologia, 12,* 323–330.

Porteus, S. D. (1965). *Porteus Maze Test: Fifty years' application.* Palo Alto, CA: Pacific Books.

Pribram, K. H. (1971). *Languages of the brain: Experimental paradoxes and principles in neuropsychology.* Englewood Cliffs, NJ: Prentice-Hall.

Pribram, K. H. (1973). The primate frontal cortex—Executive of the brain. In K. K. H. Pribram & A. R. Luria (Eds.), *Psychophysiology of the frontal lobes* (pp. 293–314). New York: Academic Press.

Pribram, K. H. (1987). The subdivisions of the frontal cortex revisited. In E. Perecman (Ed.), *The frontal lobes revisited* (pp. 11–39). Hillsdale, NJ: Lawrence Erlbaum Associates.

Pribram, K. H., Plotkin, H. C., Anderson, R. M., & Leong, D. C. Q. (1977). Information sources in the delayed alternation task for normal and "frontal" monkeys. *Neuropsychologia, 15,* 329–340.

Prigatano, G., & Parsons, O. (1976). Relationship of age and education to Halstead Test performance in different patient populations. *Journal of Consulting and Clinical Psychology, 44,* 527–533.

Reitan, R. M. (1958). Validity of the Trail Making Test as an indicator of organic brain damage. *Perceptual and Motor Skills, 8,* 271–276.

Reitan, R. M., & Wolfson, D. (1993). *The Halstead–Reitan Neuropsychological Battery: Theory and clinical interpretation* (2nd ed.). Tucson: Neuropsychology Press.

Robinson, A. L., Heaton, R. K., Lehman, R. A. W., & Stilson, D. W. (1980). The utility of the Wisconsin Card Sorting Test in detecting and localizing frontal lobe lesions. *Journal of Consulting and Clinical Psychology, 48,* 605–614.

Robinson, L. J., Kester, D. B., Saykin, A. J., Kaplan, E. F., & Gur, R. C. (1991). Comparison of two short forms of the Wisconsin Card Sorting Test. *Archives of Clinical Neuropsychology, 6,* 27–33.

Ruff, R. M., Light, R. H., & Evans, R. (1987). The Ruff Figural Fluency Test: A normative study with adults. *Developmental Neuropsychology, 3,* 37–51.

Shallice, T. (1988). *From neuropsychology to mental structure.* Cambridge, England: Cambridge University Press.

Smith, A. (1960). Changes in Porteus Maze scores of brain operated schizophrenics after an eight year interval. *The Journal of Mental Science, 106,* 967–978.

Smith, A., & Kinder, E. F. (1959). Changes in psychological test performances of brain-operated schizophrenics after eight years. *Science, 129,* 149–150.

Spreen, O., & Benton, A. L. (1965). Comparative studies of some psychological tests for cerebral damage. *Journal of Nervous and Mental Disease, 140,* 323–333.

Spreen, O., & Strauss, E. (1991). *A compendium of neuropsychological tests: Administration, norms, and commentary.* New York: Oxford University Press.

Stuss, D. T., & Benson, D. F. (1984). Neuropsychological studies of the frontal lobes. *Psychological Bulletin, 95,* 3–28.

Stuss, D. T., & Benson, D. F. (1986). *The frontal lobes.* New York: Raven Press.

Stuss, D. T., Kaplan, E. F., Benson, D. F., Weir, W. S., Chiulli, S., & Sarazin, F. F. (1982). Evidence for the involvement of orbitofrontal cortex in memory functions: An interference effect. *Journal of Comparative and Physiological Psychology, 96,* 913–925.

Stuss, D. T., Stethem, L. L., & Poirier, C. A. (1987). Comparison of three tests of attention and rapid information processing across six age groups. *The Clinical Neuropsychologist, 1,* 139–152.

Thurstone, L. L. (1938). *Primary mental abilities.* Chicago: University of Chicago Press.

Trenerry, M. R., Crosson, B., DeBoe, J., & Leber, W. R. (1989). *Stroop Neuropsychological Screening Test: Manual.* Odessa, FL: Psychological Assessment Resources.

Vik, P., & Ruff, R. M. (1988). Children's figural fluency performance: Development of strategy use. *Developmental Neuropsychology, 4,* 63–74.

Walsh, K. (1977). Neuropsychological aspects of modified leucotomy. In W. H. Sweet, S. Orbrador, & J. G. Martin-Rodriguez (Eds.), *Neurosurgical treatment in psychiatry, pain, and epilepsy* (pp. 163–174). Baltimore: University Park Press.

Wetzel, L., & Boll, T. J. (1987). *Short Category Test—Booklet Format—Manual.* Los Angeles: Western Psychological Services.

Wheeler, L., Burke, C. J., & Reitan, R. M. (1963). An application of discriminant functions to the problem of predicting brain damage using behavioral variables. *Perceptual and Motor Skills, 16,* 417–440.

Malingering

Malingering is defined in DSM III-R as "intentional production of false or grossly exaggerated physical or psychological symptoms, motivated by external incentives" (American Psychiatric Association, 1987, p. 360). *Factitious disorders* with physical or psychological symptoms involve the intentional production of symptoms due to a psychological need to assume the sick role in the absence of external incentives (American Psychiatric Association, 1987). In contrast to malingering and factitious disorders, a *conversion disorder* is an alteration of physical functioning that suggests physical disorder, but is an expression of a psychological conflict or need (American Psychiatric Association, 1987). The symptoms are *not* intentionally produced and cannot be explained by any physical disorder.

The determination of malingering may be extremely difficult (McMahon & Satz, 1981). It is important to note that malingering, or conscious feigning, and nonconscious feigning are at the ends of a continuum and that a mixture may also be noted (Walsh, 1991). Brandt (1988, p. 81) has stated that "there are no scientifically valid and reliable clinical techniques for determining with certainty whether an individual is feigning amnesia." Experts have performed poorly in studies designed to assess their ability to detect malingering (Heaton *et al.*, 1978; Wylie & Ruff, 1990). Therefore, the label of "malingering" should be applied only with great care.

Several methods are available to assess malingering. Some instruments such as the MMPI contain scales (F, L, and K Scales) that may provide evidence of malingering. Heaton *et al.* (1978) found that malingerers exhibited elevations of Scales F, 1, 3, 6, 7, and 8 relative to nonlitigating head-trauma patients. Berry *et al.* (1991) concluded from their meta-analysis that the best scales for detecting malingering are T-scaled, raw F, the original Dissimulation scale, and the F–K index. Assessment of malingering on the MMPI-2 has been reviewed by Pope *et al.* (1993).

The patient's performance may be compared to that of individuals who were attempting to malinger in controlled studies. Studies include those by: (1) Goebel (1983) of the WAIS, HRNB, LM-WMS-R, and MF; (2) Heaton *et al.* (1978) of the MMPI, WAIS, and HRNB; (3) Benton and Spreen (1961) of the BVRT; and (4) Mittenberg *et al.* (1993) of the WMS-R.

The following patterns of performance should alert the practitioner to the possibility of malingering (Orsini *et al.*, 1988):

1. Inconsistencies are noted across test performances.
2. Inconsistencies are noted between formal test results and daily functioning.
3. Test results and symptom profile are incompatible with neurological disorders.

4. Scores are depressed on sensory and motor tests, while scores of tests especially sensitive to brain dysfunction are normal.
5. Recognition memory is found to be poorer than free recall.

Several tests that have been reported to be useful in detecting malingering are reviewed below.

Symptom Validity Test (SVT)

Microdescription. An ability is assessed in a forced-choice format.

Primary Assessment Area. Malingering—sensory, memory, and other areas of functioning assessable in a two-alternative, forced-choice format (Pankratz, 1979, 1983, 1988).

Secondary Assessment Area. Verbal comprehension.

Presentation Modalities. (1) Depends on the area of functioning to be assessed; (2) auditory–verbal for instructions.

Response Modalities. (1) Speech; (2) untimed.

Description. Each test is constructed specifically for the patient's complaint. A reproducible stimulus is identified for which the patient claims a deficit. Using a two-alternative, forced-choice technique, over a large number of trials (e.g., 100), a hit rate of 50% is expected if the patient is completely unable to identify the correct stimulus. If the patient is malingering and attempting to look bad, he or she may tend to make too many misses and perform below chance. This is an indication that the patient can do the task. In some cases, the patient may begin to do well, and the test may be cast as "training" or "therapy" in the area of claimed impairment (Pankratz, 1979).

Hiscock and Hiscock (1989) developed a variation to assess memory. The test consists of eight stimulus cards, each containing a 5-digit number. For each stimulus card, there is a response card with two 5-digit numbers. The target number matches the number on the stimulus card. The foil differs from the target in at least two digits, one of which is either the first or the last digit. Four sets of response cards are made. Sets A and B differ in the numbers used as foils. Sets C and D are identical to A and B, except that the positions of the target and foil are reversed. A stimulus card is presented for 5 sec. The response card is presented after a delay of 5 sec in the first block of 24 trials, 10 sec in the second block, and 15 sec in the third and final block. The patient is told that the task is a "memory test." Feedback on the correctness of each response is provided. Following the first and second blocks of trials, the patient is told that he or she is doing well and that the interval is being increased to make the task more difficult. This procedure may increase the patient's effort to perform poorly, if he or she is malingering. Performance in the separate blocks can be compared. Guilmette *et al.* (1993) have suggested that due to the easiness of this task for neurological or psychiatric patients, even a few errors should raise the suspicion level that effort or motivation may not be optimal. Hall *et al.* (1991) have developed and studied Explicit Alternative Testing, a form of the SVT. Binder (1993a,b) has developed the Portland Digit Recognition Test.

Localization. May vary according to the symptom area assessed.

Source. Pankratz (1979, 1983, 1988).

Dot Counting Test (DCT)

Microdescription. Requires the patient to count sets of ungrouped dots.

Primary Assessment Area. Malingering—impaired general intelligence and visual–spatial ability (Lezak, 1983).

Secondary Assessment Areas. (1) Counting; (2) visual scanning.

Presentation Modalities. (1) Visual–nonverbal; (2) auditory–verbal for instructions.

Response Modalities. (1) Speech; (2) timed, but sequence of times is the primary measure.

Description. The test materials consist of six serially numbered cards. Card (1) is printed with 7 ungrouped dots, and (2) with 11, (3) with 15, (4) 19, (5) 23, and (6) 27 dots. The cards are presented in the order (2), (4), (3), (5), (6), and (1). The patient is asked to count the dots and report their number as quickly as he or she can, and response times are noted. Time should increase with increase in the number of dots. According to Lezak (1983), more than one pronounced deviation from this pattern raises the possibility of malingering. The test may be used with individuals complaining of general impaired intellectual or visual–spatial functioning.

Localization. No information is available.

Norms. Percentile norms are available in Lezak (1983).

Source. Lezak (1983).

Memorization of Fifteen Items (MFI)

Microdescription. Requires the patient to recall 15 separate but conceptually related figures.

Primary Assessment Area. Malingering—memory disorder (Lezak, 1983).

Secondary Assessment Areas. (1) Memory; (2) visual letter and number recognition; (3) verbal comprehension.

Presentation Modalities. (1) Visual–verbal; (2) visual–nonverbal; (3) auditory–verbal for instructions.

Response Modalities. (1) Speech; (2) untimed.

Description. The patient is presented with a paper containing three parallel columns of figures. The first column contains the figures "A," "1," "a," a circle, and a vertical line. The second column contains "B," "2," "b," a square, and two vertical lines. The third column contains "C," "3," "c," a triangle, and three vertical lines. The test is presented as requiring the memorization of 15 different items. Since the items in each row (e.g., ''A,'' ''B,'' ''C'') form meaningful units, the test's difficulty appears greater than it is. The patient sees the paper for 10 sec and is asked to respond after a delay of 10–15 sec (Lezak, 1983; Pankratz, 1988).

Localization. No information is available.

Norms. Goldberg and Miller [(1986) cited in Pankratz, 1988] found all of 50 psychiatric patients able to remember at least 9 of the 15 items. Of 16 mentally retarded persons, 37.5% recalled fewer than 9 items.

Sources. Rey (1964), Lezak (1983), and Pankratz (1988).

REFERENCES

American Psychiatric Association (1987). *Diagnostic and statistical manual of mental disorders* (3rd ed.– rev.). Washington, DC: American Psychiatric Association.

Benton, A., & Spreen, O. (1961). Visual memory test: The simulation of mental incompetence. *Archives of General Psychiatry, 4,* 79–83.

Berry, D. T. R., Baer, R. A., & Harris, M. J. (1991). Detection of malingering on the MMPI: A meta-analysis. *Clinical Psychology Review, 11,* 585–598.

Binder, L. M. (1993a). An abbreviated form of the Portland Digit Recognition Test. *The Clinical Neuropsychologist, 7,* 104–107.

Binder, L. M. (1993b). Assessment of malingering after mild head trauma with the Portland Digit Recognition Test. *Journal of Clinical and Experimental Neuropsychology, 15,* 170–182.

Brandt, J. (1988). Malingered amnesia. In R. Rogers (Ed.), *Clinical assessment of malingering and deception* (pp. 65–83). New York: Guilford Press.

Goebel, R. A. (1983). Detection of faking on the Halstead–Reitan Neuropsychological Test Battery. *Journal of Clinical Psychology, 39,* 731–742.

Guilmette, T. J., Hart, K. J., & Giuliano, A. J. (1993). Malingering detection: The use of a forced-choice method in identifying organic versus simulated memory impairment. *The Clinical Neuropsychologist, 7,* 59–69.

Hall, H. V., Shooter, E. A., Craine, J., & Paulsen, S. (1991). Explicit Alternative Testing: A trilogy of studies on faked memory deficits. *Forensic Reports, 4,* 259–279.

Heaton, R. K., Smith, H. H., Lehman, R. A. W., & Vogt, A. T. (1978). Prospects for faking believable deficits on neuropsychological testing. *Journal of Consulting and Clinical Psychology, 46,* 892–900.

Hiscock, M., & Hiscock, C. K. (1989). Refining the forced-choice method for the detection of malingering. *Journal of Clinical and Experimental Neuropsychology, 11,* 967–974.

Lezak, M. D. (1983). *Neuropsychological assessment* (2nd. ed). New York: Oxford University Press.

McMahon, E. A., & Satz, P. (1981). Clinical neuropsychology: Some forensic applications. In S. Filskov & R. Boll (Eds.), *Handbook of clinical neuropsychology* (pp. 686–701). New York: Wiley.

Mittenberg, W., Azrin, R., Millsaps, C., & Heilbronner, R. (1993). Identification of malingered head injury on the Wechsler Memory Scale—Revised. *Psychological Assessment, 5,* 34–40.

Orsini, D. L., Van Gorp, W. G., & Boone, K. B. (1988). *The neuropsychology casebook.* New York: Springer-Verlag.

Pankratz, L. (1979). Symptom validity testing and symptom retraining: Procedures for the assessment and treatment of functional sensory deficits. *Journal of Consulting and Clinical Psychology, 47,* 409–410.

Pankratz, L. (1983). A new technique for the assessment and modification of feigned memory deficit. *Perceptual and Motor Skills, 57,* 367–372.

Pankratz, L. (1988). Malingering on intellectual and neuropsychological measures. In R. Rogers (Ed.), *Clinical assessment of malingering and deception* (pp. 169–192). New York: Guilford Press.

Pope, K. S., Butcher, J. N., & Seelen, J. (1993). *The MMPI, MMPI-2, and MMPI-A in court: A practical guide for expert witnesses and attorneys.* Washington, DC: American Psychological Association.

Rey, A. (1964). *L'examen clinique en psychologie*. Paris: Presses Universitaires de France.

Walsh, K. W. (1991). *Understanding brain damage: A primer of neuropsychological evaluation*. Edinburgh: Churchill-Livingston.

Wylie, T. F., & Ruff, R. M. (1990). Detection of simulated malingering on neuropsychological tests. Poster presented at the 18th annual meeting of the International Neuropsychological Society, Orlando, FL.

Personality

Neuropsychological evaluation of a patient with a neurological disorder should include an assessment of the patient's adjustment to the disorder. Measures of personality and emotional functioning may be helpful in this regard. Comprehensive, objective measures of personality such as the MMPI may be useful in providing an overall assessment. The Personality Assessment Inventory (Morey, 1991) appears to be a promising new comprehensive, objective assessment instrument; however, research with neurological patients is limited. Projective instruments such as the Rorschach (R), the Thematic Apperception Test (TAT) (Murray, 1943), the Hand Test (HT) (Wagner, 1983), and the Draw-a-Person Test may be especially useful in evaluating the personality and emotional functioning of individuals with limited verbal abilities.

Minnesota Multiphasic Personality Inventory (MMPI)

Microdescription. Objective, true–false assessment of personality.

Primary Assessment Areas. (1) Personality; (2) emotional functioning.

Secondary Assessment Area. Verbal comprehension.

Presentation Modality. (1) Visual–verbal or (2) auditory–verbal if the test is read to the patient.

Response Modalities. (1) Simple upper extremity movements—marking answers or (2) speech; (3) untimed.

Description. The MMPI consists of 566 true–false questions. An optional shorter version of 399 items will yield the original 14 scales. The full version must be administered to obtain additional scales. Numerous handbooks (Dahlstrom & Welsh, 1960, 1975; Graham, 1987; Greene, 1980) and a voluminous literature are available.

Care must be taken in interpreting the MMPI in patients with neurological disorders. Neurological symptoms may elevate selected scales in the patient's profile and suggest emotional dysfunction where there is none. This phenomenon has been demonstrated for both multiple sclerosis (Meyerink *et al.*, 1988) and head injury (Gass & Russell, 1991), and methods for correcting this tendency have been proposed. Alfano *et al.* (1990) have developed the MMPI-NC44, which corrects for 44 items that were judged to reflect neurological symptoms.

Although the use of abbreviated forms of the MMPI with neurologically impaired patients has been criticized (Alfano & Finlayson, 1987), the use of such measures may sometimes be the only way to obtain a measure of personality functioning using an objective test (Sbordone & Jennison, 1983). Sbordone and Caldwell (1979) developed the Organic Brain Disorder—168 (OBD-168) patterned after the MMPI-168. The MMPI-168 uses the first 168 items of the MMPI and produces scores highly correlated with the full MMPI scales (Overall & Gomez-Mont, 1974). Regression equations allow estimation of full clinical scale scores. The OBD-168 simplifies presentation of the items while retaining their meaning. The items are posed as questions requesting a ''Yes'' or ''No'' response rather than as statements requiring a ''True'' or ''False'' response. The language is simplified in some items.

The MMPI-2 (the revised MMPI) contains 567 items. It is the same as the old MMPI except for the addition of two new validity scales, 15 content scales, and deletion or modernization of some items (Butcher, 1990; Graham, 1990).

Localization. Elevations may be noted on Scales 1, 2, 3, and 8, since a number of items on these scales may reflect neurological symptoms (Dikmen & Reitan, 1974). However, there is no profile diagnostic of brain damage (Franzen, 1989). Although numerous studies have attempted to detect MMPI patterns associated with dysfunction at particular brain loci, these studies have not yielded reliable, consistent results (Dikmen & Reitan, 1977; Gass & Russell, 1986; Franzen, 1989; Woodward *et al.*, 1984). Numerous scales have been developed to distinguish functional disorders or schizophrenia from brain damage (Hovey, 1964; Shaw & Matthews, 1965; Watson, 1971; Watson & Plemel, 1978). None of these measures has been found to distinguish brain damage from schizophrenia better than Scale 8 (Golden *et al.*, 1979). For example, Russell (1977) found that schizophrenic patients obtained higher elevations on 8 and that a cutoff of 80 correctly classified 78% of brain damaged vs. schizophrenic patients.

Norms. T-score norms are automatically obtained via the profile form. These norms are not corrected for age or education. Colligan *et al.* (1989) have collected norms for the age groups 18–19, 20–29, 30–39, 40–49, 50–59, 60–69, and 70+ crossed with gender.

Source. National Computer Systems.

Rorschach (R)

Microdescription. Requires the patient to interpret inkblots.

Primary Assessment Areas. (1) Personality; (2) emotional functioning; (3) cognitive functioning.

Secondary Assessment Areas. (1) Attention; (2) visual recognition and integration; (3) naming; (4) ability to formulate an oral–verbal expressive response (Franzen, 1989).

Presentation Modalities. (1) Visual–nonverbal; (2) auditory–verbal for instructions.

Response Modalities. (1) Speech and pointing; (2) untimed (response latencies are recorded).

Description. The materials consist of 10 stimulus cards containing symmetrical black or color inkblots printed on white. The patient is told to tell the examiner what he or she sees. The cards are presented one at a time. Response latency and position of the card are recorded. The response is recorded verbatim. After all the cards have been presented, the cards are again reviewed and the patient is asked to locate each response, and the determinants of each response are subtly queried. All responses are recorded verbatim. A guide to scoring may be found in Exner (1974, 1978, 1982, 1985).

Localization. Several systems have been proposed for the use of the Rorschach in the assessment of brain dysfunction (Dorken & Kral, 1952; Piotrowski, 1937). None of these systems has been sufficiently validated to justify clinical use (Goldfried *et al.,* 1971).

Norms. The Exner scoring system is based on data from a nonpatient group and four psychiatric groups (Exner, 1974, 1978).

Source. Psychological Assessment Resources.

REFERENCES

Alfano, D. P., & Finlayson, M. A. (1987). Comparison of standard and abbreviated MMPIs in patients with head injury. *Rehabilitation Psychology, 32,* 67–76.
Alfano, D. P., Finlayson, M. A., Stearns, G. M., & Neilson, P. M. (1990). The MMPI and neurologic dysfunction: Profile configuration and analysis. *The Clinical Neuropsychologist, 4,* 69–79.
Butcher, J. N. (1990). *The MMPI-2 in psychological treatment.* New York: Oxford University Press.
Colligan, R. C., Osborne, D., Swenson, W. M., & Offord, K. P. (1989). *The MMPI: A contemporary normative study of adults.* Odessa, FL: Psychological Assessment Resources.
Dahlstrom, W. G., & Welsh, G. S. (1960). *An MMPI handbook: A guide to use in clinical practice and research,* Vol. 1. Minneapolis: University of Minnesota Press.
Dahlstrom, W. G., & Welsh, G. S. (1975). *An MMPI handbook: A guide to use in clinical practice and research,* Vol. 2. Minneapolis: University of Minnesota Press.
Dikmen, S., & Reitan, R. M. (1974). MMPI correlates of localized cerebral lesions. *Perceptual and Motor Skills, 39,* 831–840.
Dikmen, S., & Reitan, R. M. (1977). MMPI correlates of adaptive ability deficits in patients with brain lesions. *Journal of Nervous and Mental Disease, 165,* 247–254.
Dorken, H., & Kral, V. A. (1952). The psychological differentiation of organic brain lesions and their localization by means of the Rorschach Test. *American Journal of Psychiatry, 108,* 764–771.
Exner, J. E. (1974). *The Rorschach: A comprehensive system,* Vol. 1. New York: Wiley.
Exner, J. E. (1978). *The Rorschach: A comprehensive system,* Vol. 2. New York: Wiley.
Exner, J. E. (1982). *The Rorschach: A comprehensive system,* Vol. 3. New York: Wiley.
Exner, J. E. (1985). *A Rorschach workbook for the comprehensive system* (2nd ed.). Asheville, NC: Rorschach Workshops.
Franzen, M. (1989). *Reliability and validity in neuropsychological assessment.* New York: Plenum Press.
Gass, C. S., & Russell, E. W. (1986). Minnesota Multiphasic Personality Inventory correlates of lateralized cerebral lesions and aphasic deficits. *Journal of Consulting and Clinical Psychology, 54,* 359–363.
Gass, C. S., & Russell, E. W. (1991). MMPI profiles of closed head trauma patients: Impact of neurologic complaints. *Journal of Clinical Psychology, 47,* 253–260.
Golden, C. J., Sweet, J. J., & Osmon, D. C. (1979). The diagnosis of brain damage by the MMPI: A comprehensive evaluation. *Journal of Personality Assessment, 43,* 138–142.
Goldfried, M. R., Stricker, G., & Weiner, I. B. (1971). *Rorschach handbook of clinical and research applications.* Englewood Cliffs, NJ: Prentice-Hall.
Graham, J. R. (1987). *The MMPI: A practical guide* (2nd ed.). New York: Oxford University Press.
Graham, J. R. (1990). *MMPI-2: Assessing personality and psychopathology.* New York: Oxford University Press.

Greene, R. L. (1980). *The MMPI: An interpretive manual.* New York: Grune & Stratton.

Hovey, H. B. (1964). Brain lesions and five MMPI items. *Journal of Consulting Psychology, 28,* 78–79.

Meyerink, L. H., Reitan, R. M., & Selz, M. (1988). The validity of the MMPI with multiple sclerosis patients. *Journal of Clinical Psychology, 44,* 764–769.

Morey, L. C. (1991). *The Personality Assessment Inventory: Professional manual.* Odessa, FL: Psychological Assessment Resources.

Murray, H. A. (1943). *Thematic Apperception Test: Manual.* Cambridge, Massachusetts: Harvard University Press.

Overall, J. E., & Gomez-Mont, F. (1974). The MMPI-168 for psychiatric screening. *Educational and Psychological Measurement, 34,* 315–319.

Piotrowski, Z. (1937). The Rorschach inkblot method in organic disturbances of the central nervous system. *Journal of Nervous and Mental Disease, 86,* 525–537.

Russell, E. W. (1977). MMPI profiles of brain-damaged and schizophrenic subjects. *Journal of Clinical Psychology, 33,* 190–193.

Sbordone, R. J., & Caldwell, A. R. (1979). The "OBD-168": Assessing the emotional adjustment to cognitive impairment and organic brain damage. *Clinical Neuropsychology, 1,* 36–41.

Sbordone, R. J., & Jennison, J. H. (1983). A comparison of the OBD-168 and MMPI to assess the emotional adjustment of traumatic brain injured inpatients to their cognitive deficits. *Clinical Neuropsychology, 5,* 87–88.

Shaw, D. J., & Matthews, C. G. (1965). Differential MMPI performance of brain-damaged vs. pseudoneurologic groups. *Journal of Clinical Psychology, 21,* 405–408.

Wagner, E. E. (1983). *The Hand Test—Revised: Manual.* Los Angeles: Western Psychological Services.

Watson, C. G. (1971). An MMPI scale to separate brain-damaged from schizophrenic men. *Journal of Consulting and Clinical Psychology, 36,* 121–125.

Watson, C. G., & Plemel, D. (1978). An MMPI scale to separate brain damaged from functional psychiatric patients in neuropsychiatric settings. *Journal of Consulting and Clinical Psychology, 46,* 1127–1132.

Woodward, J. A., Bisbee, C. T., & Bennett, J. E. (1984). MMPI correlates of relatively localized brain damage. *Journal of Clinical Psychology, 40,* 961–969.

IV

Deficits, Competencies, and Disabilities

The heart of the neuropsychological evaluation and report involves the analysis and interpretation of the interview and test data. The results of the testing are summarized and strengths and weaknesses are noted. Examination of the pattern of test deficits in the context of information from the history and interview is essential for diagnosis. Deficit determination is fundamental to the process. The diagnosis and the patient's strengths and weaknesses are translated into recommendations for therapy.

In addition to diagnosis and recommendations for therapy, the neuropsychologist is often requested to draw conclusions from interviews, records, and test data about the patient's capability to perform in a number of arenas. These arenas include the capacity for self-care and independent living, driving ability, vocational functioning, and academic functioning. It may be necessary to assess specific aspects of competence in civil competency evaluations, Social Security disability evaluations, and workers' compensation evaluations. Part IV addresses these issues.

Deficit Determination

Deficits are determined by comparing the patient's performance with a standard. The standard may be the normative performance of a patient-equivalent population on relevant variables such as age, education, or gender (*normative comparison standard*). When *individual comparison standards* are used, the patient's performance is compared to his or her previous test performances or to estimates of premorbid performance. The patient's performance may be compared to the level required to perform an activity such as managing one's finances or driving (*competence comparison standard*).

NORMATIVE COMPARISON STANDARDS

Lezak (1983) has suggested that normative comparisons are most useful in evaluating functions not closely tied to general intellectual ability, i.e., functions largely mediated by subcortical structures, such as memory, learning, and attention. Normative comparisons may be useful for functions that are generally present in all intact adults, such as the ability to speak, count change, draw a recognizable person, read a map, and use basic tools and utensils. Certain basic motor, sensory, and perceptual functions are also appropriately evaluated via normative comparisons. For example, fine tactile discrimination tends to vary in a narrow range and to be somewhat all-or-none in pattern of functioning (Russell, 1980). Of course, even for these functions, determination of the patient's previous level of functioning, through history-taking or other means, is essential. It should be noted that normative data and statistical distributions are also used in making intra-individual comparisons and comparisons to competence levels.

There are several classification schemas used to describe performance levels and deficits relative to norms. The schemas used by Benton *et al.* (1983), Heaton *et al.* (1991), and Wechsler (1981) are presented in Appendix A. Tables for conversions between z-scores, T-scores, percentiles, and WAIS-R IQs and a graphic representation of these and other relationships are also presented in Appendix A.

INDIVIDUAL COMPARISON STANDARDS

Deficits may be determined by comparing a patient's current level of functioning with his or her premorbid level. If previous test results are available, as in serial neuropsychological testing, comparisons are relatively straightforward, although practice effects may confound interpretation. If testing is not available, then premorbid performance levels must be estimated. A thorough history is essential for making these estimates. Background information can be obtained by interviewing the patient and significant others. Relevant information should include an educational, occupational, and leisure history and information about household activities the patient performed prior to any morbidity. Educational and occupational records should be obtained if feasible.

A number of techniques have been developed for estimating premorbid IQ. One technique involves the comparison of performance on tests purported to be insensitive to brain injury with those purported to be sensitive. The WAIS Vocabulary (V) and Information (I) subtests have been believed to be among the best indicators of premorbid intelligence. However, impaired performance on the subtest may be misleading. It may be depressed due to limited educational opportunities. V may be depressed in even mild aphasia. Wechsler (1958) proposed the WAIS Deterioration Quotient calculated on the basis of "Hold" (V, I, OA, and PC) and "Don't Hold" (BD, DSym, DS, and S) subtests. The formula is as follows:

$$\text{Deterioration Quotient} = \text{Hold} - (\text{Don't Hold/Hold})$$

Since the Hold subtests can be impaired in a variety of neurological conditions, this method may underestimate impairment (Vogt & Heaton, 1977). Klesges et al. (1981) report that research assessing the Wechsler "Hold–Don't Hold" quotient has been mixed, but recommend that "use of the 'hold-don't' quotients is not advisable on a routine basis" (p. 37).

Lezak (1983) proposed that the patient's best performance be can used as a standard for judging all other current performance. Empirical assessment has found that this "best performance method" is likely to result in a significant overestimation of the patient's premorbid IQ and performance on neuropsychological tests (Mortensen et al., 1991). Matarazzo (1990) has warned the practitioner that use of the highest and lowest subtest scores as indices of the patient's premorbid level of cognitive functioning and degree of impairment is not justified when isolated from life history and current medical findings.

It is important to take into account the standard error of measurement in interpreting scores. Test scatter alone does not prove brain injury. When interpreting VIQ–PIQ differences, it should be noted that Mattarazzo and Herman (1984, 1985) found a standard deviation of 11.12 and a range of −43 to +49 in the WAIS-R standardization sample.

The NART (Nelson, 1982; Nelson & O'Connell, 1978), NAART (Blair & Spreen, 1989), and an American version of the NART (AMNART) (Grober & Sliwinski, 1991) are reading tests that appear to provide a better estimate of premorbid IQ than Vocabulary test scores (Spreen & Strauss, 1991). Wiens et al. (1993) found the NAART to underestimate the IQ of higher IQ groups and overestimate the IQ of lower IQ groups.

Demographic measures have had limited success as estimators of premorbid IQ. Equations are available for the WAIS (Wilson et al., 1978) and the WAIS-R (Barona & Chastain, 1986; Barona et al., 1984). Karzmark et al. (1985) found the Wilson regression equation to be the most useful multivariate approach for estimation of WAIS FSIQ. Klesges and Troster (1987) noted that only weak correlations have been found between predicted and obtained IQ scores using the Wilson equation. Promising findings have been reported for the Intellectual Correlates Scale, a scale of items reflecting interests, attitudes, personal values, and personality characteristics correlated with WAIS-R IQs (Schlottmann & Johnsen, 1991). The scale was a better predictor of FSIQ and PIQ but a worse predictor of VIQ than the Barona equations.

Karzmark et al. (1984) developed a regression equation to predict premorbid Halstead–Reitan Average Impairment Ratings. Cross-validation resulted in an impressive multiple squared correlation of 0.59. Klesges and Troster (1987) computed the correlation between the difference of actual vs. predicted Average Impairment Rating and the presence vs. absence of brain damage. The correlation was modest but significant. They concluded that no premorbid formula should be the sole or primary determinant of cerebral dysfunction. They suggest that using the Barona and Karzmark equations together might yield improved results. "Premorbid estimates based on multiple assessments tapping various abilities should provide increased sensitivity, reliability, and validity" (Klesges & Troster, 1987, p. 9).

COMPETENCE COMPARISON STANDARDS

Deficits may be determined by comparison to the level of performance required on a task to enable one to perform an activity. Competencies may include the cognitive ability to live alone safely, the ability to manage one's finances, and driving fitness. Research on the relationship of test results to everyday functioning and competencies is in its infancy. A summary of some of these relationships may be found in Chapters 28–32.

REFERENCES

Barona, A., & Chastain, R. L. (1986). An improved estimate of premorbid IQ for blacks and whites on the WAIS-R. *International Journal of Clinical Neuropsychology, 8,* 169–173.

Barona, A., Reynolds, C. R., & Chastain, R. (1984). A demographically based index of premorbid intelligence for the WAIS-R. *Journal of Consulting and Clinical Psychology, 52,* 885–887.

Benton, A. L., Hamsher, K., Varney, N. R., & Spreen, O. (1983). *Contributions to neuropsychological assessment: A clinical manual.* New York: Oxford University Press.

Blair, J. R., & Spreen, O. (1989). Predicting premorbid IQ: A revision of the National Adult Reading Test. *Clinical Neuropsychologist, 3,* 129–136.

Grober, E., & Sliwinski, M. (1991). Development and validation of a model for estimating premorbid verbal intelligence in the elderly. *Journal of Clinical and Experimental Neuropsychology, 13,* 933–949.

Heaton, R. K., Grant, I., & Matthews, C. G. (1991). *Comprehensive norms for an expanded Halstead-Reitan Battery: Demographic corrections, research findings, and clinical applications.* Odessa, FL: Psychological Assessment Resources.

Karzmark, P., Heaton, R. K., Grant, I., & Matthews, C. G. (1984). Use of demographic variables to predict overall level of performance on the Halstead–Reitan Battery. *Journal of Consulting and Clinical Psychology, 52,* 663–665.

Karzmark, P., Heaton, R. K., Grant, I., & Matthews, C. G. (1985). Use of demographic variables to predict Full Scale IQ: A replication and extension. *Journal of Clinical and Experimental Neuropsychology, 7,* 412–420.

Klesges, R. C., & Troster, A. I. (1987). A review of premorbid indices of intellectual and neuropsychological functioning: What have we learned in the past five years? *International Journal of Clinical Neuropsychology, 9,* 1–10.

Klesges, R. C., Wilkening, G. N., & Golden, C. J. (1981). Premorbid indices of intelligence: A review. *Clinical Neuropsychology, 3,* 32–39.

Lezak, M. (1983). *Neuropsychological assessment* (2nd ed.). New York: Oxford University Press.

Matarazzo, J. D. (1990). Psychological assessment versus psychological testing: Validation from Binet to the school, clinic, and courtroom. *American Psychologist, 45,* 999–1016.

Matarazzo, J. D., & Herman, D. O. (1984). Base-rate data for the WAIS-R: Test–retest stability and VIQ–PIQ differences. *Journal of Clinical Neuropsychology, 6,* 351–366.

Matarazzo, J. D., & Herman, D. O. (1985). Clinical uses of the WAIS-R: Base rates of differences between VIQ and PIQ in the WAIS-R standardization sample. In B. B. Wolman (Ed.), *Handbook of intelligence: Theories, measurements, and applications* (pp. 899–932). New York: Wiley.

Mortensen, E. L., Gade, A., & Reinisch, J. M. (1991). A critical note on Lezak's "Best Performance Method" in clinical neuropsychology. *Journal of Clinical and Experimental Psychology, 13,* 361–371.

Nelson, H. E. (1982). *National Adult Reading Test (NART): Test Manual.* Windsor, UK: NFER Nelson.

Nelson, H. E., & O'Connell, A. (1978). Dementia: The estimation of pre-morbid intelligence levels using the new adult reading test. *Cortex, 14,* 234–244.

Russell, E. W. (1980). Tactile sensation, an all-or-none effect of cerebral damage. *Journal of Clinical Psychology, 36,* 858–864.

Schlottmann, R. S., & Johnsen, D. E. (1991). The Intellectual Correlates Scale and the prediction of premorbid intelligence in brain-damaged adults. *Archives of Clinical Neuropsychology, 6,* 363–374.

Spreen, O., & Strauss, E. (1991). *A compendium of neuropsychological tests: Administration, norms, and commentary.* New York: Oxford University Press.

Vogt, A. T., & Heaton, R. K. (1977). Comparison of Wechsler Adult Intelligence Scale indices of cerebral dysfunction. *Perceptual and Motor Skills, 45,* 607–615.

Wechsler, D. (1958). *The measurement and appraisal of adult intelligence* (4th ed.). Baltimore: Williams & Wilkins.

Wiens, A. N., Byran, J. E., & Crossen, J. R. (1993). Estimating WAIS-R FSIQ from the National Adult Reading Test—Revised in normal subjects. *The Clinical Neuropsychologist, 7,* 70–84.

Wilson, R. S., Rosenbaum, G., Brown, G., Rourke, D., Whitman, D., & Grisell, J. (1978). An index of premorbid intelligence. *Journal of Consulting and Clinical Psychology, 46,* 1554–1555.

Self-Care and Independent Living

The ability of the individual to perform activities of daily living (ADLs) and to live independently without supervision may be at issue in a neuropsychological evaluation. On the basis of interviews with patient, family, and staff, review of available records, behavioral observations, and test data, the neuropsychologist may need to assess the patient's ability to care for his or her needs without assistance.

A judgment about the patient's ability to function independently must often be made when a patient who has had an illness that has affected cognitive functioning is being discharged from the hospital. For inpatients in the process of being discharged, there is usually highly relevant information available from nurses, physical therapists, occupational therapists, speech therapists, and physicians about safety awareness, judgment, and the patient's ability to perform ADLs. In such cases, the decision about the level of assistance and supervision needed on discharge is usually a team decision. If support is available from responsible family or friends, it is prudent to provide the maximal support possibly required when the patient is first discharged and to remove this support gradually as the patient exhibits increasingly capable and responsible behavior. If support is not available, discharge may be delayed until the patient is capable of living independently or until a suitable placement is found. Determinations of the ability of outpatients to live independently may be more difficult due to a lack of direct behavioral observation data and data from other health care and rehabilitation professionals.

Activities of daily living may include the following: dressing, eating, cleaning, shopping, cooking, taking public transportation, paying bills, maintaining a residence, grooming, hygiene, using telephones, and using a post office (J. M. Williams, 1988; Social Security Administration, 1986). A distinction is sometimes made between more basic ADLs such as dressing and eating and more complex ADLs such as using a post office. A distinction may also be made between the patient's ability to perform various ADLs and the patient's ability to know his or her own limitations and to utilize available resources appropriately. A patient may be extremely physically impaired, yet be able to use those resources available intelligently and safely, and attain maximum independence within his or her limitations.

Neuropsychological test scores may be of assistance in making judgments about self-care abilities. They have been demonstrated to be related to current self-care abilities in stroke patients and are of some value in predicting improvement in self-care and ambulation (Heaton & Pendleton, 1981). Lorenze and Cancro (1962) found that the sum of BD-WAIS-R and OA-WAIS-R correlated highly with independent dressing and independent grooming in stroke patients. N. Williams (1967) has reported significant correlations between dressing and copying. Anderson *et al.* (1974) found that the WMS, PIQ, and PMT had some predictive validity for improvement in self-care in stroke patients. Lehmann *et al.* (1975) found a statistically significant correlation in stroke patients between a sum of scores of WAIS DSym, BD, and PC and a functional measure of self-care, ambulation, and mobility.

Klonoff *et al.* (1970) found that ambulatory chronic schizophrenic patients did better than hospitalized chronic schizophrenic patients on all measures of the HRNB except the FTT (dominant hand) and TMTB. Winograd (1984) compared ratings on the Self-Care Scale, a scale that assesses dressing, eating, and ambulation, with the Short Portable Mental Status Questionnaire (SPMSQ), a 10-item test of orientation, recent memory, long-term memory, and serial calculation, and with the Mental Competence Scale, a structured interview. Winograd (1984) found a correlation of $r = 0.37$ ($p < 0.05$) between the Self-Care Scale and the SPMSQ and a correlation between the Self-Care Scale and the Mental Competence Scale of $r = 0.58$ ($p < 0.0001$). She noted that a substantial number of patients who had poor scores on the SPMSQ were nevertheless able to perform ADLs in the nursing home setting. This observation and the lesser correlation of the SPMSQ with the Self-Care Scale are not surprising, since the SPMSQ assesses cognition and memory, while the Self-Care Scale assesses overlearned motor habits.

Tests of visual–perceptual, motor, and memory skills have often been found to be significantly correlated with everyday functioning (Acker, 1990). The VIQ, PIQ, TMTA&B, WMS, and Motor Free Visual Perception Test, administered at 6–12 months after head injury, were found to be significantly correlated with the Disability Rating Scale (which rates Arousability, Awareness, Responsibility, Cognitive Ability for Self-Care Activities, Dependence on Others, and Psychosocial Adaptability) at 1 year and Social Status Outcome at 2 years after injury (Acker, 1986). No correlation was found with Community Skills. In a long-term follow-up study of head injury, Acker (1990) reported highly significant correlations ($p < 0.001$) between the BVMGT, Motor Free Visual Perception Test, Quick Test, RPM, WMS Memory Quotient, and Social Status Outcome.

Pollack *et al.* (1968) reported that higher PIQ and VIQ were related to higher levels of independence and social and occupational function on follow-up in adult schizophrenics. Lezak (1983) was able to distinguish dependent from independent brain-damaged patients using the TTT.

Klonoff *et al.* (1986) found quality of life as reported by head-injury patients on the Sickness Impact Profile to correlate with tests of memory and constructional ability. For patients with chronic obstructive pulmonary disease, McSweeny *et al.* (1985) found that Average Impairment Rating correlated modestly with measures of everyday functioning (Life Quality Indices). They found the quality of life, as reported on the Sickness Impact Profile, to be predicted by GS, GP Time, and TMTB.

Although group studies demonstrating correlations and predictive validity for neuropsychological tests may provide useful guidelines for making inferences in individual cases, there are many factors specific to each individual case that must be taken into account (Rappaport *et al.,* 1991). ADLs specific to a patient may need to be analyzed in terms of clusters of skills needed for the task (Tupper & Cicerone, 1990). These skills, in turn, may be related to the patient's performance on neuropsychological tests. Chelune and Moehle (1986) have developed a table relating everyday activities to skills and skills to tests.

In addition to cognitive and personality testing, interviews supplemented by questionnaires and rating scales are essential to the evaluation and prediction of everyday functioning. Acker (1990) has provided an extensive list of questionnaires and rating scales for the assessment of everyday functioning. Gilewski and Zelinski (1986) may be consulted for a listing of everyday memory questionnaires. The environment and the environmental demands on the patient must also be evaluated when making a thorough assessment of everyday functioning (Naugle & Chelune, 1990).

An alternative approach to the assessment of self-care skills and independence is the use of tests specifically designed to assess everyday functioning. The Cognitive Competency Test includes Practical Reading Skills, Management of Finances, Route Learning, Spatial Orientation, Card Arrangement, Picture Interpretation, and Memory (Wang & Ennis, 1986). The Rivermeade Behavioral Memory Test (Wilson *et al.*, 1985) was developed to provide an assessment of memory relevant to everyday functioning.

REFERENCES

Acker, M. B. (1986). Relationships between test scores and everyday life functioning. In B. Uzzell & Y. Gross (Eds.), *Clinical neuropsychology of intervention* (pp. 85–117). Boston: Martins Nijhoff.

Acker, M. B. (1990). A review of the ecological validity of neuropsychological tests. In D. E. Tupper & K. D. Cicerone (Eds.), *The neuropsychology of everyday life: Assessment and competencies* (pp. 19–55). Boston: Kluwer Academic Publishers.

Anderson, T. P., Bourestom, N., Greenberg, F. R., & Hildyard, V. G. (1974). Predictive factors in stroke rehabilitation. *Archives of Physical Medicine and Rehabilitation, 55,* 545–553.

Chelune, G. J., & Moehle, K. A. (1986). Neuropsychological assessment and everyday functioning. In D. Wedding, A. M. Horton, Jr., & J. Webster (Eds.), *The neuropsychology handbook: Behavioral and clinical perspective* (pp. 489–525). New York: Springer.

Gilewski, M. J., & Zelinski, E. M. (1986). Questionnaire assessment of memory complaints. In L. W. Poon (Ed.), *Handbook for clinical memory assessment of older adults* (pp. 93–107). Washington, DC: American Psychological Association.

Heaton, R. K., & Pendleton, M. G. (1981). Use of neuropsychological tests to predict adult patients' everyday functioning. *Journal of Consulting and Clinical Psychology, 49,* 807–821.

Klonoff, H., Fibiger, C. H., & Hutton, G. H. (1970). Neuropsychological patterns in chronic schizophrenia. *Journal of Nervous and Mental Disease, 150,* 291–300.

Klonoff, P. S., Costa, L. D., & Snow, W. G. (1986). Predictors and indicators of quality of life in patients with closed-head injury. *Journal of Clinical and Experimental Psychology, 8,* 469–485.

Lehmann, J. F., De Lateur, B. J., Fowler, R. S., Warren, C. G., Arnhold, R., Schertzer, G., Hurka, R., Whitmore, J. J., Masock, A. J., & Chambers, K. H. (1975). Stroke rehabilitation: Outcome and prediction. *Archives of Physical Medicine and Rehabilitation, 56,* 383–389.

Lezak, M. D. (1983). *Neuropsychological assessment* (2nd ed.). New York: Oxford University Press.

Lorenze, E. J., & Cancro, R. (1962). Dysfunction in visual perception with hemiplegia: Its relation to activities of daily living. *Archives of Physical Medicine and Rehabilitation, 43,* 514–517.

McSweeney, A. J., Grant, I., Heaton, R. K., Prigatano, G. P., & Adams, K. M. (1985). Relationship of neuropsychological status to everyday functioning in healthy and chronically ill persons. *Journal of Clinical and Experimental Neuropsychology, 7,* 281–291.

Naugle, R. I., & Chelune, G. J. (1990). Integrating neuropsychological and "real-life" data: A neuropsychological model for assessing everyday functioning. In D. E. Tupper & K. D. Cicerone (Eds.), *The neuropsychology of everyday life: Assessment and competencies* (pp. 57–73). Boston: Kluwer Academic Publishers.

Pollack, M., Levenstein, D. D. S. W., & Klein, D. F. (1968). A three-year posthospital follow up of adolescent and adult schizophrenics. *American Journal of Orthopsychiatry, 38,* 94–110.

Rappaport, A., Allworth, E., & Thomas, K. (1991). The validity of neuropsychological tests in the prediction of functional activities. In W. R. Levick, B. G. Frost, M. Watson, & H. P. Pfister (Eds.), *Brain impairment: Advances in applied research.* Newcastle, Australia: Australian Society for the Study of Brain Impairment.

Social Security Administration (1986). *Disability evaluation under Social Security* (SSA Publication No. 05-10089). Washington, DC: U.S. Department of Health and Human Services.

Tupper, D. E., & Cicerone, K. D. (1990). Introduction to the neuropsychology of everyday life. In D. E. Tupper & K. D. Cicerone (Eds.), *The neuropsychology of everyday life: Assessment and competencies* (pp. 3–18). Boston: Kluwer Academic Publishers.

Wang, P. L., & Ennis, K. E. (1986). Competency assessment in clinical populations: An introduction to the Cognitive Competency Test. In B. Uzzell & Y. Gross (Eds.), *Clinical neuropsychology of intervention* (pp. 119–133). Boston: Martins Nijhoff.

Williams, J. M. (1988). Everyday cognition and the ecological validity of intellectual and neuropsychological tests. In J. M. Williams & C. J. Long (Eds.), *Cognitive approaches to neuropsychology* (pp. 123–141). New York: Plenum Press.

Williams, N. (1967). Correlation between copying ability and dressing activities in hemiplegia. *American Journal of Physical Medicine, 46,* 4.

Wilson, B., Cockburn, J., & Baddeley, A. (1985). *The Rivermeade Behavioural Memory Test.* Reading, England: Thames Valley Test Co.

Winograd, C. H. (1984). Mental status tests and the capacity for self-care. *Journal of the American Geriatrics Society, 32,* 49–55.

Driving

The neuropsychologist may be expected to arrive at conclusions about driving fitness based on results of the neuropsychological evaluation. Legal precedents suggest that there may be a duty to inform the patient, the patient's family, and in some cases even relevant authorities if it is determined that the patient may not be capable of driving safely (Bracy *et al.*, 1990). If the patient refuses to consent to the release of such information to authorities, a conflict between the ethical values of "confidentiality" and "duty to warn" may arise. The neuropsychologist should be familiar with the law governing this issue in his or her locality (Hopewell & van Zomeren, 1990).

Studies linking neuropsychological test results to driving fitness are limited in number and scope. For healthy individuals, reaction time is not related to driver quality. "The efficient driver is not the one who reacts quickly, but the one who avoids situations in which only his fast reaction can save him from disaster" (van Zomeren *et al.*, 1987, p. 701). However, reaction time has been found to correlate moderately high with driving a slalom course (Stokx & Gaillard, 1986). IQ is not related to driving skills in healthy individuals. However, van Zomeren *et al.* (1987) have suggested that "an IQ below 80 may have consequences for insight on the strategic and tactical levels of driving" (p. 702). One study has suggested that degree of aphasia has no predictive value for driving fitness (Golper *et al.*, 1980). Visual perceptual deficits resulting from a right CVA may result in impaired driving ability (Bardach, 1971). Lack of self-criticism, poor judgment, and impulsivity may have negative implications for safe driving (van Zomeren *et al.*, 1987). Simulator scores tend to correlate poorly with fitness for driving in traffic (van Zomeren *et al.*, 1987).

Research on the relationship of neuropsychological test results and driving fitness is sparse and has suggested the possibility of only very limited inferences. Therefore, if the issue of driving fitness is to be addressed by a neuropsychological evaluation, special tests may need to be included (Bracy *et al.*, 1990). The Cognitive Behavioral Driver's Inventory was created for this purpose. Subtests of this instrument include: (1) brake reaction time, (2) visual acuity, (3) peripheral vision, (4) PC-WAIS-R, (5) DSym-WAIS-R, (6) TMTA&B, and (7) several computerized tests assessing attention, reaction time, sustained attention, and the ability to shift attention. This instrument has been demonstrated to predict the likelihood of passing a road test. It is available from Psychological Software Services, 6555 Carrollton Ave., Indianapolis, IN 46220.

Hopewell (1988) has suggested that evaluation of driving fitness should focus on executive functions. Driving can be conceptualized as involving operational, tactical, and strategic levels. The *operational* level involves controlling the vehicle, attending to and scanning the relevant driving environment, steering, perceiving, and taking evasive action. The *tactical* level includes decisions made while driving in traffic such as reducing one's speed when entering a residential area or deciding when to pass another vehicle. At the *strategic* level, driving decisions are usually made without time pressure prior to the excursion and may involve the assessment and acceptance of risk such as choice of route and evaluation of risks of traffic. This model emphasizes the importance of executive decision-making in driving. Decisions made at higher levels can decrease demands on lower levels (Hopewell, 1988).

Hopewell (1988) has proposed an outline for driving assessment and remediation: (1) notification of the Medical Board of injury status (varies by state); (2) adaptive driving referral; (3) vision testing; (4) hearing screening; (5) reaction-time assessment; (6) range-of-motion assessment, manual muscle test, and functional strength; (7) neuropsychological assessment; (8) psychiatric, neurological, or substance abuse referral; (9) simulator or small-vehicle evaluation; (10) full-scale vehicle evaluation; (11) driver training; (12) family counseling; (13) Medical Board recontact; (14) Department of Public Safety or Motor Vehicles road test; and (15) periodic retest by neuropsychologist or rehabilitation team. Hopewell emphasizes that recommendations about driving should be team decisions. Successful passage of assessment or training should lead to testing by state authorities.

Neuropsychologists who refer patients for driving training should be aware of the success rate of such programs. Studies have suggested that physical handicaps per se are not related to an increased accident or violation rate (van Zomeren *et al.*, 1987). Rehabilitation center driving courses have reported high return-to-driving rates with patients having impairments other than brain damage (90% in spinal-cord-injured patients). A rate of only 50% was found in brain-injured patients (Shore *et al.*, 1980).

Given the formative nature of assessment and prediction of driving fitness, great care should be made in drawing conclusions from neuropsychological assessments, even with ancillary tests. Costs vs. benefits as well as complex ethical and legal duties must be factored into any recommendations.

REFERENCES

Bardach, J. L. (1971). Psychological factors in the handicapped drivers. *Archives of Physical Medicine and Rehabilitation, 52*, 328–332.

Bracy, O. L., Engum, E. S., & Lambert, E. W. (1990). *Manual for the Cognitive Behavioral Driver's Inventory.* Indianapolis: Psychological Software Services.

Golper, L. A. C., Rau, M. T., & Marshall, R. C. (1980). Aphasic adults and their decisions on driving: Evaluation. *Archives of Physical Medicine and Rehabilitation, 61*, 34–40.

Hopewell, C. A. (1988). *Head injury rehabilitation: Adaptive driving after TBI.* Houston: HDI Publishers.

Hopewell, C. A., & van Zomeren, A. H. (1990). Neuropsychological aspects of motor vehicle operation. In D. E. Tupper & K. D. Cicerone (Eds.), *The neuropsychology of everyday life: Assessment and competencies* (pp. 307–334). Boston: Kluwer Academic Publishers.

Shore, D., Gurgold, G., & Robbins, S. (1980). Handicapped driving: Overview of assessment and training. *Archives of Physical Medicine and Rehabilitation, 65*, 163–167.

Stokx, L. C., & Gaillard, A. W. K. (1986). Task and driving performance of patients with a severe concussion of the brain. *Journal of Clinical and Experimental Psychology, 8*, 421–436.

Van Zomeren, A. H., Brouwer, W. H., & Minderhoud, J. M. (1987). Acquired brain damage and driving: A review. *Archives of Physical Medicine and Rehabilitation, 68*, 697–705.

30

Academic and Vocational Functioning

ACADEMIC FUNCTIONING

For patients who wish to return to school or who would like to learn a new occupation because of an inability to return to a previous occupation due to injury, the likelihood of success in an educational setting is a crucial issue. The kind of course work, the instructional method and social setting of the educational institution, and the cognitive and emotional attributes of the patient must be taken into account in addressing this issue.

IQ provides some information about a patient's likelihood of academic success. Matarazzo (1972) has reported a correlation of approximately 0.50 between intelligence and academic success. Verbal IQ is a good predictor of academic success (Chelune & Moehle, 1986). Of course, more direct measures of academic achievement are provided by tests such as the WRAT-R. For example, if the patient's performance level on the WRAT-R is significantly below that of the course of study he or she intends to undertake, remedial courses or a reevaluation of goals would be recommended. Distractibility and impaired attention may suggest that tutoring in a quiet environment is more likely to result in successful learning than a classroom environment. Severe deficits in memory or learning may prohibit return to or entry into a standard classroom setting.

History, interview of the patient and significant others, behavioral observation, and personality testing are important for determining the patient's ability to respond appropriately to the social setting of an educational institution. A patient may have intact academic skills but may exhibit disinhibited, socially inappropriate behavior. Such behavior, unless remediated, might disrupt the reintegration of the patient into a standard educational environment.

VOCATIONAL FUNCTIONING

The ability of the patient to return to work is often at issue in a neuropsychological evaluation. Neuropsychological tests, especially in combination with personality assessment, appear to have some predictive validity for return to work. Reviews may be found in Heaton and Pendelton (1981) and in Chelune and Moehle (1986). For patients with non-rapidly progressing neurological disorders, Newnan *et al.* (1978) found a multiple correlation of 0.53 between chronic unemployment and its 10 most sensitive predictor variables. Average Impairment Rating was the strongest predictor, followed by Perceptual Errors, HCT, TPT-Memory, and SSPT. An AIR cutoff of 1.61 classified 78% of the patients correctly as employed or unemployed. Wage income was largely a function of performance on the Story Memory Test (Heaton *et al.,* 1991) and TPT-Time. Average wage was best predicted by Story Memory Test, WAIS PIQ, MMPI L Scale, HCT, TPT-Time, AIR, and WAIS FSIQ. Total hours worked was best predicted by the MMPI 3, 8, 4, 7, 1, 2, and 6 Scales and Spatial Relations Errors.

Heaton *et al.* (1978) found significant differences on nearly all test measures between full-time employed and unemployed patients. By the standards of Russell *et al.* (1970), unemployed group means were in the mildly impaired range for the AIR and all HRNB scores except for moderate impairment on TMTB and no impairment on TPT-Memory. More personality disturbance was noted for the unemployed group MMPI F Scale and all clinical scales. T-scores of the unemployed group were above 70 on the MMPI 8 and 2 Scales. A discriminant function based on an extended HRNB and MMPI was able to classify 83.7% of the patients correctly. Bayless *et al.* (1989) found that TTT performance as measured by a revised version of Lezak's Complexity score is related to employment after head injury. The performance of nearly half of 25 patients who did not return to work was impaired, while the performance of only one of 25 patients who did return to work was impaired.

Although the general correlations and predictive relationships reported in studies such as those cited above provide a framework within which judgments may be made about the appropriateness of return to work, each case is unique. The patient's pattern of strengths and weaknesses and the ability requirements of the work for which return is being considered are diverse. Each case must therefore be judged according to its unique attributes.

If the neuropsychologist is treating the patient as well as doing an evaluation for the patient, it may be appropriate for him or her to actively assist the patient's efforts to return to work. Phone conversations or meetings with the employer (with the patient's consent, of course) to provide information about the patient's special needs and to assist the employer in understanding the patient's residual problems may be appropriate in some cases. Ongoing therapy with the patient and follow-up discussions with the employer can assist the patient and employment setting in mutually adjusting to one another.

Neuropsychological evaluations are often requested by vocational rehabilitation counselors to aid in determining the kind of employment appropriate for the patient and to provide recommendations about how impaired skills might be remediated. Although vocational rehabilitation counselors may request neuropsychological evaluations, they may not understand many of the issues involved in the rehabilitation of neurologically impaired patients or neuropsychological concepts (Kay & Silver, 1988). Reports should therefore be accessible to the lay person. The counselor is likely to benefit from information about pitfalls that may surface during the process of vocational rehabilitation. Although the counselor will usually have information about the medical and physical status of the client, he or she may benefit from information about sensory and motor functioning relevant to job performance. The evaluation should provide an accounting of the client's cognitive strengths and weaknesses and whether these attributes would make the client competitive in the workplace. Qualitative observations about the way in which items or tests are failed may be particularly helpful to the counselor in designing a rehabilitation program (Kay & Silver, 1988). In addition to the evaluation of cognitive functioning, the counselor needs to know about the client's interpersonal skills, reaction to stress or failure, level of confidence, emotional stability, social support network, and level of self-insight.

REFERENCES

Bayless, J. D., Varney, N. R., & Roberts, R. J. (1989). Tinker Toy Test performance and vocational outcome in patients with closed head injuries. *Journal of Clinical and Experimental Neuropsychology, 11,* 913–917.

Chelune, G. J., & Moehle, K. A. (1986). Neuropsychological assessment and everyday functioning. In D. Wedding, A. M. Horton, Jr., & J. Webster (Eds.), *The neuropsychology handbook: Behavioral and clinical perspective* (pp. 489–525). New York: Springer.

Heaton, R. K., & Pendleton, M. G. (1981). Use of neuropsychological tests to predict adult patients' everyday functioning. *Journal of Consulting and Clinical Psychology, 49,* 807–821.

Heaton, R. K., Chelune, G. J., & Lehman, R. A. W. (1978). Using neuropsychological and personality tests to assess the likelihood of patient employment. *Journal of Nervous and Mental Disease, 166,* 408–416.

Heaton, R. K., Grant, I., & Matthews, C. G. (1991). *Comprehensive norms for an extended Halstead–Reitan Battery: Demographic corrections, research findings, and clinical applications.* Odessa, FL: Psychological Assessment Resources.

Kay, T., & Silver, S. M. (1988). The contribution of the neuropsychological evaluation to the vocational rehabilitation of the head-injured adult. *Journal of Head Trauma Rehabilitation, 3,* 65–76.

Matarazzo, J. D. (1972). *Wechsler's measurement and appraisal of adult intelligence* (5th ed.). Baltimore: Williams & Wilkins.

Newnan, O. S., Heaton, R. K., & Lehman, R. A. (1978). Neuropsychological and MMPI correlates of patients' future employment characteristics. *Perceptual and Motor Skills, 46,* 635–642.

Russell, E. W., Neuringer, C., and Goldstein, G. (1970). *Assessment of brain damage: A neuropsychological key approach.* New York: Wiley.

Civil Competency Evaluations

Civil competency is a legal concept and can be determined only by a judge (Appelbaum & Gutheil, 1991). Nevertheless, information provided by mental health professionals is often crucial to a judge's decision. Neuropsychologists are often requested in such circumstances to determine whether individuals have the capacity to make decisions about and manage their own affairs. An extended mental status examination or neuropsychological evaluation can provide information essential to the decision-making process. The decision is serious because a person found incompetent can be deprived of rights. A surrogate decision-maker such as a guardian or conservator may be appointed. "Guardians and conservators are 'fiduciaries' who are legally bound to act only in the best interests of the person" (Stromberg *et al.*, 1988, p. 607). On the other hand, an inappropriate determination of competency for a truly incompetent individual could allow that person to suffer financial hardship or even serious physical injury.

Competence can be conceptualized as a threshold requirement for persons to retain the power to make decisions for themselves. One may distinguish between general and specific competence: "General competence is that state, described in many of the statutes governing guardianship procedures, determined by the ability to handle all one's affairs in an adequate manner. Specific competence is defined only in relation to a particular act: whether one is competent to write a will, make a contract, testify in court, or stand trial for murder" (Appelbaum & Gutheil, 1991, p. 219).

Practitioners performing evaluations for competency hearings will usually find that the law provides little guidance or specific criteria. There is a great deal of variability in the statutes from state to state (Grisso, 1986). Appelbaum and Gutheil (1991) have suggested some standards, but each practitioner should consult the relevant laws in his or her locale. It should be noted that the mere presence of mental illness or disability does not constitute incompetence. Competence is not a fixed attribute of an individual that is invariant across environments. For example, the standard of competence for a person who possesses a large and financially complex estate is likely to be different from that of one whose sole support is his or her disability check that is exchanged for room and board in a supported living situation. Competence should be assessed functionally within the context of the individual's environment. This is accomplished by assessing the individual's cognitive capacity through extended mental status or neuropsychological testing, records review, and interviews with the individual, significant others, or other relevant knowledgeable individuals. The evaluation should assess and take into account both the demands and the supports inherent in the individual's environment. It should assess the individual's awareness of his or her living situation, significant supportive relationships, sources of financial support, physical or intellectual limitations, physical safety issues, and threats to financial security. The individual's understanding of these considerations should be compared with information available in records and information provided by significant others and professionals. The use of hypothetical examples is essential for assessing the individual's ability to make appropriate decisions and to understand the consequences of these decisions. Hypothetical business transactions or emergency situations are posed to the individual, who then describes the decision or course of action he or she would take. The individual's ability to explore alternative decisions and to understand the consequences of those decisions should be assessed.

Deficits noted on neuropsychological testing should be related to functional deficits relevant to the patient's living situation. If, for example, an impairment is found in calculational ability, it should be determined whether this impairment affects the individual's ability to function financially or whether there are any readily available supports that might supplement the individual's calculational ability. Hypothetically posed problem situations that depend on the area of cognitive functioning exhibiting a deficiency may be used to assess the relevance of cognitive deficits to real-life functioning.

The neuropsychologist should have a basic understanding of the legal concepts and laws relevant to the competency hearing for which the evaluation is being prepared. These considerations may include concepts such as "guardianship," "durable power of attorney," and "conservatorship." A more detailed discussion of these issues is beyond the scope of this book. The neuropsychologist should also be aware of the seriousness of a competency hearing and the effect that the legal finding of incompetence may have on the individual and family. Such a finding can lead to a tendency of the family to "infantilize" the individual and to encourage dependence rather than autonomy. The individual may feel anger and resentment directed at the family and involved professionals. He or she may suffer a significant loss of self-esteem (Appelbaum & Gutheil, 1991).

REFERENCES

Appelbaum, P. S., & Gutheil, T. G. (1991). *Clinical handbook of psychiatry and the law.* Baltimore: Williams & Wilkins.

Grisso, T. (1986). *Evaluating competencies: Forensic assessments and instruments.* New York: Plenum Press.

Stromberg, C. D., Haggarty, D. J., Leibenluft, R. F., McMillian, M. H., Mishkin, B., Rubin, B. L., & Trilling, H. R. (1988). *The psychologist's legal handbook.* Washington, DC: Council for the National Register of Health Service Providers in Psychology.

Disability Evaluations

Neuropsychologists are often requested to perform disability evaluations for Social Security (Puente, 1984, 1987) or Workers' Compensation. Generally, these evaluations require the practitioner to establish a diagnosis, to depict the patient's functional impairments, to relate the functional impairments to the diagnosis, and to determine the patient's capacity to work. For Workers' Compensation evaluations, the practitioner may be additionally required to determine the degree to which the diagnosis and impairments were caused by work-related factors. It should be noted that the brief descriptions that follow do not provide sufficient information from which one could proceed with these evaluations. For Social Security disability evaluations, one should consult publications of the Social Security Administration (SSA) such as *Disability Evaluation Under Social Security* (Social Security Administration, 1986) and one's local Social Security Disability Determination Branch. Each jurisdiction has its own Workers' Compensation system. Local Workers' Compensation agencies and representatives should be contacted regarding eligibility requirements, benefit levels, claims procedures, and relevant rules, regulations, and laws.

SOCIAL SECURITY DISABILITY

The individual applies for benefits at the local SSA office. Social Security Disability (SSD) is potentially available for individuals who made sufficient FICA contributions to Social Security while working. Supplemental Security Income (SSI) may be available for individuals in financial need who do not qualify for SSD due to insufficient work-related contributions (Kodimer, 1988). Hulley (1991) has described the application process from the patient's point of view.

The determination of disability by the SSA involves the determination of "the inability to engage in *any* substantial gainful activity by reason of any medically determinable physical or mental impairment which can be expected to result in death or has lasted or can be expected to last for a continuous period of not less than 12 months" (Social Security Administration, 1986, p. 1). Consultants "do not define disability but provide documentation as to a patient's medical status" (Kodimer, 1988, p. 79). The SSA utilizes the data in making decisions about disability awards.

Broad categories of mental disorders recognized by the SSA are (1) organic mental disorders; (2) schizophrenic, paranoid and other psychotic disorders; (3) affective disorders; (4) mental retardation and autism; (5) anxiety-related disorders; (6) somatoform disorders; (7) personality disorders; and (8) substance addiction disorders. Specific criteria for these disorders may be found in SSA publications. A comprehensive review, updated with pocket parts, of medical issues in Social Security disability determination has been authored by Morton (1983).

It is important for the consultant to be specific in communicating findings. Inferences and reasoning should be communicated clearly and findings translated into SSA criteria. Psychological testing may be limited due to direct requests for specific tests or time and funding limitations. According to Kodimer (1988, p. 79), "typically a Wechsler Adult Intelligence Scale—Revised (WAIS-R), possibly the Wechsler Memory Scale, and a Bender-Gestalt will be ordered to accompany the interview." Although SSA does refer to the HRNB and the LNNB in its publications, according to Kodimer (1988, p. 79), "never will adequate funds be provided for any form of even moderately comprehensive neuropsychological assessment and/or report." Test results should be reported in a readily understandable fashion. Tests, test results, and their consequences should be explained in detail. It is especially important to do so if the neuropsychologist uses tests that may be unfamiliar to SSA personnel (Kodimer, 1988).

Test results should be interpreted in terms of degree of impairment and consequences for everyday functioning, especially functioning in a work environment (Krajeski & Lipsett, 1987). Functional areas include (1) activities of daily living (ADLs); (2) social functioning; (3) concentration, persistence, and pace; and (4) deterioration or decompensation in work or worklike settings (Social Security Administration, 1986). ADLs include such activities as cleaning, shopping, taking public transportation, paying bills, and maintaining a residence. Social functioning involves the ability to get along with other individuals. Concentration, persistence, and pace comprise the ability to sustain focused attention sufficiently long to permit the timely completion of tasks commonly found in work settings. "Deterioration or decompensation in work or work-like settings refers to repeated failure to adapt to stressful circumstances which cause the individual either to withdraw from that situation or to experience exacerbation of signs and symptoms" (Social Security Administration, 1986, p. 65). The consultant must address all these functional areas in his or her report.

WORKERS' COMPENSATION

If part of a worker's claim alleges emotional stress or the presence of a mental disorder, the claimant may be referred to a mental health professional for evaluation. The referral may come from the individual's attorney or from an insurance carrier or defense attorney. A significant percentage of claims are litigated (Brodsky, 1987). The consultant is usually asked to address a number of issues in the evaluation. These issues are usually specified in the referral letter and often include: (1) whether the individual has a mental disorder, (2) the duration and pattern of the disorder, (3) the cause of the disorder (e.g., work), (4) the need for treatment and likelihood of recovery, (5) the ability of the individual to return to work, (6) the need for rehabilitation, (7) the individual's preinjury level of functioning, and (8) whether the individual is stable or is likely to improve or deteriorate.

Before the patient is seen, records should be reviewed. When seeing the patient, the examiner should describe his or her professional status. The fact that the examination is being conducted in the context of the workers' compensation claim, that there is no confidentiality, that a report will be sent to the referring source, and that the examiner will provide no treatment and make no direct referrals to other health providers for treatment should be explained to the patient (Brodsky, 1987). The referral source should be identified. The interview may follow the general outline provided in Chapter 12. Emphasis is placed on questions the answers to which may assist the consultant in addressing issues stated in the referral letter. Brodsky (1987) has suggested a detailed set of questions. Neuropsychological testing (including personality assessment) may be diagnostically useful and may assist in clarifying cognitive deficits. Either ruling out or confirming the existence of a personality disorder is important because a personality disorder may be viewed as a preexisting condition (Lasky, 1993). The report should be detailed and the reasoning through which conclusions are reached should be documented.

Familiarity with the *Guides to the Evaluation of Permanent Impairment* (American Medical Association, 1990) is essential. The *Guides* provide precise definitions of terms such as "impairment," "disability," and "employability" and the logical relationships between them. Guidelines are presented for determining whether a patient is stable and ratable and, if the patient is ratable, for calculating the percentage of impairment. Of special interest to clinical neuropsychologists are the sections on the nervous system, mental and behavioral disorders, and pain.

Jarvis and Hamlin (1984) have provided a list of pitfalls to be avoided in compensation evaluations:

1. Since claimants are often involved in litigation, great care should be taken to avoid even minor errors in scoring. These errors can be used by an attorney to discredit the report and testimony of the consultant even though they might not result in any meaningful difference.
2. Since some medications can alter test performance, the neuropsychologist should be aware of all the medications a patient is taking.
3. Malingering should be assessed. This assessment is discussed in Chapter 25.

Further relevant information on neuropsychological evaluation in Workers' Compensation cases may be found in "Workers' Compensation and Clinical Neuropsychological Assessment" (Puente and Gillespie, 1991).

REFERENCES

American Medical Association (1990). *Guides to the evaluation of permanent impairment* (3rd ed. rev.). Chicago: American Medical Association.

Brodsky, C. M. (1987). The psychiatric evaluation in workers' compensation. In A. T. Meyerson & T. Fine (Eds.), *Psychiatric disability: Clinical, legal, and administrative dimensions* (pp. 313–332). Washington, DC: American Psychiatric Press.

Hulley, W. (1991). So you believe you are qualified for Social Security Income? *Journal of Head Injury, 2*(3), 6–7.

Jarvis, P. E., & Hamlin, D. (1984). Avoiding pitfalls in compensation evaluations. *International Journal of Clinical Neuropsychology, 6,* 214–216.

Kodimer, C. (1988). Neuropsychological assessment and Social Security disability: Writing meaningful reports and documentation. *Journal of Head Trauma Rehabilitation, 3,* 77–85.

Krajeski, J., & Lipsett, M. (1987). The psychiatric consultation for Social Security Disability Insurance. In A. T. Meyerson & T. Fine (Eds.), *Psychiatric disability: Clinical, legal, and administrative dimensions* (pp. 287–311). Washington, DC: American Psychiatric Press.

Lasky, H. (1993). *Psychiatric claims in Workers' Compensation and civil litigation,* Volume 1. New York: Wiley.

Morton, D. A., III (1983). *Medical proof of Social Security disability.* St. Paul: West Publishing.

Puente, A. E. (1984). Social Security disability determinations: A neglected area for clinical neuropsychology. *International Journal of Clinical Neuropsychology, 6,* 89.

Puente, A. E. (1987). Social Security disability and clinical neuropsychological assessment. *The Clinical Neuropsychologist, 1,* 353–363.

Puente, A. E., & Gillespie, J. B. (1991). Workers' Compensation and clinical neuropsychological assessment. In J. Dywan, R. D. Kaplan, & F. J. Pirozzolo (Eds.), *Neuropsychology and the law* (pp. 39–63). New York: Springer-Verlag.

Social Security Administration (1986). *Disability evaluation under Social Security* (SSA Publication No. 05-10089). Washington, DC: U.S. Department of Health and Human Services.

V

Psychosocial Therapies

Part V summarizes some of the primary psychological treatments of neuropsychiatric disorders. The descriptions provided are not intended to be at all comprehensive. They are intended to outline to the neuropsychologist some of the psychotherapeutic options that are available and that may be recommended in a neuropsychological evaluation. With appropriate modifications for patients suffering from specific neurological disorders, some of the traditional psychotherapeutic approaches may be adapted for patients with neurobehavioral disorders. A brief mention is made and references provided for these therapies. Bare-bones outlines of some therapeutic techniques specifically relevant to neurobehavioral disorders are provided; these include coma stimulation, behavior modification for behavioral problems associated with neurobehavioral disorders, and cognitive rehabilitation. Applications of the therapies in specific disorders will be found in Part VI.

It should be noted that the therapies cited in this part do not exhaust the psychosocial supports appropriate for many patients. Psychosocial intervention may also include assisting the patient and family in locating financial resources such as Social Security, vocational rehabilitation resources, support groups and agencies, and a variety of other social supports. This intervention is likely to involve networking with numerous community professionals and agencies. Support groups and agencies are described at the end of each chapter in Part VI.

Coma Stimulation

Although consciousness is suppressed in deep coma, sensorial stimulation may affect vegetative functions such as sweating, variations in pupil size, cardiac rhythms, and respiration. Reactions to the presence of family members or empathetic nurses may sometimes be observed (Mazaux *et al.,* 1989). Studies of patients' recollections of posttraumatic coma have reported themes of imprisonment, sensory experiences, and death (Schnaper, 1975; Tosch, 1988). On the basis of these considerations, the following recommendations have been made (Tosch, 1988):

1. Patients in coma may be spoken to, be handled gently, and be oriented.
2. They may be told that they may experience unusual sensations while unconscious. La Puma *et al.* (1990) have reported some of the benefits of talking to comatose patients. They should be spoken to as one would speak to other patients. Doing so may help others to respect the patient.
3. Ominous prognostic and other medical discussions should not be held in the presence of the patient.
4. Patients should be encouraged to discuss recollections of coma when consciousness is regained.
5. If noxious stimuli are used, the least noxious stimulus that elicits behavior should be used.

If there are no medical contraindications (e.g., increased intracranial pressure), a sensory stimulation program may increase input to the reticular activating system and increase arousal to the threshold necessary for responsiveness, increase the likelihood of monitoring for functional responsiveness, and provide environmental richness for patients exhibiting minimal awareness (Whyte & Glenn, 1986; Wilson *et al.,* 1991). A stimulation program may include the following:

1. Environmental distractions should be controlled.
2. A variety of stimuli should be applied in each modality, followed by requests for responses. Due to slowed information processing, ample time must be allowed for the patient to respond. Sessions should be brief.
3. Stimuli having emotional significance, such as tape recordings of family members' voices (Yanko, 1985) or favorite musical selections, are most likely to elicit responses. The family may be an important asset to the treatment team in providing care and meaningful stimulation (Jacobs *et al.,* 1986).
4. Responses may be reinforced by social rewards, preferred music, or other inducements (Boyle & Greer, 1983).

5. Once a measurable response has been identified, efforts can focus on refining the response. Gianutsos (1987) has published a software program designed to assist in this task. Gianutsos (1990) suggests that the goal of training should be for the patient to be able to: (a) respond in less than 1 sec, (b) release the response, (c) inhibit the response, and (d) sustain responding for 20 trials.

6. As the response is mastered, the patient may progress through a number of cognitive "milestones" (Gianutsos, 1990).

REFERENCES

Boyle, M. E., & Greer, R. D. (1983). Operant procedures and the comatose patient. *Journal of Applied Behavioral Analysis, 16*, 3–12.

Gianutsos, R. (1987). *Computer programs for cognitive rehabilitation,* Volume 5, *Software tools for use with the individual emerging from coma into consciousness.* Bayport, NY: Life Science Associates.

Gianutsos, R. (1990). Response system analysis: What the neuropsychologist can contribute to the rehabilitation of individuals emerging from coma. *Neuropsychology Review, 1*, 21–30.

Jacobs, H. E., Muir, C. A., & Cline, J. D. (1986). Family reactions to persistent vegetative state. *Journal of Head Trauma Rehabilitation, 1*, 55–62.

La Puma, J., Schiedermayer, D. L., Gulyas, A. E., & Siegler, M. (1990). Talking to comatose patients. *Neurotrauma Medical Report, 4*(2), 1–3.

Mazaux, J. M., Gagnon, M., & Barat, M. (1989). Management of neuropsychological impairment after severe head injury. In E. Perecman (Ed.), *Integrating theory and practice in clinical neuropsychology* (pp. 337–357). Hillsdale, NJ: Laurence Erlbaum Associates.

Schnaper, N. (1975). The psychological implications of severe trauma: Emotional sequelae to unconsciousness. *Journal of Trauma, 15*, 94–98.

Tosch, P. (1988). Patients' recollections of their posttraumatic coma. *Journal of Neuroscience Nursing, 20*, 223–228.

Whyte, J., & Glenn, M. B. (1986). The care and rehabilitation of the patient in a persistent vegetative state. *Journal of Head Trauma Rehabilitation, 1*, 39–53.

Wilson, S. L., Powell, G. E., Elliot, K., & Thwaites, H. (1991). Sensory stimulation in prolonged coma: Four single case studies. *Brain Injury, 5*, 393–400.

Yanko, J. (1985). Nursing and the continuum of recovery: The acute phase. In M. Ylvisikar (Ed.), *Head injury rehabilitation: Children and adolescents* (pp. 141–147). San Diego: College Hill Press.

Behavior Modification

Behavioral problems may be associated with disorders of the central nervous system. The therapy of choice for such problems is often a behavior modification program possibly supplemented by psychoactive medications. Behavior modification should be done by health care personnel with appropriate training and competence. It is essential that all staff involved in a behavior-change program have a clear understanding of the theoretical principles of behavioral techniques and a commitment to their use (Turnbull, 1988).

Numerous ethical and legal issues, which may vary according to locality, attend the use of behavior modification (Czyzewski *et al.,* 1986; Turnbull, 1988). Examples of issues include (1) informed consent, (2) the right to receive or refuse therapy, (3) privacy, (4) personal property, (5) communications, (6) the right to a safe and humane environment, and (7) the use of punishment, seclusion, and restraint procedures. Individuals designing and implementing behavior-change programs should be thoroughly familiar with accepted ethical and legal standards regarding these issues in their community.

In the following discussion, a summary of behavioral problems and treatment techniques is presented. First, the principles of operant conditioning and derivative techniques are summarized. Behavioral problems are then described and applications of the techniques suggested. It should be noted that this summary does not supply sufficient information to guide appropriate use of these techniques. They should be used only by individuals with appropriate training or under appropriate supervision.

BEHAVIORAL ASSESSMENT

Defining the Target Behavior

The target behavior or behavior to be modified should be operationally defined in language understandable by the individuals administering the behavior program. If possible, it should also be understandable by the patient.

Identifying Antecedents and Consequents

A record is made of the patient's behavior and of the events preceding and following the behavior to determine which events may be precipitating or reinforcing. Continuous recording at regular intervals may be useful if a token economy is in place or if the behavior is high in frequency. If the behavior is low in frequency, critical-event sampling, in which recording is performed only when the target behavior has been produced, may require less staff time and result in better staff compliance (Franzen & Lovell, 1987).

Establishing a Baseline

The frequency of the target behavior is recorded prior to any intervention for comparison with its frequency during or after treatment (Seron, 1987).

Identifying Reinforcers

Reinforcers may be identified by asking the patient about personal preferences, by observing the patient's preferences, and by determining the patient's high-frequency, high-probability behaviors and applying the Premack principle (Milby, 1982). Care must be taken to select reinforcers that do not compromise the patient's rights (Turnbull, 1988).

Identifying Adaptive and Incompatible Behaviors

If the target behavior is to be reduced or eliminated, adaptive behaviors (e.g., more appropriate behaviors for gaining staff attention) should be identified. Reinforcing these behaviors provides the patient with an alternative means for obtaining rewards. Reinforcement of adaptive responses that are incompatible with the target response may reduce the frequency of the target behavior.

PROCEDURES TO INITIATE NEW BEHAVIOR

Shaping

Reinforcement is contingent on an approximation to the target response. Closer approximations are required until the target response is achieved (Milby, 1982).

Modeling

The behavior is modeled and the patient imitates the model. Feedback and reinforcement are given immediately after the imitated response (Milby, 1982).

Instruction, Prompts, and Cues

Verbal instruction describing the behavior may assist the patient in performing the desired act. Prompts and cues may assist the patient in initiating a behavior in the appropriate circumstances. As the patient's performance improves, the prompts and cues are faded (Seron, 1987).

Physical Guidance

Physically directing the patient's movements may sometimes help the patient to initially produce and to learn the behavior (Foxx, 1982a).

PROCEDURES TO INCREASE OR MAINTAIN BEHAVIOR

Reward Conditioning

Reinforcement is contingent on an increase in the number or rate of the target response (Milby, 1982).

Self-Monitoring

If the patient is motivated, self-recording of the target behavior may result in increased frequency of the behavior (Milby, 1982).

Modeling

Modeling in individual or group settings may increase the frequency of the target behavior, especially if this modeling is combined with feedback and reinforcement (Milby, 1982).

PROCEDURES TO REDUCE OR ELIMINATE BEHAVIOR

Modification of Antecedents

Reduction or elimination of antecedents that elicit the target behavior may lessen the frequency of the behavior (Franzen & Lovell, 1987).

Differential Reinforcement of Other Behavior

The patient is reinforced for any behavior other than the target behavior. This technique provides the patient with the freedom to choose from a wide variety of more adaptive behaviors (Franzen & Lovell, 1987; Repp & Brulle, 1981).

DIFFERENTIAL REINFORCEMENT OF INCOMPATIBLE BEHAVIOR

Incompatible behaviors or behaviors that are topographically incompatible with the target behavior are reinforced (Franzen & Lovell, 1987; Repp & Brulle, 1981).

Overcorrection

After the target behavior occurs, the patient is required to practice a behavior incompatible with the target behavior (Franzen & Lovell, 1987).

Extinction

Reinforcement is withheld following the target behavior, which has previously been reinforced. The target behavior may initially increase.

Punishment

Aversive conditioning or the application of an aversive consequence after the target behavior may modify the target behavior, but may also have disadvantages: (1) production of emotional behavior, (2) aggression, (3) negative modeling, and (4) attempt by the patient to escape or to avoid the situation or person (Foxx, 1982b).

Response Cost

If the patient emits the target behavior, he or she loses previously acquired reinforcers (Repp & Brulle, 1981).

Time-Out

The patient's access to reinforcement is removed for a short period of time (Repp & Brulle, 1981). Time-out on the spot involves immediate withdrawal of reinforcement, e.g., staff attention.

Seclusion and Restraint

Methods of seclusion and physical restraint are different from time-out in that time-out involves removal from a positive situation, but does not involve the application of an aversive stimulus (Franzen & Lovell, 1987). Seclusion and restraint are more likely to be perceived as punishment and may lead to adjunctive aggressive behaviors. For these reasons, special treatment, ethical, and legal issues apply to seclusion and restraint (Tardiff, 1989). Restraint can become reinforcing if a substantial amount of attention is associated with the implementation of the procedure. There is a danger that the procedure may be used in an arbitrary or punitive fashion for the staff's convenience. Since the patient may become combative, the use of restraint may endanger the staff members implementing the procedure (Foxx, 1982b). Common standards for the use of seclusion and restraint procedures include: (1) use only in emergencies or for the prevention of injury to self or others; (2) documentation that less restrictive procedures have been tried or at least considered and ruled out; (3) a maximum time limit; (4) written documentation of parameters such as date, duration, evaluation, periodic checks, and behavior; (5) written procedures and policies; and (6) a prohibition of use for convenience of staff or as a substitute for treatment (Czyzewski et al., 1986). Since standards vary with locality, the practitioner is urged to become knowledgeable about local standards.

ENVIRONMENTAL MODIFICATION

Environmental modification often refers to a global modification of the antecedents of behavior. For example, a quiet room may be provided to reduce stimulation for an agitated, head-injured patient.

TOKEN ECONOMIES

A token economy is a complex, systematic behavioral program that uses tokens (conditioned reinforcers such as chips or points). The tokens can be exchanged for backup reinforcers such as consumables and activities. Token programs have been used in a variety of treatment and rehabilitation settings (Blackerby, 1988; Kazdin, 1977). An excellent description of a token economy in a brain injury rehabilitation setting may be found in *Brain Injury Rehabilitation* (Wood, 1987). The *Journal of Head Trauma Rehabilitation* (1988), Vol. 3, N. 3, also contains useful information on the use of behavior modification and token economies with head-injured individuals.

STRESS INOCULATION

Stress inoculation may be conceptualized as a three-step procedure: (1) cognitive preparation—presentation of rationale, (2) skills acquisition—learning relaxation techniques and adaptive cognitions, and (3) application training—practice in progressively stronger target-behavior-evoking situations (Lira *et al.*, 1983). Stress inoculation may be effective in anger management (Novaco, 1977).

BEHAVIORAL PROBLEMS IN NEUROPSYCHIATRIC DISORDERS

Impaired Arousal, Alertness, and Awareness

Impaired arousal and alertness may occur in a variety of neurological disorders. Generalized brain impairment, bilateral frontal lobe damage, or brainstem damage may be causative (Wood, 1987). Although stimulation should be provided for patients with these symptoms, care should be taken to respect increases in patients' fatigue levels. In head-injury patients, overstimulation may result in confusion and agitation, leading to increased lethargy (Howard, 1988). Recording the length of time and time of day that patients were able to participate in activities can help establish optimum levels of stimulation.

Agitation

Patients with impaired cerebral functioning may exhibit agitation, head-injured patients being especially susceptible (Howard, 1988). Head-injured patients may have isolated episodes of quick, irritable outbursts and exhibit hyperactivity and hypersensitivity. Modification of antecedents may be effected by controlling stimulation in situations in which agitated outbursts are likely. Agitation is commonly attended by disorientation, confusion, impaired immediate memory, and sharply decreased attention span. Impaired memory and decreased attention span may allow the patient to be more easily redirected because he or she has more difficulty in forming and sustaining an intention. Calm, controlled, nonthreatening verbal or gestural redirection with empathy for and validation of the patient's feelings can defuse situations the patient finds threatening and can minimize disruption of unit activities when the patient wanders. Confrontation and emotional escalation may be avoided.

Therapists should avoid reinforcing outbursts, but should immediately label and reward self-control behaviors (Howard, 1988).

Aggression

Aggressive behavior may be defined as behavior that is (1) harmful to people or property, (2) intimidating or threatening, or (3) in the rehabilitation setting, intentionally disruptive of rehabilitation activities and social reintegration (Wood, 1987). Wood (1987) has distinguished several distinct varieties of aggression in brain-injured patients. *Episodic aggression* may result from paroxysmal electrical discharges secondary to damage to the medial portions of the frontal lobes. Treatment of this form of aggression is likely to require medication in addition to behavioral management (Wood, 1987).

Disinhibited aggression may occur when a patient lacks emotional control and the ability to inhibit aggressive impulses due to frontal lobe damage. A combination of behavioral techniques may assist patients in gaining increased control (Wood, 1987).

Since aggressive behavior usually elicits attention from the staff, these forms of aggression may evolve into *learned aggression.* Learned aggression is often purposeful, related to reinforcement, and premeditated. Franzen and Lovell (1987) suggest time-out, differential reinforcement of other behavior, differential reinforcement of incompatible behavior, modeling, extinction, and overcorrection as possible techniques for decreasing aggressive behavior. Punishment is not recommended because it may elicit aggressive behaviors (Franzen & Lovell, 1987). Extinction may be inappropriate for treating violent behavior due to the possibility that violent behavior may initially increase. Time-out may not be feasible if the behavior is physically violent; the patient may not be safe in or remain in time-out, and medication or restraint or both may have to be considered. Stress inoculation has been used successfully (Lira *et al.,* 1983). Goldstein and Keller (1987) have described a detailed approach to the assessment and treatment of aggression in the general population.

Disinhibited and Socially Inappropriate Behavior

Diffuse cortical or frontal lobe lesions can result in disinhibited, impulsive behavior. Socially inappropriate behavior, especially inappropriate sexual behavior due to impulsivity and impaired social perception, may be upsetting to both staff and family and can substantially retard reintegration of the patient into society. Impulsivity can also seriously compromise a patient's safety. Time-out has been used successfully in the treatment of sexually inappropriate behavior (Wood, 1987).

Ainitia and Lack of Motivation

Brain-injured patients may exhibit a lack of activity, interest, and initiative—ainitia. This behavioral symptom may follow diffuse cortical or bilateral frontal damage (Wood, 1987). Motivation and hedonic responsiveness may also be affected. The discovery of relevant, powerful reinforcers is essential for treating these problems (Wood, 1987). A variety of operant paradigms can be employed in improving motivational performance (Ince, 1976).

Impaired Living Skills

Patients having neurological impairments may exhibit physical or cognitive deficits or both, which may in turn compromise activities of daily living and social and job skills. Treatment programs designed using behavior modification may be more effective in remediating these behavioral deficits (Ince, 1976; Wood, 1987).

Additional Psychological and Psychophysiological Disorders

In addition to the behavioral disorders previously mentioned, patients with neurological disorders may have any of the psychological or psychophysiological disorders found in the nonneurological population. These disorders may be exacerbated by the neurological condition.

REFERENCES

Blackerby, W. F. (1988). Practical token economies. *Journal of Head Trauma Rehabilitation, 3,* 33–45.

Czyzewski, M. J., Sheldon, J., & Hannah, G. T. (1986). Legal safety in residential treatment environments. In F. J. Fuoco & W. P. Christian (Eds.), *Behavior analysis and therapy in residential programs* (pp. 194–230). New York: Van Nostrand Reinhold.

Foxx, R. M. (1982a). *Increasing behaviors of severely retarded and autistic persons.* Champaign, IL: Research Press.

Foxx, R. M. (1982b). *Decreasing behaviors of severely retarded and autistic persons.* Champaign, IL: Research Press.

Franzen, M. D., & Lovell, M. R. (1987). Behavioral treatments of aggressive sequelae of brain injury. *Psychiatric Annals, 17,* 389–396.

Goldstein, A. P., & Keller, H. R. (1987). *Aggressive behavior: Assessment and intervention.* New York: Pergamon.

Howard, M. E. (1988). Behavior management in the acute care rehabilitation setting. *Journal of Head Trauma Rehabilitation, 3,* 14–22.

Ince, L. P. (1976). *Behavioral modification in rehabilitative medicine.* Springfield, IL: Charles C. Thomas.

Kazdin, A. E. (1977). *The token economy: A review and evaluation.* New York: Plenum Press.

Lira, F. T., Carne, W., & Masri, A. M. (1983). Treatment of anger and impulsivity in a brain damaged patient: A case study applying stress inoculation. *Clinical Neuropsychology, 5,* 159–160.

Milby, J. B. (1982) Operant conditioning. In D. M. Doleys, R. L. Meredith, & A. R. Ciminero (Eds.), *Behavioral medicine: Assessment and treatment strategies* (pp. 19–43). New York: Plenum Press.

Novaco, R. (1977). Stress inoculation: A cognitive therapy for anger and its application to a case of depression. *Journal of Consulting and Clinical Psychology, 45,* 600–608.

Repp, A. C., & Brulle, A. R. (1981). Reducing aggressive behavior of mentally retarded persons. In J. L. Matson & J. R. McCartney (Eds.), *Handbook of behavior modification with the mentally retarded* (pp. 177–210). New York: Plenum Press.

Seron, X. (1987). Operant procedures and neuropsychological rehabilitation. In M. J. Meier, A. L. Benton, and L. Diller (Eds.), *Neuropsychological rehabilitation* (pp. 132–161). Edinburgh: Churchill-Livingston.

Tardiff, T. (1989). *Concise guide to assessment and management of violent patients.* Washington, DC: American Psychiatric Press.

Turnbull, J. (1988). Perils (hidden and not so hidden) of the token economy. *Journal of Head Trauma Rehabilitation, 3,* 46–52.

Wood, R. L. (1987). *Brain injury rehabilitation: A neurobehavioral approach.* Rockville, MD: Aspen.

Cognitive Rehabilitation

Cognitive rehabilitation may be conceptualized as involving three approaches: (1) *retraining* the impaired ability, (2) compensating for the loss of the impaired ability by a modified use of a preserved ability (*behavioral compensation*), and (3) compensating for the loss of the impaired ability by the use of cognitive prostheses (*prosthetic compensation*).

RETRAINING

Craine and Gudeman (1981) listed eight principles of neurotraining:

1. Recovery of function following cortical damage is possible.
2. The organization of the cerebral cortex is an ''open system'' and is highly adaptive and malleable.
3. Environmental influences can reorganize the functions of the cerebral cortex.
4. Neurotraining must recapitulate the original acquisition of the skill being trained.
5. Since higher cortical functions integrate sensory modalities, therapy should combine various modalities.
6. Neurotraining should focus on developing processes that underlie learning rather than specific content areas.
7. Neurotraining should be aimed at the patient's specific deficit.
8. Patients must be provided with direct specific feedback.

Retraining of attention is an example of successful retraining of a function (Sohlberg & Mateer, 1987).

Cognitive rehabilitation may be more efficacious when combined with other therapeutic modalities. Rattok *et al.* (1992) have reported that a therapeutic mix containing cognitive rehabilitation and small-group interpersonal communication training is more effective than mixes lacking in either of these components.

The mechanisms of recovery of function in the nervous system have been reviewed in detail elsewhere (Gouvier *et al.*, 1986; Rothi & Horner, 1983) and will not be reviewed here. The relevance of retraining to this process continues to be investigated.

BEHAVIORAL COMPENSATION

If the impaired ability does not respond to retraining, a preserved ability may sometimes be used to serve the purpose of the old ability. An example is the use of writing or sign language by a severely dysarthric patient.

PROSTHETIC COMPENSATION

Sometimes a cognitive prosthesis may be used to take over the function of an irreversibly impaired ability. An example is the use of an appointment book and a diary by an amnesic patient (Sohlberg & Mateer, 1989b).

ISSUES AND GUIDELINES

Although research appears to be accumulating that attests to the efficacy of some forms of cognitive rehabilitation, issues of efficacy continue to be controversial (Berrol, 1990; Levin, 1990; Volpe & McDowell, 1990). Guidelines have been developed by an American Psychological Association Division 40 (Clinical Neuropsychology) Task Force for computer-assisted neuropsychological rehabilitation and cognitive remediation (Matthews *et al.,* 1991).

There are many cognitive rehabilitation programs and materials, both computerized and noncomputerized, available for purchase. The efficacy of most of these programs and materials has not been tested. They usually do not even have norms for the therapist to use to assess the patient's performance and to set performance goals.

The cognitive rehabilitation methods summarized below have some empirical support, but much more research is needed. Cognitive rehabilitation is reviewed for the areas of orientation, attention, memory, communication, visuospatial functioning, and executive functioning.

ORIENTATION

Reality orientation programs are used to systematically reacquaint patients with salient features of the environment (time, location, circumstance) and to redirect attention from internal stimuli to external events (McNeny & Dise, 1990). Reality orientation is pursued 24 hr a day (Holden & Woods, 1982). Each time staff interact with the patient, they remind him or her of time, place, and person and provide a commentary on events. Confused thinking and rambling speech are not reinforced. This activity is supplemented by reality-orientation group sessions. Sessions are daily and may be $\frac{1}{2}$–1 hr in duration. Reality-orientation groups are sometimes created at different levels (Holden & Woods, 1982). A basic group may emphasize repetition of basic information (reading from a board, writing in a diary) with many clues provided to guarantee successful performance. A more advanced group may provide basic information and additionally explore past experiences. Research suggests that reality orientation may increase verbal orientation in elderly patients (Holden & Woods, 1982).

Although the ability of reality-orientation therapy to improve the orientation of traumatically brain-injured patients has not been demonstrated, Corrigan *et al.* (1987) have found reality-orientation groups to be useful in monitoring recovery. Patients were rated on orientation to time and place, identification of therapists and group members, repetition of paired associates, report of significant daily events, and use of planning and scheduling aids. Scores were useful in determining readiness for neuropsychological testing and more advanced cognitive rehabilitation or placement in a long-term-care facility.

ATTENTION

Evidence appears to be accumulating that practice of attentional tasks of graded difficulty can improve attentional abilities. Reinforcement of attentional behavior has been found to improve attention (Wood, 1987). Several training approaches have been developed for the remediation of impairments in attention.

Orientation Remedial Module

The Orientation Remedial Module is part of the cognitive rehabilitation program developed at the New York University Medical Center (Ben-Yishay *et al.*, 1980, 1987; Piasetsky *et al.*, 1982). Exercises require the patient to press a button to turn on a light, release a button to stop a sweep hand at a designated location, identify numbers and colors at various horizontal locations in the visual field, estimate the passage of time, and press a key to match a rhythm. The performance of brain-injured patients tended to improve on all tasks and appeared to generalize to improved performance on tests of attention (Ben-Yishay *et al.*, 1987).

Attention Process Training

Sohlberg and Mateer (1987) trained patients on tasks corresponding to five types of attentional processes: (1) *focused* attention—the patient is trained on reaction time tasks and detection of auditorily presented numbers; (2) *sustained* attention—the patient is trained on auditory tasks, number manipulation, and time estimation; (3) *selective* attention—training is provided on auditory tasks with background noise, tasks requiring inhibition of responses, and visuomotor tasks with distractors; (4) *alternating* attention—training is provided on calculational flexibility exercises (addition/subtraction, before/after) and simultaneous sequencing exercises; (5) *divided* attention—the patient masters a simultaneous multiple attention exercise, multilevel card sort, and an auditory/visual dual task. Patients improved on independent measures of attention (Sohlberg & Mateer, 1987).

MEMORY

Memory Retraining

Repetitive memory drills have been performed under the assumption that practice will strengthen damaged memory processes (memory muscle theory). There is no evidence to support the efficacy of this procedure (Schacter & Glisky, 1986; Wilson, 1989).

Mnemonic Strategies

Strategies such as semantic categorization (Baddeley, 1982), semantic elaboration (Gianutsos & Gianutsos, 1979), visual imagery (Gasparrini & Satz, 1979; Wilson, 1987), and the

PQRST learning strategy (Grafman, 1984; Wilson, 1987) may have limited effectiveness. The techniques do not readily generalize (Schacter & Glisky, 1986). Patients with severe intellectual and memory impairments are likely to have difficulty in mastering the strategies (Schacter & Glisky, 1986). Patients with less severe impairments may experience some limited benefits (Wilson, 1987). Patients whose memory impairment is due primarily to attentional impairment may benefit from strategies designed to improve attention (Webster & Scott, 1988).

Memory Prostheses

Environmental modification, external memory aids, domain-specific knowledge, and learned behavior patterns have been used to facilitate the patient's performance in situations that usually make demands on memory. Environmental modification may include orientation boards containing a calendar, name of location, weekly schedule, family photos, biography and accident history, and therapy schedule (Grafman, 1984). Labels and building design can facilitate orientation in a residential facility (Wilson, 1989).

Notebooks, timers, programmable digital watches, and computers have been used as external memory aids. The use of such methods has been criticized on the grounds that they cannot code enough environmental complexity, are too cumbersome, and may be lost or misplaced (Webster & Scott, 1988). Despite these drawbacks, external memory aids may be the best alternative for memory-impaired individuals (Corvitz, 1989; Zencius et al., 1990). External memory devices should: (1) be portable, (2) be useful in a wide variety of situations, (3) store many cues for a long period of time, and (4) be easy to use (Harris, 1978). Cues should: (1) be given as close as possible to the time action is required, (2) be active rather than passive (e.g., a diary is passive), and (3) be specific reminders for particular actions.

Timers have been used to remind patients to boost from a wheelchair to avoid decubiti (Klein & Fowler, 1981). Digital watches have been used to compensate for impaired memory (Gouvier, 1982). Multiple-alarm digital watches such as the Casio Module No. 563 Data Bank watch can be programmed for multiple alarm times over a span of weeks and to display a brief verbal reminder at the alarm (Naugle et al., 1988).

Sohlberg and Mateer (1989b) have described the successful use of a memory book by a severely memory-impaired patient. The book was divided into several sections: (1) Orientation; (2) Memory Log—diary of hourly activities and information; (3) Calendar for scheduling appointments; (4) Things To Do; (5) Transportation—maps, bus information, and directions; (6) Feelings Log; (7) Names and identifying information of new people; and (8) Today At Work—information necessary to perform job duties. The patient learned to use the book in three stages. In the Acquisition phase, the patient developed declarative knowledge of the sections of the memory book through repetition. In the Application phase, a record was kept of the patient's hourly writing in his Memory Log and of the degree of cueing necessary to remind the patient to write. The patient was engaged in role plays simulating real-life events requiring the use of the memory book. In the final, Adaptation phase, the patient was given assignments to use the memory book in the hospital and in the community.

Schacter and Glisky (1986) have reported some success in training amnesic patients to use computers. Patients were first taught rudimentary computer terminology using the method of vanishing cues (Glisky et al., 1986). Cues consisting of letter fragments of the words to be learned were systematically reduced across trials. Patients were also able to learn to perform simple commands on the computer and to write simple programs. There was a substantial retention of these abilities over periods of up to 9 months, suggesting the possibility that this domain-specific knowledge might allow patients to use the computer as a memory prosthesis (Glisky & Schacter, 1988).

Although the usefulness of external memory prostheses is yet to be proven, preliminary studies are promising. They suggest that external memory aids may be useful if domain-specific knowledge is provided through a behavioral learning program using repetition and fading of cues. The patient can then be taught to use the memory aid in the community.

COMMUNICATION

Although numerous aphasia therapies have been developed and have been in use for years, controversy persists about the efficacy of aphasia therapy in general and about the relative value of specific therapies (Basso, 1989; Kitselman & Wertz, 1985; Kotten, 1989). Both negative and positive outcome studies have been reported. Nevertheless, many authorities in the area generally believe that aphasia therapy promotes recovery (Basso, 1989; Benson, 1979; Darley, 1979; Kitselman & Wertz, 1985).

Stimulation–Facilitation Therapy

Schuell *et al.* (1964) maintained that disrupted neurolinguistic processes are strengthened through stimulation. Patients are provided with intensive linguistic stimulation, especially in the auditory modality. Stimulation must be clear, of adequate amplitude, and have a high probability of eliciting a response. Stimulation may be repetitive. A response must be evoked by each stimulus. Emphasis is on stimulation of linguistic responses rather than on correction of errors.

Programmed-Operant Therapy

Operant conditioning principles are applied in the programmed-operant approach (Holland, 1970; LaPoint, 1983). Baseline measures are obtained to identify responses to be modified. The responses are then shaped and modified via feedback and reinforcement. After modified responses have been established in therapy, discriminative stimuli are faded and the responses are elicited in and generalized to more natural communicative settings.

Visual Action Therapy

Visual Action Therapy (Helm-Estabrooks *et al.,* 1982) trains global aphasics to use symbolic gestures to represent visually absent objects. It is conceptualized as a program to train limb praxis. Tasks involve associating pictures with everyday objects, manipulating real objects, and producing symbolic gestures that represent objects.

Melodic Intonation Therapy

In Melodic Intonation Therapy, the patient is taught to produce sentences by singing an intonational pattern that approximates a natural prosodic pattern (Sparks & Holland, 1976). Therapy begins with the patient tapping out the rhythm as the therapist sings the sentence. Gradually, the patient joins the therapist in singing the sentence. The therapist's speaking is gradually faded. The response is then shaped toward normal prosody. Sparks *et al.* (1974) reported some success with patients who had shown no improvement prior to therapy.

Functional Communication Therapy

The procedures of Functional Communication Therapy are designed to coincide closely with natural conversation (Davis, 1983; Davis & Wilcox, 1981, 1985). It utilizes the turn-taking that is a feature of normal conversation, the communication of new information by using stimuli that are not known to the receiver, any communicative modality, and feedback on the success with which information has been communicated. The results of several studies have suggested that this approach may have some efficacy (Aten *et al.*, 1982).

Amerind Sign Language

American Indian Sign Language (Amerind) has been used to provide patients with an alternative means of communication and as a step in learning spoken language (Skelly *et al.*, 1974). An adaptation is available for hemiplegic patients. The patient is first taught commonly used signs by imitation. The sign is presented and the corresponding word is spoken. Gradually, the sign is faded. Amerind may be an effective technique in selected cases (Rao *et al.*, 1980).

Speech/Language Prostheses

If the patient is unable to speak or write, communication may be assisted by specially designed devices. In the simplest device, pictures or pictorial representations can be provided and the patient can communicate by pointing (Silverman, 1989). Communication boards may be constructed using pictures, symbols, words, or letters. Computer programs and peripheral devices are available that allow a patient to "type" letters to the monitor using a microswitch. The words "typed" to the computer may be converted to speech using a speech synthesizer. Words can also be "typed" to a monitor or other device using switches triggered by muscle action potentials (Silverman, 1989).

VISUOSPATIAL FUNCTIONING

Many patients who are experiencing visual neglect may benefit from a variety of training procedures. The staff at the New York University Institute of Rehabilitation Medicine has developed a scanning machine that has a target that traverses the perimeter of a board 78" L × 8" W (Diller & Weinberg, 1977). The board is also studded with two rows of 10 colored lights. The patient practices scanning by following the target and by searching for the lights. Weinberg *et al.* (1977) found that practice on this apparatus along with practice in cancellation and in reading specially prepared materials resulted in improved reading at posttesting. Training in scanning has also been demonstrated to improve abilities to navigate a wheelchair obstacle course in patients who exhibit left-sided homonymous hemianopsia and left hemi-inattention (Gouvier *et al.*, 1984; Webster *et al.*, 1984).

Training in skills involving visual–perceptual organization may also be efficacious. Weinberg *et al.* (1982) trained right-brain-damaged stroke patients, who did not exhibit neglect but did exhibit deficits on visuocognitive testing, on tasks designed to establish a systematic strategy for organizing complex visual material. Training involved learning the locations of words in a paragraph, forming meaningful gestalts from dots, and observing the irregular perimeter of stimulus figures. Posttesting revealed improvement relative to controls on 8 of 12 visuocognitive tests. Young *et al.* (1983) found that left hemiplegic patients who received cancellation training, scanning training, and Block Design training did significantly better than patients who received routine occupational therapy on posttesting on the BD-WAIS-R subtest, a letter cancellation task, and the WRAT Reading subtest.

EXECUTIVE FUNCTIONING

Although numerous programs for the remediation of executive-functioning and problem-solving impairments in brain have been developed, research on these programs has been limited (Goldstein & Levin, 1987). Von Cramon and Matthes-von Cramon (1990) investigated the effects of a 6-week cognitive training program. On the basis of tests reported to be sensitive to frontal lobe dysfunction, they divided brain-damaged patients into good and poor problem-solvers. The poor problem-solvers were divided into a problem-solving training group and a memory-training group. Problem-solving training was done in a group setting and consisted of four modules. The first module focused on developing the ability to generate goal-directed ideas through brainstorming and weighing the consequences of ideas generated. In the second module, the patients were required to distinguish relevant from irrelevant information in practical situations. The third module required patients to use multiple timetables and schedules to plan a trip. The fourth module focused on drawing inferences. The patients read and analyzed short detective stories. Von Cramon and Matthes-von Cramon (1990) found that the problem-solving treatment group improved more on a Planning Test and the Tower of Hanoi puzzle than the memory treatment group.

Sohlberg and Mateer (1989a) have developed a model for treating executive dysfunctions. Major treatment areas are Selection and Execution of Cognitive Plans, Time Management, and Self-Regulation. Each of these areas is broken down into subcomponents, each of which has corresponding training tasks. The model is illustrated with a case study.

Cicerone and Wood (1987) reported the successful treatment of a head-injured patient who exhibited impaired planning ability and self-control. The patient was taught to verbalize a plan of behavior before and during the execution of a task. Verbalization was gradually faded. Craine (1982) has reported a detailed case study of the retraining of a patient with frontal lobe dysfunction.

Lack of initiation, disinhibition, and emotional dyscontrol can result from impaired executive functioning. The treatment of these problems is addressed in Chapter 34.

REFERENCES

Aten, J. L., Caligiuri, M. P., & Holland, A. L. (1982). The efficacy of functional communication therapy for chronic aphasic patients. *Journal of Speech and Hearing Disorders, 47,* 93–96.

Baddeley, A. (1982). *Your memory: A user's guide.* New York: Macmillan.

Basso, A. (1989). Spontaneous recovery and language rehabilitation. In X. Seron & G. Deloche (Eds.), *Cognitive approaches in neuropsychological rehabilitation* (pp. 17–37). Hillsdale, NJ: Laurence Erlbaum Associates.

Benson, D. F. (1979). Aphasia rehabilitation. *Archives of Neurology, 36,* 187–189.

Ben-Yishay, Y., Rattok, J., Ross, B., Lakin, P., Cohen, J., & Diller, L. (1980). A remedial module for the systematic amelioration of basic attentional disturbances in head trauma patients. In Y. Ben-Yishay (Ed.), *Working approaches to remediation of cognitive deficits in brain damaged persons* (pp. 70–127). New York: NYU Medical Center.

Ben-Yishay, Y., Piasetsky, E. B., & Rattok, J. (1987). A systematic method for ameliorating disorders in basic attention. In M. J. Meier, A. L. Benton, & L. Diller (Eds.), *Neuropsychological rehabilitation* (pp. 165–181), Edinburgh: Churchill-Livingston.

Berrol, S. (1990). Issues in cognitive rehabilitation. *Archives of Neurology, 47,* 221–220.

Cicerone, K. D., & Wood, J. C. (1987). Planning disorder after closed head injury: A case study. *Archives of Physical Medicine and Rehabilitation, 68,* 111–115.

Corrigan, J. D., Arnett, J. A., Houck, L. J., & Jackson, R. D. (1987). Reality orientation for brain injured patients: Group treatment and monitoring of recovery. *Archives of Physical Medicine and Rehabilitation, 66,* 626–630.

Corvitz, H. F. (1989). Memory retraining: Everyday needs and future prospects. In L. W. Poon, D. C. Rubin, & B. A. Wilson (Eds.), *Everyday cognition in adulthood and late life* (pp. 681–691). Cambridge, England: Cambridge University Press.

Craine, J. F. (1982). The retraining of frontal lobe dysfunction. In L. E. Trexler (Ed.), *Cognitive rehabilitation: Conceptualization and intervention* (pp. 239–262). New York: Plenum Press.

Craine, J. F., & Gudeman, H. E. (1981). *The rehabilitation of brain functions: Principles, procedures, and techniques of neurotraining.* Springfield, IL: Charles C. Thomas.

Darley, F. (1979). Treat or neglect. *ASHA, 21,* 628–631.

Davis, G. A. (1983). *A survey of adult aphasia.* Englewood Cliffs, NJ: Prentice-Hall.

Davis, G. A., & Wilcox, M. J. (1981). Incorporating parameters of natural conversation in aphasia treatment. In R. Chapey (Ed.), *Language intervention strategies in adult aphasia* (pp. 169–193). Baltimore: Williams & Wilkins.

Davis, G. A., & Wilcox, M. J. (1985). *Adult aphasia rehabilitation: Applied pragmatics.* San Diego: College-Hill Press.

Diller, L., & Weinberg, J. (1977). Hemi-inattention in rehabilitation: The evolution of a rational remediation program. In E. A. Weinstein & R. P. Friedland (Eds.), *Advances in neurology,* Volume 18 (pp. 63–82). New York: Raven Press.

Gasparrini, B., & Satz, P. (1979). A treatment for memory problems in left hemisphere CVA patients. *Journal of Clinical Neuropsychology, 1,* 137–150.

Gianutsos, R., & Gianutsos, J. (1979). Rehabilitating the verbal recall of brain-damaged patients by mnemonic training: An experimental demonstration using single-case methodology. *Journal of Clinical Neuropsychology, 1,* 117–135.

Glisky, E. L., & Schacter, D. L. (1988). Long-term retention of computer learning by patients with memory disorders. *Neuropsychologia, 26,* 173–178.

Glisky, E. L., Schacter, D. L., & Tulving, E. (1986). Learning and retention of computer-related vocabulary in memory-impaired patients: Method of vanishing cues. *Journal of Clinical and Experimental Neuropsychology, 8,* 292–312.

Goldstein, F. C., & Levin, H. S. (1987). Disorders of reasoning and problem-solving ability. In M. J. Meier, A. L. Benton, & L. Diller (Eds.), *Neuropsychological rehabilitation* (pp. 327–354). Edinburgh: Churchill-Livingston.

Gouvier, W. (1982). Using the digital alarm chronograph in memory retraining. *Behavioral Engineering, 7,* 134.

Gouvier, W. D., Cottam, G., Webster, J. S., Beissel, G. F., & Wofford, J. D. (1984). Behavioral interventions with stroke patients for improving wheelchair navigation. *International Journal of Clinical Neuropsychology, 6,* 186–190.

Gouvier, W. D., Webster, J. S., & Blanton, P. D. (1986). Cognitive training with braindamaged patients. In D. Wedding, A. M. Horton, Jr., & J. Webster (Eds.), *The neuropsychology handbook: Behavioral and clinical perspectives* (pp. 278–324). New York: Springer.

Grafman, J. (1984). Memory assessment and remediation in brain-injured patients. In B. A. Edelstein & E. Couture (Eds.), *Behavior assessment and rehabilitation of the traumatically brain-damaged* (pp. 151–189). New York: Plenum Press.

Harris, J. E. (1978). External memory aids. In M. M. Gruneburg, P. E. Morris, & R. N. Sykes (Eds.), *Practical aspects of memory* (pp. 172–179). London: Academic Press.

Helm-Estabrooks, N., Fitzpatrick, P. M., & Barresi, B. (1982). Visual action therapy for aphasia. *Journal of Speech and Hearing Disorders, 47,* 385–389.

Holden, U. P., & Woods, R. T. (1982). *Reality orientation: Psychological approaches to the confused elderly.* Edinburgh: Churchill-Livingston.

Holland, A. L. (1970). Case studies in aphasia rehabilitation using programmed instruction. *Journal of Speech and Hearing Disorders, 35,* 377–390.

Kitselman, K. P., & Wertz, R. T. (1985). The treatment of aphasia. In J. K. Darby (Ed.), *Speech and language evaluation in neurology: Adult disorders* (pp. 217–244). Orlando, FL: Grune & Stratton.

Klein, R. M., & Fowler, R. S. (1981). Pressure relief training device: The microcalculation. *Archives of Physical and Medical Rehabilitation, 62,* 500–501.

Kotten, A. (1989). Aphasia therapy: A multidimensional process. In E. Perecman (Ed.), *Integrating theory and practice in clinical neuropsychology* (pp. 293–315). Hillsdale, NJ: Laurence Erlbaum Associates.

LaPoint, L. L. (1983). Aphasia intervention with adults: Historical, present, and future approaches. In D. F. Johns (Ed.), *Clinical management of neurogenic communicative disorders* (pp. 129–190). Boston: Little, Brown.

Levin, H. S. (1990). Cognitive rehabilitation: Unproved but promising. *Archives of Neurology, 47,* 223–224.

Matthews, C. G., Harley, J. P., & Malec, J. F. (1991). Guidelines for computer-assisted neuropsychological rehabilitation and cognitive remediation. *The Clinical Neuropsychologist, 5,* 3–19.

McNeny, R., & Dise, J. (1990). Reality orientation therapy. In M. Rosenthal, M. R. Bond, E. R. Griffith, & J. D. Miller (Eds.), *Rehabilitation of the adult and child with traumatic brain injury* (2nd ed.) (pp. 366–373). Philadelphia: F. A. Davis.

Naugle, R., Naugle, C., Prevey, M., & Delaney, R. (1988). New digital watch as a compensatory device for memory dysfunction. *Cognitive Rehabilitation, 6*(4), 22–23.

Piasetsky, E. B., Ben-Yishay, Y., Weinberg, J., & Diller, L. (1982). The systematic remediation of specific disorders: Selected application of methods derived in a clinical research setting. In L. E. Trexler (Ed.), *Cognitive rehabilitation: Conceptualization and intervention* (pp. 205–222), New York: Plenum Press.

Rao, P., Basil, A. G., Koller, J. M., Fullerton, B., Diener, S., & Burton, P. (1980). The use of American Indian Code by severe aphasic adults. In M. Burns & J. Andrews (Eds.), *Neuropathologies of speech and language diagnosis and treatment: Selected papers.* Evanston, IL: Institute for Continuing Education.

Rattok, J., Ben-Yishay, Y., Ezrachi, O., Lakin, P., Piatsetsky, E., Ross, B., Silver, S., Vakil, E., Zide, E., & Diller, L. (1992). Outcome of different treatment mixes in a multidimensional neuropsychological rehabilitation program. *Neuropsychology, 6,* 395–415.

Rothi, L. J., & Horner, J. (1983). Restitution and substitution: Two theories of recovery with application to neurobehavioral treatment. *Journal of Clinical Neuropsychology, 5,* 73–81.

Schacter, D. L., & Glisky, E. L. (1986). Memory remediation: Restoration, alleviation, and the acquisition of domain specific knowledge. In B. Uzzell & Y. Gross (Eds.), *Clinical neuropsychology of intervention* (pp. 257–282). Boston: Martinus Nijhoff.

Schuell, H., Jenkins, J. J., & Jimenez-Pabon, E. (1964). *Aphasia in adults: Diagnosis, prognosis, and treatment.* New York: Harper & Row.

Silverman, F. H. (1989). *Communication for the speechless: An introduction to augmentative communication for the severely communicatively impaired* (2nd ed.). Englewood Cliffs, NJ: Prentice Hall.

Skelly, M., Schinsky, L., Smith, R. W., & Fust, R. S. (1974). American Indian Sign (Amerind) as a facilitator of verbalization for the oral verbal apraxic. *Journal of Hearing and Speech Disorders, 39,* 445–456.

Sohlberg, M. M., & Mateer, C. A. (1987). Effectiveness of an attention-training program. *Journal of Clinical and Experimental Neuropsychology, 9,* 117–130.

Sohlberg, M. M., & Mateer, C. A. (1989a). *Introduction to cognitive rehabilitation: Theory and practice.* New York: Guilford Press.

Sohlberg, M. M., & Mateer, C. A. (1989b). Training use of compensatory memory books: A three stage behavioral approach. *Journal of Clinical and Experimental Neuropsychology, 11,* 871–891.

Sparks, R. W., & Holland, A. L. (1976). Method: Melodic intonation therapy for aphasia. *Journal of Speech and Hearing Disorders, 41,* 287–297.

Sparks, R., Helm, N., & Albert, M. (1974). Aphasia rehabilitation resulting from melodic intonation therapy. *Cortex, 10,* 303–316.

Volpe, B. T., & McDowell, F. H. (1990). The efficacy of cognitive rehabilitation in patients with traumatic brain injury. *Archives of Neurology, 47,* 220–222.

Von Cramon, D. Y., & Matthes-von Cramon, G. (1990). Frontal lobe dysfunctions in patients—Therapeutical approaches. In R. L. Wood & I. Fussey (Eds.), *Cognitive rehabilitation in perspective* (pp. 164–179). London: Taylor & Francis.

Webster, J. S., & Scott, R. R. (1988). Behavioral assessment and treatment of the brain-injured patient. In M. Hersen, R. M. Eisler, & P. M. Miller (Eds.), *Progress in behavior modification 1988,* Volume 22 (pp. 48–87). Newbury Park, CA: Sage Publications.

Webster, J. S., Jones, S., Blanton, P., Gross, R., Beissell, G. F., & Wofford, J. (1984). Visual scanner training with stroke patients. *Behavior Therapy, 15,* 129–143.

Weinberg, J., Diller, L., Gordon, W., Gerstman, L. J., Lieberman, A., Lakin, P., Hodges, G., & Ezrachi, O. (1977). Visual scanning training effect on reading-related tasks in acquired right brain damage. *Archives of Physical Medicine and Rehabilitation, 58,* 479–486.

Weinberg, J., Piasetsky, E., Diller, L., & Gordon, W. (1982). Treating perceptual organization deficits in nonneglecting RBD stroke patients. *Journal of Clinical Neuropsychology, 4,* 59–75.

Wilson, B. A. (1987). *Rehabilitation of memory.* New York: Guilford Press.

Wilson, B. A. (1989). Coping strategies for memory dysfunction. In E. Perecman (Ed.), *Integrating theory and practice in clinical neuropsychology* (pp. 155–174). Hillsdale, NJ: Laurence Erlbaum Associates.

Wood, R. L. (1987). *Brain injury rehabilitation: A neurobehavioral approach.* Rockville, MD: Aspen.

Young, G. C., Collins, D., & Hren, M. (1983). Effect of pairing scanning training with block design training in the remediation of perceptual problems in left hemiplegics. *Journal of Clinical Neuropsychology, 5,* 201–212.

Zencius, A., Wesolowski, M. D., & Burke, W. H. (1990). A comparison of four memory strategies with traumatically brain-injured clients. *Brain Injury, 4,* 33–38.

Psychotherapy: Individual, Family, and Group

This chapter refers briefly to some of the psychotherapeutic approaches available in treating patients with neurological disorders. Often, an appropriate mix of individual, family, and group therapies is required to provide the patient with maximum benefit. Mention is also made of therapy programs that address pain management and posttraumatic stress disorder (PTSD). A detailed presentation is beyond the scope of this book. The reader is referred to citations in the text for further information.

INDIVIDUAL THERAPY

Patients who are stricken with a neurological disorder may experience anger, depression, anxiety, and loss of self-esteem (Grimm & Bleiberg, 1986). Psychotherapy is often a vital component of patients' rehabilitation. Problems unique to doing therapy with patients with neurological disorders include the necessity of distinguishing between emotional reactions secondary to awareness of altered function and emotional disorders that directly result from a central nervous system (CNS) lesion. For example, the emotional lability sometimes associated with right hemisphere stroke can be very disconcerting to both the patient and the patient's family. An understanding of the physical basis of the lability is essential in this instance. The neuropsychologist–therapist must be able to make this distinction for a variety of neurological disorders.

An understanding of the evolution of emotional concomitants of neurological disorders is also important. For example, emotional distress may increase 6 months after a head injury (Fordyce *et al.,* 1983). Psychotherapy must take into account any intellectual impairments the patient may have due to the neurological disorder. Severe memory deficits, severe apathy, and confusion may limit the applicability of many traditional psychotherapies (Grimm & Bleiberg, 1986).

Regardless of the therapeutic approach and modalities used with the patient, it is important to have an understanding of the psychosocial stress associated with disability and impairment (Burdon, 1990). Cohn (1961) has described a five-stage process of adjustment to disability. In the first stage (Shock), the patient may express disbelief and even deny the existence of the disorder or disability. This may change when the patient becomes aware of the limitations to his or her performance. In the second stage (Expectancy for Recovery), the patient is aware of the disorder, but expects a quick and complete recovery. Total recovery is the only acceptable goal. This expectation may change if recovery does not occur quickly or if the patient leaves the inpatient setting for the community and becomes further aware of the extent of his or her disabilities. In the third stage (Mourning), the patient becomes acutely aware of the seriousness of the disability and feels the loss so deeply that he or she feels that all is lost or hopeless. The patient may experience suicidal ideation or even become actively suicidal. In this stage, the patient may lack motivation and come to be viewed by therapy staff as a problem patient. In the fourth stage (Defense), the patient may be beginning to adjust to disability and may see his or her role as becoming increasingly independent or may fall back into denial. Adjustment is the fifth and final stage. In this stage, the patient feels adequate and can accept the disability as simply one of his or her characteristics. The stages are not invariable and may not always occur in this order. It is important for the therapist to determine the way in which the patient is perceiving his or her disability and attempting to cope. Appropriate therapeutic interventions may then be attempted.

Cognitive–Behavioral, Dynamic, and Supportive Therapies

A variety of cognitive–behavioral methods (Kanfer & Goldstein, 1986) are available to treat numerous problems, symptoms, and syndromes (Bellack *et al.*, 1990; Tarlow, 1989; Tarlow & Maxwell, 1989). Traditional dynamic (Grimm & Bleiberg, 1986) and supportive therapies may also be appropriate for some patients.

Biofeedback

In some cases, patients with neurological disorders may benefit from relaxation training or biofeedback or both. Patients with severe attentional or cognitive deficits may have difficulty in participating in relaxation exercises. If extremely severe attentional–cognitive impairment or agitation is not present and if there are no other contraindications, relaxation training may provide some benefit.

Neurological disorders may involve or be accompanied by multiple systems involvement or multiple injuries. Acute or chronic pain may result from the neurological disorder or these additional involvements. Stress management and biofeedback may be useful in treating some forms of pain (Isele, 1990; Schwartz, 1987). Biofeedback has also been used successfully in neuromuscular reeducation (Fogel, 1987; Krebs, 1987) and in treating headache (Blanchard & Andrasik, 1985) and essential hypertension (Olson & Kroon, 1987). Schwartz (1987) has put together an excellent guide to biofeedback therapy. Numerous specific applications of biofeedback have been reported in *Biofeedback: Principles and Practice for Clinicians* (Basmajian, 1989).

Hypnosis

Hypnosis has been found to be an effective treatment modality for a variety of problems common to some populations of patients with neurological disorders. Pain, anxiety disorders, and addictive disorders have been treated with hypnosis (Hammond, 1990). A variety of theoretical and practical approaches are available (Araoz, 1985; Araoz & Negley-Parker, 1988; Erickson & Rossi, 1979; Golden *et al.*, 1987).

FAMILY THERAPY

In her International Neuropsychology Society presidential address, ''Brain Damage Is a Family Affair,'' Lezak (1988) described the significant emotional and practical burdens that often befall a brain-damaged patient's close family members. Cognitive and behavioral changes in the patient may place substantial stresses on the family system (Rosenthal & Geckler, 1986). The family members may respond with disbelief and denial, anxiety, and depression. Education and family therapy are likely to assist the family in coping with behavioral changes and adapting to the patient's needs (Rosenthal & Geckler, 1986).

Traditional family assessment instruments and therapies may be appropriate when the therapist is knowledgable about the therapy and the behavioral and family problems specific to a given neuropsychiatric disorder. Jacob and Tennenbaum (1988) have reviewed a variety of methods of family assessment. Numerous approaches to family therapy have been developed. A small subset of the theories is as follows: (1) conjoint family therapy (Satir, 1967), systemic family therapy (Hoffman, 1981), structural family therapy (Umbarger, 1983), and psychodynamic family therapy (Ackerman, 1958).

GROUP THERAPY

Group therapy may be an effective therapeutic modality for some brain-damaged patients and their families (Hill & Carper, 1985; Imes, 1984; Sohlberg & Mateer, 1989) and for medical patients in general (Lonergan, 1983). Participation in group therapy allows the patient to see that he or she is not alone, that there are other individuals suffering from the same malady. Patients can share their feelings, provide one another with emotional support, and learn each other's coping skills. If denial is a problem for a patient or a family member, it may not survive the scrutiny of the group. A group setting may also help motivate patients to perform better in therapy activities. Group therapy and activities may help inpatients cope with hospitalization.

Group therapy may not be appropriate for patients with severe acting-out tendencies who may disrupt the group and become further alienated as a result (Grimm & Bleiberg, 1986). Special precautions may have to be taken if the group includes patients who are easily confused, vulnerable to anxiety, or extremely sensitive to feedback.

Yalom (1985) has provided a detailed description of group therapy with both outpatient and inpatient (Yalom, 1983) populations. Some patients may benefit from referral to community self-help groups such as local head-injury or stroke clubs in addition to participation in therapist-led group therapy.

PAIN MANAGEMENT

Acute or chronic pain may be a correlate of neurological disorders. Because pain is a biopsychosocial phenomenon (Karoly & Jensen, 1987), a multimodal approach to pain management is likely to be most effective. Numerous treatment programs have been described (Abram et al., 1990; Hanson & Gerber, 1990; Turk et al., 1983). A thorough overview of the assessment and treatment of chronic pain is available in Chronic Pain (Miller, 1990).

POSTTRAUMATIC STRESS DISORDER (PTSD) TREATMENT

When traumatic injury occurs, PTSD sometimes results (Scrignar, 1988). Studies have suggested that imaginal exposure is an effective treatment for PTSD (Barlow, 1988). Scrignar

(1988) has described a variety of approaches to the treatment of PTSD. Although evidence is sparse (Herbert & Mueser, 1992), preliminary reports suggest that the technique of Eye Movement Desensitization and Reprocessing may be an efficacious treatment model for PTSD (Shapiro, 1991).

REFERENCES

Abram, S. E., Haddox, J. D., & Kettler, R. E. (1990). *The pain clinic manual.* Philadelphia: J. B. Lippincott Co.
Ackerman, N. W. (1958). *The psychodynamics of family life: Diagnosis and treatment of family relationships.* New York: Basic Books.
Araoz, D. L. (1985). *The new hypnosis.* New York: Brunner/Mazel.
Araoz, D. L., & Negley-Parker, E. (1988). *The new hypnosis in family therapy.* New York: Brunner/Mazel.
Barlow, D. H. (1988). *Anxiety and its disorders: The nature and treatment of anxiety and panic.* New York: Guilford Press.
Basmajian, J. V. (Ed.). (1989). *Biofeedback: Principles and practice for clinicians.* Baltimore: Williams & Wilkins.
Bellack, A. S., Hersen, M., & Kazdin, A. E. (Eds.). (1990). *International handbook of behavior modification and therapy* (2nd ed.). New York: Plenum Press.
Blanchard, E. B., & Andrasik, F. (1985). *Management of chronic headaches: A psychological approach.* New York: Pergamon Press.
Burdon, G. (1990). Psychosocial aspects and adjustment during various phases of neurological disability. In D. A. Umphred (Ed.), *Neurological rehabilitation* (pp. 163–180). St. Louis: C. V. Mosby.
Cohn, N. (1961). Understanding the process of adjustment to disability. *Journal of Rehabilitation, 27*(6), 16–22.
Erickson, M. H., & Rossi, E. L. (1979). *Hypnotherapy: An exploratory casebook.* New York: Irvington.
Fogel, E. R. (1987). Biofeedback-assisted musculoskeletal therapy and neuromuscular reeducation. In M. S. Schwartz (Ed.), *Biofeedback: A practitioner's guide* (pp. 377–409). New York: Guilford Press.
Fordyce, D. J., Roueche, J. R., & Prigatano, G. P. (1983). Enhanced emotional reactions in chronic head trauma patients. *Journal of Neurology, Neurosurgery, and Psychiatry, 46,* 620–624.
Golden, W. L., Dowd, E. T., & Friedberg, F. (1987). *Hypnotherapy: A modern approach.* New York: Pergamon Press.
Grimm, B. H., & Bleiberg, J. (1986). Psychological rehabilitation in traumatic brain injury. In S. B. Filskov & T. J. Boll (Eds.), *Handbook of clinical neuropsychology,* Volume 2 (pp. 495–560). New York: Wiley-Interscience.
Hammond, D. C. (Ed.). (1990). *Handbook of hypnotic suggestions and metaphors.* New York: W. W. Norton.
Hanson, R. W., & Gerber, K. E. (1990). *Coping with chronic pain: A guide to patient self-management.* New York: Guilford Press.
Herbert, J. D., & Mueser, K. (1992). Eye movement desensitization: A critique of the evidence. *Journal of Behavior Therapy and Experimental Psychiatry, 23,* 169–174.
Hill, J., & Carper, M. (1985). Greenery: Group therapeutic approaches with the head injured. *Cognitive Rehabilitation, 3,* 18–29.
Hoffman, L. (1981). *Foundations of family therapy.* New York: Basic Books.
Imes, C. (1984). Interventions with stroke patients: EMG biofeedback, group activities, cognitive retraining. *Cognitive Rehabilitation, 2,* 4–17.
Isele, F. W. (1990). Biofeedback and hypnosis: Multifaceted approaches in the management of pain. In T. W. Miller (Ed.), *Chronic pain,* Volume 2 (pp. 489–431). Madison, CT: International Universities Press.
Jacob, T., & Tennenbaum, D. L. (1988). *Family assessment: Rationale, methods, and future directions.* New York: Plenum Press.
Kanfer, F. H., & Goldstein, A. P. (Eds.). (1986). *Helping people change: A textbook of methods* (3rd ed.). New York: Pergamon Press.
Karoly, P., & Jensen, M. P. (1987). *Multimethod assessment of chronic pain.* Oxford: Pergamon Press.
Krebs, D. E. (1987). Biofeedback in neuromuscular re-education and gait training. In M. S. Schwartz (Ed.), *Biofeedback: A practitioner's guide* (pp. 343–376). New York: Guilford Press.
Lezak, M. D. (1988). Brain damage is a family affair. *Journal of Clinical and Experimental Psychology, 10,* 111–123.

Lonergan, E. C. (1983). Groups for medical patients: Coping mechanisms mobilized and revealed. In L. R. Wolberg & M. L. Aronson (Eds.), *Group and family therapy: 1982* (pp. 63–77). New York: Brunner/Mazel.

Miller, T. W. (1990). *Chronic pain,* Volumes 1 & 2. Madison, CT: International Universities Press.

Olson, R. P., & Kroon, J. S. (1987). Biobehavioral treatment of essential hypertension. In M. S. Schwartz (Ed.), *Biofeedback: A practitioner's guide* (pp. 316–339). New York: Guilford Press.

Rosenthal, M., & Geckler, C. (1986). Family therapy issues in neuropsychology. In D. Wedding, A. M. Horton, Jr., & J. Webster (Eds.), *The neuropsychology handbook: Behavioral and clinical perspectives* (pp. 325–344). New York: Springer.

Satir, V. (1967). *Conjoint family therapy* (2nd ed.). Palo Alto, CA: Science and Behavior Books.

Schwartz, M. S. (1987). *Biofeedback: A practitioner's guide.* New York: Guilford Press.

Scrignar, C. B. (1988). *Post-traumatic stress disorder: Diagnosis, treatment, and legal issues* (2nd ed.). New Orleans: Bruno Press.

Shapiro, F. (1991). Eye movement desensitization and reprocessing procedure: From EMD to EMD/R—A new treatment model for anxiety and related trauma. *The Behavior Therapist, 14,* 133–135.

Sohlberg, M. M., & Mateer, C. A. (1989). *Introduction to cognitive rehabilitation: Theory and practice.* New York: Guilford Press.

Tarlow, G. (1989). *Clinical handbook of behavior therapy: Adult medical disorders.* Cambridge, MA: Brookline Books.

Tarlow, G., & Maxwell, A. (1989). *Clinical handbook of behavior therapy: Adult psychological disorders.* Cambridge, MA: Brookline Books.

Turk, D. C., Meichenbaum, D., & Genest, M. (1983). *Pain and behavioral medicine.* New York: Guilford Press.

Umbarger, C. C. (1983). *Structural family therapy.* New York: Grune & Stratton.

Yalom, I. D. (1983). *Inpatient group therapy.* New York: Basic Books.

Yalom, I. D. (1985). *The theory and practice of group psychotherapy* (3rd ed.). New York: Basic Books.

VI

Disorders

Part VI contains brief descriptions of some of the disorders commonly encountered by clinical neuropsychologists. The disorders are analyzed according to the outline presented below.

Description

A brief description is provided.

Incidence and Risk Factors

Incidence is usually given as the number of new cases per 100,000 per year. *Prevalence* is the number of individuals having a disorder (per 100,000) at a given time. Risk factors are also listed.

Etiology and Pathology

The causation and underlying pathology of the disorder are sketched.

Medical Assessment

Some basic medical assessment procedures are reviewed: neurological examination, laboratory findings, CT, MRI, and EEG.

Neuropsychological Assessment

The rationale for neuropsychological assessment is reviewed. Expected results are summarized by functional area: Attention, Memory, Intelligence, Speech/Language, Arithmetic, Visuospatial Functioning, Sensory Functioning, Motor Functioning, Executive Functioning, and Personality. The LNNB is treated separately.

Medical Treatment

Common medical treatments are summarized.

Psychosocial Therapies

Applications of cognitive rehabilitation, behavior therapy, and individual, family, and group psychotherapy are briefly reviewe 1.

Prognosis

The expected cognitive and physical outcome is summarized.
For some disorders, subclasses of the disorder are identified with further subheadings.

Closed Head Injury

DESCRIPTION

Closed head injury is an acceleration–deceleration injury to the brain that may result in a loss of consciousness. Closed head injuries are contrasted with open head injuries such as penetrating missile injuries of the brain.

Severe closed head injury is associated with a Glasgow Coma Scale (GCS) of 0–8 and a posttraumatic amnesia (PTA) of greater than 1 day (Bond, 1986; W. R. Russell, 1932).

Moderate closed head injury is associated with a GCS of 9–12 and PTA of 1–24 hr (Bond, 1986; W. R. Russell, 1932).

Mild closed head injury is an acceleration–deceleration injury to the brain that results in a loss of consciousness of less than 20 min., a GCS of 13–15 on hospital admission, and PTA of less than 1 hr (Bond, 1986; Rimel *et al.,* 1981; W. R. Russell, 1932; Rutherford, 1989).

INCIDENCE AND RISK FACTORS

Closed Head Injury

Gender

The ratio of males to females is approximately 2:1, with the greatest difference in the age range 15–24 years (Rimel *et al.,* 1990).

Age

The incidence of head injury has been found to be greatest for the age ranges 10–30 and 75 and over (Rimel *et al.,* 1990).

External Causes

The majority of head-injured patients have been involved in motor vehicle accidents, with falls being the second major category (Rimel *et al.,* 1990). This proportion varies somewhat with location and culture.

Previous Head Injuries

Individuals who have sustained a head injury are at a greater risk of incurring a subsequent head injury. Annegers *et al.* (1980) found that after a head injury, the incidence of a second head injury was 3 times that of a first head injury. After a second head injury, the incidence was 8 times that of a first head injury.

Alcohol Use

Alcohol consumption has been implicated as a risk factor for head injury (Rimel & Jane, 1983).

Mild Closed Head Injury

Gender

The ratio of males to females is approximately 2:1, except for the very young and those over 45 (Kraus and Nourjah, 1989; Rimel *et al.,* 1981). Kraus and Nourjah (1989) found a rate of 175 males and 85 females per 100,000 with an overall incidence of 131/100,000 for hospitals in San Diego County, California.

Age

The average age was 27 for a sample of central Virginia residents (Rimel *et al.,* 1981). Mildly head-injured subjects over 50 years sometimes exhibit severe neuropsychological sequelae (Mazzucchi *et al.,* 1992).

External Causes

In the San Diego study (Kraus & Nourjah, 1989), 42% involved a motor vehicle accident (MVA), 23% were due to falls, 13% to assaults, 6% to non-MVA bicycle accidents, and 6% to sports and recreation activities. These proportions vary somewhat with location. Assault was found to be the predominant cause of mild head injury (31%) in the Bronx (Levin *et al.,* 1987c).

Previous Head Injuries

Rimel *et al.* (1981) reported that 31% of their series had been hospitalized previously for head injuries.

Alcohol Use

Rimel *et al.* (1981) reported that 35% of their series had a blood alcohol level greater than the level of legal intoxication.

ETIOLOGY AND PATHOLOGY

Severe Head Injury

Local damage may occur at the site of the impact (J. D. Miller *et al.*, 1990). It may take the form of a contusion or laceration. Edema may occur in the area, resulting in swelling and a space-occupying lesion. When the head is subjected to acceleration–deceleration, the brain can impact against the walls of the anterior and middle cranial fossae, and contusion or laceration damage to the tips and undersurface of the temporal and frontal lobes, may occur. Hemorrhage may occur, resulting in intracranial mass lesions. Shearing of axons within their myelin sheaths may occur. Coma may result from impairment of function in the reticular activating system in the brainstem. A number of secondary factors can affect the injured brain—arterial hypoxemia and hypotension, anemia, hyponatremia, intracranial infection, cerebral arterial vasospasm, hydrocephalus, and posttraumatic epilepsy. Posttraumatic epilepsy may affect about 5% of head-injured patients. A variety of factors are predictive of risk for posttraumatic epilepsy (Bennett, 1987b).

In addition to brain injury, head injury may result in injury to cranial nerves (Narayan *et al.*, 1990). The head-injury survivor may also suffer multitrauma such as injuries to a variety of organ systems, spinal cord, or orthopedic injuries (Griffith & Mayer, 1990; Horn & Garland, 1990).

Mild Head Injury

Axonal injury is a consistent feature of mild to moderate head injury (Povlishock & Coburn, 1989). A small proportion (1–3%) of patients develop potentially serious intracranial sequelae such as subdural or epidural hematomas (Dacey, 1989).

MEDICAL ASSESSMENT

Severe Head Injury

Late CT scans may detect ventricular enlargement (Van Dongen & Braakman, 1980). Ventricular enlargement, when detected at least 1 month after injury, has been related to disability and to impaired cognitive and memory functioning (Levin *et al.*, 1981; Meyers *et al.*, 1983). MRI appears to be significantly more sensitive to the brain damage resulting from head injury. In a sample of mild to moderate closed head-injured patients, Levin *et al.* (1987b) found 85% to have lesions that were visualized by MRI but undetected by CT.

Although CT may be less sensitive than MRI, CT may be more useful in evaluation of the acutely head-injured patient (Ruff *et al.*, 1989a). Acutely head-injured patients may have metallic surgical clips or shunts that rule out exposure to a strong magnetic field. If the patient is confused or agitated, he or she may not remain motionless for the longer image-acquisition time required by MRI. CT scan is sufficiently sensitive to detect mass lesions warranting neurosurgical intervention (Luerssen *et al.*, 1986).

Mild Head Injury

Since neurosurgical complications are unusual in patients who have sustained mild concussive injuries, most physicians rely on a period of close observation. However, patients who have altered levels of consciousness, neurological deficits, or open or penetrating injuries are commonly admitted to the hospital for further treatment and evaluation. Alternative criteria for hospitalization and CT scans have been reviewed by Dacey (1989). Abnormal CT findings are associated with older age, white race, signs of basilar skull fracture, and being either a pedestrian hit by a motor vehicle or a victim of an assault (Jeret *et al.*, 1993).

NEUROPSYCHOLOGICAL ASSESSMENT

Severe Head Injury

Neuropsychological assessment of head injury varies depending on the severity of the head injury and the stage of recovery. Patients with severe to moderate head injuries generally progress through a series of stages. The Rancho Los Amigos Scale of Cognitive Levels (RLASCL) defines eight levels of cognitive functioning (Adamovich *et al.*, 1985; Malkmus *et al.*, 1980):

Level I (no response)—unresponsive to all stimuli

Level II (generalized responses)—inconsistent and nonspecific responses

Level III (localized responses)—inconsistent responses directly related to the stimulus

Level IV (confused–agitated)—disoriented, inappropriate, agitated, and sometimes aggressive behavior

Level V (confused, inappropriate nonagitated)—distractible, responds to simple commands

Level VI (confused–appropriate)—inconsistently oriented, appropriate responses to simple commands

Level VII (automatic–appropriate)—appropriate and oriented in hospital and home, impaired insight, judgment, and emotional control

Level VIII (purposeful–appropriate)—oriented, learns new material, impaired tolerance for stress

Although there is great variability in severity and type of head injury and all do not progress through these stages, the RLASCL has provided rehabilitation team members with a conceptualization of head injury and a means for interdisciplinary communication.

Cripe (1987) has distinguished four phases of recovery: (1) loss of consciousness, (2) posttraumatic amnestic phase, (3) rapid recovery phase, and (4) long-term plateau stage. During the coma phase (RLASCL I–III), progress is monitored with the GCS (Teasdale & Jennett, 1974). The GCS rates coma depth on the basis of degree of eye-opening, best motor response, and best verbal response.

During the PTA phase (RLASCL IV and V), progress may be monitored with brief mental status evaluations such as the MMSE, NCSE, or GOAT. Behavior checklists may also assist in monitoring patients' problems and progress. Behavior observation may be used in designing behavior modification programs.

During the rapid recovery phase (RLASCL VI and VII), a comprehensive neuropsychological evaluation can provide detailed information about deficits and strengths essential for rehabilitation planning (Dikmen, 1989). Further issues that might also be addressed are likely long-term behavioral outcome, behavioral changes resulting from interventions or complications, living situation at discharge, and likely vocational options (Dikmen, 1989).

When recovery has stabilized (long-term plateau stage), comprehensive neuropsychological assessment may be performed to predict long-term residual effects of head injury (Cripe, 1987, 1989).

A variety of posttraumatic headaches may occur following head injury (Bennett, 1988).

Orientation

Orientation during recovery is commonly tracked using the GOAT (Levin *et al.*, 1982).

Attention

Self-report inventories often reveal reduced concentration. At 6 months after severe head injury, McKinlay *et al.* (1983) found 40% of patients reporting impaired concentration. At 12 months, the percentage dropped to 9%. Relatives, however, reported the incidence of problems of concentration to be 25%.

DS, especially DS Backwards, may be impaired both early and later in recovery (Bigler *et al.*, 1981; Drudge *et al.*, 1984). DSym is also likely to be impaired (Bigler *et al.*, 1981; Drudge *et al.*, 1984).

Performance on the PASAT is impaired (Gronwall & Sampson, 1974; O'Shaughnessy *et al.*, 1984; Stuss *et al.*, 1989). Peck and Mitchell (1990) found the PASAT unable to distinguish mild, moderate, and severe head-injury patients. They attributed this result to the extreme sensitivity of the PASAT to brain injury. Slowing is found on the SCWT, but a specific effect is not expected on the interference trial (Stuss *et al.*, 1985; Van Zomeren, 1981). Choice reaction time appears to be more sensitive to head injury than simple reaction time (Van Zomeren, 1981).

General Intelligence and Social Understanding

Performance may be impaired on any or all subscales of the WAIS or WAIS-R. I- and C-WAIS may be impaired (Bigler *et al.*, 1981; Drudge *et al.*, 1984). FSIQ, VIQ, PIQ, and PA-WAIS may be impaired both early and late in recovery (Bigler *et al.*, 1981; Drudge *et al.*, 1984). PIQ is generally depressed more after head injury than VIQ, but this discrepancy diminishes over the first year (Mandleberg, 1975; Mandleberg & Brooks, 1975), although this diminution may not hold in cases of acute aphasia (Levin *et al.*, 1979). WAIS-R FSIQ, VIQ, and PIQ may distinguish mild, moderate, and severe head-injury patients (Peck & Mitchell, 1990).

Memory

Memory is one of the cognitive domains most sensitive to closed head injury (Capruso & Levin, 1992). Performance on the ACT is impaired (Stuss *et al.*, 1985, 1989). Crosson *et al.* (1989) were able to divide subjects into three nearly equal groups on the basis of CVLT performance. Groups were defined on the basis of having made: (1) decreased correct recognitions and increased false recognitions, (2) decreased correct recognitions and normal false recognitions, or (3) normal correct and false recognitions. Paniak *et al.* (1989) found SRT performance impaired within 6 months and after more than 1 year. A preponderance of random long-term retrieval vs. consistent long-term retrieval was noted. Performance on the WMS-R may be impaired on all indexes (Wechsler, 1987). ROCFT:M may distinguish mild, moderate, and severe head-injury patients (Peck & Mitchell, 1990). The RAVLT may distinguish mild, moderate, and severe head-injury patients on the fifth learning trial and on the delayed recall trial (Peck & Mitchell, 1990).

Speech/Language

Impairment may be noted on the SR and SSPT (Drudge *et al.*, 1984). V- and S-WAIS may be impaired (Bigler *et al.*, 1981; Drudge *et al.*, 1984).

Arithmetic

A-WAIS may be impaired early in recovery (Bigler *et al.*, 1981; Drudge *et al.*, 1984).

Visuospatial Functioning

Performance is slowed on TMTA early and later in recovery (Bigler *et al.*, 1981; Drudge *et al.*, 1984; Peck & Mitchell, 1990; Stuss *et al.*, 1989). PC-, BD-, and OA-WAIS may be impaired (Bigler *et al.*, 1981; Drudge *et al.*, 1984). ROCFT:C may distinguish mild, moderate, and severe head-injury patients (Peck & Mitchell, 1990).

Sensory Functioning

Impairment may be noted on the RKSPE, excluding Tactile Form Recognition (Bigler *et al.*, 1981; Drudge *et al.*, 1984). TPT performance may be impaired for Time, Memory, and Location (Drudge *et al.*, 1984).

Motor Functioning

Performance may be impaired on the FTT both early and later in recovery (Bigler *et al.*, 1981; Drudge *et al.*, 1984) and on GS (Drudge *et al.*, 1984). GP may distinguish mild, moderate, and severe head-injury patients (Peck & Mitchell, 1990).

Executive Functioning

Performance may be impaired on the TMTB (Drudge *et al.*, 1984; Peck & Mitchell, 1990; Stuss *et al.*, 1989) and on the Halstead CT (Bigler *et al.*, 1981; Drudge *et al.*, 1984). Increased perseverative errors are expected on the WCST (Stuss, 1987). The COWAT may distinguish mild, moderate, and severe head-injured patients (Peck & Mitchell, 1990). The RFFT is impaired in head-injured patients. It may distinguish moderately from severely head-injured patients (Ruff *et al.*, 1986).

Halstead Impairment Index

Impairment may be noted both early and late in recovery (Drudge *et al.*, 1984).

Personality

A variety of personality disturbances are common after brain injury: (1) anxiety and catastrophic reaction, (2) denial of illness, (3) paranoia, (4) psychomotor, (5) agitation, and (6) depression and social withdrawal (Parker, 1990; Prigatano, 1987). In the early stages of brain injury, the patient may be confused, restless, agitated, and combative and may have limited insight and exhibit paranoid ideation. Preexisting personality traits may contribute to paranoid ideation. As their recovery progresses, patients often underestimate their residual neuropsychological deficits and may attempt to return to work or social activities. They may tend to acknowledge their physical symptoms but deny cognitive or functional disability (Cicerone, 1989). Failure and social rejection may lead to depression and social withdrawal. Although depression is common after head injury, it is not necessarily directly related to the severity of brain injury or the level of neuropsychological impairment (Prigatano, 1987). Social withdrawal may be related to severity of injury (Levin & Grossman, 1978) and neuropsychological impairment (Prigatano, 1985, 1987). Amotivational states and lack of initiation may result from bilateral frontal lobe dysfunction. Although amotivational states are often viewed by rehabilitation staff as a disturbance in feeling states, they may be due to an impairment in the cognitive ability to form and initiate plans.

Self-awareness may be impaired after head injury (Prigatano, 1991). Emotional dysphoria has been found to be positively correlated with awareness of sensory and cognitive change (Gasquoine, 1992).

Studies of head-injured patients' performance on the MMPI have yielded inconsistent results. Dikmen and Reitan (1977) found elevations on Scales 1, 2, 3, 7, and 8 more likely for severely head-injured patients than for mildly head-injured patients. In contrast, Novack *et al.* (1984) found mildly head-injured patients to be more likely than severely head-injured patients to exhibit elevations on Scales 1 and 3. Gass and Russell (1991) found that neurologically related items had significant effects on Scales 1, 2, 3, 7, and 8. They recommended the use of the Harris–Lingoes subscales to determine the symptomatic areas that contribute to scores on the basic clinical scales.

On the Katz Adjustment Scale—Relatives Form (Hogarty & Katz, 1971), ratings of moderately head-injured patients by relatives exhibited elevations on the subscales verbal expansiveness, helplessness, suspiciousness, anxiety, withdrawal and retardation, psychopathology, confusion, and bizarreness (Stambrook *et al.,* 1990). In addition to these scales, for severely head-injured patients, there were also elevations on belligerence, negativism, nervousness, and hyperactivity.

The Behavior Change Inventory (Hartlage, 1989), which may be completed by the patient or a significant other, may provide useful information about behavior changes pre–post injury.

Mild Head Injury

Following mild head injury, patients report a variety of complaints—headaches, fatigue, dizziness, sensitivity to bright light and noise, insomnia, difficulty concentrating, irritability, memory difficulties, and anxiety. Headaches may occur in 30–90% of patients (Evans, 1992). Dikmen *et al.* (1986) found mildly head-injured patients to endorse complaints of "bothered by noise," "insomnia," and "memory difficulties" significantly more than controls. In a three-center study, Levin *et al.* (1987c) ranked postconcussional symptoms according to frequency: (1) headaches, (2) fatigability, (3) dizziness, (4) sleep, (5) recent memory, (6) depression, (7) anxiety, (8) appetite, (9) thinking, (10) concentration, (11) blurred vision, (12) coordination, (13) noise sensitivity, (14) patience, and (15) vertigo (Levin *et al.,* 1987c). Patients often complain of symptoms more numerous and more severe than those found on neuropsychological testing.

Although some cognitive impairment may be noted in the first week after a mild head injury, for most patients, little impairment is expected at 1 month (Levin *et al.,* 1987a). A subset of mildly head-injured patients may exhibit continued impairment (Leininger *et al.,* 1990). In some patients, deficits in attention and information processing may be noted on complex and demanding tasks 6 months after uncomplicated mild head injury (Bohnen *et al.,* 1992). Short periods of PTA are unreliably reported and difficult to assess (Gronwall & Wrightson, 1980).

Orientation

At 3 days postinjury, impairment may be noted on the GOAT orientation items (McLean *et al.,* 1983).

Attention

Performance on the SR exhibited significant impairment relative to controls at 1 month but not at 1 year postinjury (Dikmen *et al.,* 1986, 1989). DS, DSym-WAIS-R, and PASAT may be impaired within 1 week but not at 1 month (Levin *et al.,* 1987a). Gentilini *et al.* (1989) found impaired performance on a distributed attention task at both 1 and 3 months. Older motor vehicle accident victims who continue to complain of symptoms may exhibit impairment on the PASAT (Leininger *et al.,* 1990).

Memory

Mild head-injury patients rarely exhibit significant retrograde amnesia (Ruff *et al.,* 1989b). Retrograde amnesia rarely extends over 30 min. (W. R. Russell & Nathan, 1946). ACT performance is likely to be impaired, especially in the first 2 weeks after injury (Stuss *et al.,* 1989). Performance on the WMS may not be impaired (Dikmen *et al.,* 1986). SRT may be impaired at 3 days postinjury, but not at 1 month, on Sum Recall, Sum Long-Term Retrieval, Sum Long-Term Storage, Sum Consistent Long-Term Retrieval, Immediate Recall, and Immediate Recognition (McLean *et al.,* 1983). Impairment has been found on the SRT (4-hr delayed recall) at 1 month, but not at 1 year, postinjury (Dikmen *et al.,* 1986, 1989). Otherwise, no impairment is expected on the SRT at 1 month (Gentilini *et al.,* 1985). Older motor vehicle accident victims who continue to complain of symptoms may exhibit impairment on the RAVLT (Leininger *et al.,* 1990). Impairment within 1 week but not at 1 month is expected on the BVRT:A (Levin *et al.,* 1987a). Older motor vehicle accident victims who continue to complain of symptoms may exhibit impairment on the ROCF:M (Leininger *et al.,* 1990). Impairments on the ROCF:M and CVLT have been reported by Zappala and Trexler (1992).

Speech/Language

Vocabulary is not likely to exhibit impairment (Leininger *et al.,* 1990).

Visuospatial Functioning

No impairment is expected on the TMTA (Stuss *et al.,* 1989) or on RPM (Gentilini *et al.,* 1985). Older motor vehicle accident victims who continue to complain of symptoms may exhibit impairment on the ROCF:C (Leininger *et al.,* 1990).

Sensory Functioning

No impairment is expected on the SSPT or the TPT (Dikmen *et al.*, 1986).

Motor Functioning

Motor functioning (FTT) is generally not compromised in mild head injury (Dikmen *et al.*, 1986).

Executive Functioning

No impairment is expected on the TMTB (Stuss *et al.*, 1989) or the CT (Dikmen *et al.*, 1986). Older motor vehicle accident victims who continue to complain of symptoms may exhibit impairment on the CT (Leininger *et al.*, 1990).

Personality

Emotional problems may arise for a variety of reasons. Patients who have experienced only minimal or no loss of consciousness and have received a minimal evaluation and little or no explanation of their symptoms may experience increased emotional distress and the feeling that they are ''losing their mind'' (O'Hara, 1988). Since the patient is usually experiencing less obvious impairments in cognitive functioning, he or she may attempt to return to work prematurely and experience performance difficulties and lack of understanding from work associates, family, and friends. The patient's relatively intact self-awareness can result in a greater emotional response to problems in attention, memory, fatigue, and emotional dyscontrol. O'Hara (1988) has identified symptom clusters: (1) Depression/''Paralysis''—feeling that self has changed but not understanding; (2) Anger/Blame—hostility, refusal of assistance; (3) Denial/Defensiveness; (4) Somatization; (5) Regression/Dependency—patient takes on dependent role and avoids risk-taking; and (6) Psychotic Disintegration. PTSD may sometimes be present (Davidoff *et al.*, 1988).

MEDICAL TREATMENT

Severe Head Injury

Acute management of head injury may require assisted ventilation, treatment of raised intracranial pressure via osmotic therapy (mannitol) or sedative therapy, and treatment of hyperthermia, hypertension, and tachycardia (J. D. Miller *et al.*, 1990). Indications for surgical treatment are to: (1) provide relief from brain compression due, for example, to an intracranial hematoma; (2) prevent infection by debridement and lavage of compound wounds; and (3) insert a device for monitoring intracranial pressure (J. D. Miller *et al.*, 1990).

PSYCHOSOCIAL THERAPIES

Severe Head Injury

Cognitive Rehabilitation

Rehabilitation of attention and memory impairments has been demonstrated to be successful in some studies. Programs are available for remediating visuospatial impairment, problem-solving deficits, and impairments in executive functioning. These programs are reviewed in Chapter 35.

Behavior Modification

Techniques of behavior modification are often employed with head-injured patients, especially in the early stages of recovery. These techniques are reviewed in Chapter 34.

Individual Psychotherapy

Individual therapy must take into account the profile of personality disturbances exhibited by the patient and the relationship of any personality disturbances to organic impairment. Cognitive impairments must be taken into account and may be treated in the course of psychotherapy. Suggestions must often be concrete, simplified, and directive. Patients with impaired attention, concentration, and memory may benefit by summarizing the main points of therapy sessions and by taking notes (Carberry & Burd, 1986; L. Miller, 1993). Patients who exhibit rigidity and inflexibility may benefit from practice in brainstorming and in constructing lists of alternatives. If empathy is impaired, the patient can be asked to verbalize the feelings of others.

Acquisition of insight into impairments that affect social and vocational performance is often a necessary step in learning how to adapt to, overcome, and compensate for impairments. Denial may be treated by providing patients with feedback about their impairments. Patients may resist "lectures" on their shortcomings. Failures in cognitive rehabilitation, in simulated situations, and in real-life situations may be more instructive. Insight into deficits may, in turn, result in anxiety, depression, withdrawal, or a "catastrophic reaction."

A variety of special supports may be required in returning to work or school (D. Russell & Sharratt, 1992). Since head injury may result in sexual dysfunction, assessment and treatment may be indicated (Blackerby, 1990; Kreutzer & Zasler, 1989).

Group Therapy

Group therapy may provide patients with insight into their problems and support from others facing similar challenges. A group setting can be used as a context for learning the use of a diary as a memory prosthesis (Sloan et al., 1989) and for practice in problem-solving (Foxx & Bittle, 1989) (see Chapter 36).

Family Therapy

The traumatic brain injury of a family member often disrupts the family and results in severe distress for family members (Lezak, 1988; Oddy et al., 1978; Thomsen, 1974). Personality changes may be most disturbing to the family. Care-takers may feel trapped and family members isolated (Lezak, 1978). The spouse's needs for companionship and affection may not be met. The family may go through stages in response to the patient's head injury: (1) shock—the family members may feel severe psychological distress, anger, frustration, confusion, and helplessness when faced with the moment-to-moment possibility of the patient's death; (2) elation—when the patient is out of immediate medical danger, an experience of relief may follow; (3) reality—the family begins to realize that many of the patient's impairments may persist and experiences a sense of loss; (4) crisis—the family experiences stress in making a long-term adaptation to caring for the patient at home; and (5) mourning and redefining the relationship—the family mourns the loss of the patient's pre–traumatic brain injury personality and acceptance of the new individual begins (Spanbock, 1987).

Lezak (1978) suggests that relatives often need to understand that the feelings of anger, frustration, and sorrow are natural emotions. If they are direct care-takers for the patient, they may need to give themselves permission to take care of themselves. Counseling may be required to assist the family in coping with role changes in the family and changes in the patient.

The family's behavior at the bedside may be misleading. To keep up appearances, family members may exhibit the "command performance syndrome" and refrain from displaying emotion when interacting with the patient or health care professionals in the rehabilitation setting (Sbordone *et al.,* 1984).

The participation of the family in the recovery process can be helpful for all involved. A handout should be available for families describing traumatic brain injury, the recovery process, and ways in which family members can participate. At RLASCL I and II, the family should be briefed on the coma. They can make an effort to make contact by talking to the patient in normal conversational tones about familiar things. At Level III, the family can to continue provide reassurance and assist in orienting the patient. Families are usually upset when they see the often bizarre and confused behavior typical of Level IV. They will usually benefit from an in-depth explanation of the patient's behavior. The family should be advised to keep the patient's environment quiet and calm, speak in simple, short phrases, and gently orient the patient. At Levels V and VI, the family can continue to take an active role in assisting in orientation, in regaining remote memories, and in relearning previous skills. At Levels VII and VIII, the family can support the patient in attending therapies, support him or her in coping with lost abilities, and encourage completion of "homework" assignments such as note-taking. Family members may be trained to assist in the patient's cognitive rehabilitation (Anderson & Parente, 1985).

Head Injury—The Facts (Gronwall *et al.,* 1990) may be useful for families. The *Brain Injury Glossary* (Lehmkuhl, 1993) may be useful to both family and health professionals. It may be helpful to refer the family to the local head-injury self-help group and to the National Head Injury Foundation, 333 Turnpike Road, Southborough, MA 01772.

Mild Head Injury

Individual Therapy

Education about the pathophysiology, the neuropsychological consequences, and the normal course of spontaneous recovery of mild brain injury is an important part of therapy (Bennett, 1987a). If specific organic impairments in personality functioning are noted, methods used for treating these problems in cases of more severe head injury may be applied. Cognitive rehabilitation may be prescribed for specific cognitive deficits. Bennett (1987a) points out that a mild head injury may offer the patient an opportunity for personal growth. During recovery, the patient may have an opportunity to assess his or her values, goals, and life directions. Being a head-injury survivor and having experienced loss, the patient may feel more sensitive to the needs of others.

Group Therapy

Group therapy with six to eight participants may assist patients to validate their experiences, to regain feelings of self-worth, and to exercise social skills (Bennett, 1987a). Neuropsychology, emotional changes, and social consequences of mild head injury, ways to cope with loss of cognitive ability, social alienation, and anger control may be covered in group.

PROGNOSIS

Severe Head Injury

Mortality is inversely related to the GCS during the first 24 hr after injury and directly related to duration of loss of consciousness. Mortality is higher for older patients.

Rate of recovery of intellectual functioning is greatest during the first 3 months. It decreases by the end of the first year. In contrast, emotional and behavioral problems may increase from 3 to 12 months after injury and may continue to increase (Richardson, 1990).

Variables related to return to work include duration of coma or PTA, age, previous personality, personality changes, posttraumatic epilepsy, and age.

Mild Head Injury

Increasing age is associated with poorer outcome (Rutherford *et al.*, 1977, 1979; Wrightson & Gronwall, 1981). Outcome is poorer with a previous head injury (Gronwall & Wrightson, 1975). Gronwall and Wrightson (1975) found that young adults sustaining a second mild head injury exhibited a greater reduction in information-processing rate and recovered more slowly than individuals who had sustained their first head injury. Higher socioeconomic status is associated with increased return to employment (Rimel *et al.*, 1981). Short periods of PTA are difficult to assess and are not a consistent predictor of symptomatology and disability (Wrightson & Gronwall, 1981).

REFERENCES

Adamovich, B. B., Henderson, J. A., & Auerbach, S. (1985). *Cognitive rehabilitation of closed head injured patients: A dynamic approach.* San Diego: College-Hill Press.

Anderson, J., & Parente, F. (1985). Training family members to work with the head injured patient. *Cognitive Rehabilitation, 3*(4), 12–15.

Annegers, J. F., Grabow, J. D., Kurland, L. T., & Laws, E. R. (1980). The incidence, causes, and secular trends of head trauma in Olmstead County, Minnesota, 1935–1974. *Neurology, 30*, 912–919.

Bennett, T. L. (1987a). Neuropsychological counseling of the adult with minor head injury. *Cognitive Rehabilitation, 5*(1), 10–16.

Bennett, T. L. (1987b). Post-traumatic epilepsy: Its nature and implications for head injury recovery. *Cognitive Rehabilitation, 6*(5), 14–18.

Bennett, T. L. (1988). Post-traumatic headaches: Subtypes and behavioral treatments. *Cognitive Rehabilitation, 7*(2), 34–39.

Bigler, E. D., Steinman, D. R., & Newton, J. S. (1981). Clinical assessment of cognitive deficit in neurologic disorder. II. Cerebral trauma. *Clinical Neuropsychology, 3*, 13–18.

Blackerby, W. F. (1990). A treatment model for sexuality disturbance following brain injury. *Journal of Head Trauma Rehabilitation, 5*, 73–82.

Bohnen, M. D., Jolles, J., & Twijnstra, A. (1992). Neuropsychological deficits in patients with persistent symptoms six months after head injury. *Neurosurgery, 30*, 692–696.

Bond, M. R. (1986). Neurobehavioral sequelae of closed head injury. In I. Grant & K. M. Adams (Eds.), *Neuropsychological assessment of neuropsychiatric disorders* (pp. 347–373). New York: Oxford University Press.

Capruso, D. X., & Levin, H. S. (1992). Cognitive impairment following closed head injury. In R. W. Evans (Ed.), *The neurology of trauma* (pp. 879–893). Philadelphia: W. B. Saunders.

Carberry, H., & Burd, B. (1986). Individual psychotherapy with the brain injured adult. *Cognitive Rehabilitation, 4*(4), 22–24.

Cicerone, K. D. (1989). Psychotherapeutic interventions with traumatically brain-injured patients. *Rehabilitation Psychology, 34,* 105–114.

Cripe, L. I. (1987). The neuropsychological assessment and management of closed head injury: General guidelines. *Cognitive Rehabilitation, 5*(1), 18–22.

Cripe, L. I. (1989). Neuropsychological and psychosocial assessment of the brain-injured person: Clinical concepts and guidelines. *Rehabilitation Psychology, 34,* 93–100.

Crosson, B., Novack, T. A., Trenerry, M. R., & Craig, P. L. (1989). Differentiation of verbal memory deficits in blunt head injury using the recognition trial of the California Verbal Learning Test: An exploratory study. *The Clinical Neuropsychologist, 3,* 29–44.

Dacey, R. G. (1989). Complications after apparently mild head injury and strategies of neurosurgical management. In H. S. Levin, H. M. Eisenberg, & A. L. Benton (Eds.), *Mild head injury* (pp. 83–101). New York: Oxford University Press.

Davidoff, D. A., Laibstain, D. F., Kessler, H. R., & Mark, V. H. (1988). Neurobehavioral sequelae of minor head injury: A consideration of post-concussive syndrome versus post-traumatic stress. *Cognitive Rehabilitation, 6*(2), 8–13.

Dikmen, S. (1989). Response to "Neuropsychological and psychosocial assessment of the brain-injured person: Clinical concepts and guidelines." *Rehabilitation Psychology, 34,* 101–103.

Dikmen, S., & Reitan, R. (1977). Emotional sequelae of head injury. *Annals of Neurology, 2,* 492–494.

Dikmen, S., McLean, A., & Temkin, N. (1986). Neuropsychological and psychosocial consequences of minor head injury. *Journal of Neurology, Neurosurgery, and Psychiatry, 49,* 1227–1232.

Dikmen, S., Temkin, N., & Armsden, G. (1989). Neuropsychological recovery: Relationship to psychosocial functioning and postconcussional complaints. In H. S. Levin, H. M. Eisenberg, & A. L. Benton (Eds.), *Mild head injury* (pp. 229–241). New York: Oxford University Press.

Drudge, O. W., Williams, J. M., Kessler, M., & Gomes, F. B. (1984). Recovery from severe closed head injuries: Repeat testings with the Halstead–Reitan Neuropsychological Battery. *Journal of Clinical Psychology, 40,* 259–265.

Evans, R. W. (1992). The postconcussion syndrome and the sequelae of mild head injury. In R. W. Evans (Ed.), *The neurology of trauma* (pp. 815–847). Philadelphia: W. B. Saunders.

Foxx, R. M., & Bittle, R. G. (1989). *Thinking it through: Teaching problem-solving strategy for community living.* Champaign, IL: Research Press.

Gasquoine, P. G. (1992). Affective state and awareness of sensory and cognitive effects after closed head injury. *Neuropsychology, 6,* 187–196.

Gass, C. S., & Russell, E. W. (1991). MMPI profiles of closed head trauma patients: Impact of neurologic complaints. *Journal of Clinical Psychology, 47,* 253–260.

Gentilini, M., Nichelli, P., Schoenhuber, R., Bortolotti, P., Tonelli, L., Falasca, A., & Merli, G. A. (1985). Neuropsychological evaluation of mild head injury. *Journal of Neurology, Neurosurgery, and Psychiatry, 48,* 137–140.

Gentilini, M., Nichelli, P., & Schoenhuber, R. (1989). Assessment of attention in mild head injury. In H. S. Levin, H. M. Eisenberg, & A. L. Benton (Eds.), *Mild head injury* (pp. 163–175). New York: Oxford University Press.

Griffith, E. R., & Mayer, N. H. (1990). Hypertonicity and movement disorders. In M. Rosenthal, M. R. Bond, E. R. Griffith, & J. D. Miller (Eds.), *Rehabilitation of the adult and child with traumatic brain injury* (2nd ed.) (pp. 127–147). Philadelphia: F. A. Davis.

Gronwall, D., & Sampson, H. (1974). *The psychological effects of concussion.* Auckland: Oxford University Press.

Gronwall, D., & Wrightson, P. (1975). Cumulative effect of concussion. *Lancet, 2,* 995–997.

Gronwall, D., & Wrightson, P. (1980). Duration of post-traumatic amnesia after mild head injury. *Journal of Clinical Neuropsychology, 2,* 51–60.

Gronwall, D., Wrightson, P., & Waddell, P. (1990). *Head injury—The facts: A guide for families and care givers.* Oxford: Oxford University Press.

Hartlage, L. C. (1989). *Behavior change inventory.* Brandon, VT: Clinical Psychology Publishing.

Hogarty, G. E., & Katz, M. M. (1971). Norms of adjustment and social behavior. *Archives of General Psychiatry, 25,* 470–480.

Horn, L. J., & Garland, D. E. (1990). Medical orthopedic complications associated with traumatic brain injury. In M. Rosenthal, M. R. Bond, E. R. Griffith, & J. D. Miller (Eds.), *Rehabilitation of the adult and child with traumatic brain injury* (2nd ed.) (pp. 107–126). Philadelphia: F. A. Davis.

Jeret, J. S., Mandell, M., Anziska, B., Lipitz, M., Vilceus, A. P., Ware, J. A., & Zesiewicz, T. A. (1993). Clinical predictors of abnormality disclosed by computed tomography after mild head trauma. *Neurosurgery, 32,* 9–16.

Kraus, J. F., & Nourjah, P. (1989). The epidemiology of mild head injury. In H. S. Levin, H. M. Eisenberg, & A. L. Benton (Eds.), *Mild head injury* (pp. 8–22). New York: Oxford University Press.

Kreutzer, J. S., & Zasler, N. D. (1989). Psychosocial consequences of traumatic brain injury: Methodology and preliminary findings. *Brain Injury, 3,* 177–186.

Lehmkuhl, L. D. (Ed.) (1993). *Brain injury glossary.* Houston: HDI Publishers.

Leininger, B. E., Gramling, S. E., Farrell, A. D., Kreutzer, J. S., & Peck, E. A. (1990). Neuropsychological deficits in symptomatic minor head injury patients after concussion and mild concussion. *Journal of Neurology, Neurosurgery, and Psychiatry, 53,* 293–296.

Levin, H. S., & Grossman, R. G. (1978). Behavioral sequelae of closed head injury: A quantitative study. *Archives of Neurology, 35,* 720–727.

Levin, H. S., Grossman, R. G., Rose, J. E., & Teasdale, G. (1979). Long-term neuropsychological outcome of closed head injury. *Journal of Neurosurgery, 50,* 412–422.

Levin, H. S., Meyers, C. A., Grossman, R. G., & Sarwar, M. (1981). Ventricular enlargement after closed head injury. *Archives of Neurology, 38,* 623–629.

Levin, H. S., Benton, A. L., & Grossman, R. G. (1982). *Neurobehavioral consequences of closed head injury.* New York: Oxford University Press.

Levin, H. S., Mattis, S., Ruff, R. M., Eisenberg, H. M., Marshall, L. F., Tabaddor, K., High, W. M., & Frankowski, R. F. (1987a). Neurobehavioral outcome following minor head injury: A three-center study. *Journal of Neurosurgery, 66,* 234–243.

Levin, H. S., Amparo, E., Eisenberg, H. M., Williams, D. H., High, W. M., Jr., McArdle, C. B., & Weiner, R. L. (1987b). Magnetic resonance imaging and computerized tomography in relation to the neurobehavioral sequelae of mild and moderate head injuries. *Journal of Neurosurgery, 66,* 706–713.

Levin, H. S., Gary, H. E., High, W. M., Mattis, S., Ruff, R. M., Eisenberg, H. M., Marshall, L. F., & Tabaddor, K. (1987c). Minor head injury and the postconcussional syndrome: Methodological issues in outcome studies. In H. S. Levin, J. Grafman, & H. M. Eisenberg (Eds.), *Neurobehavioral recovery from head injury* (pp. 262–275). New York: Oxford University Press.

Lezak, M. D. (1978). Living with the characterologically altered brain injured patient. *Journal of Clinical Psychiatry, 39,* 592–598.

Lezak, M. D. (1988). Brain damage is a family affair. *Journal of Clinical and Experimental Neuropsychology, 10,* 111–123.

Lishman, W. A. (1973). The psychiatric sequelae of head injury: A review. *Psychological Medicine, 3,* 304–318.

Luerssen, T. G., Hesselink, J. R., Ruff, R. M., Healy, M. E., & Grote, C. A. (1986). Magnetic resonance imaging of craniocerebral injury. *Concepts in Pediatric Neurosurgery, 8,* 190–208.

Malkmus, D., Booth, B. J., & Kodemer, C. (1980). *Rehabilitation of the head injured adult: Comprehensive cognitive management.* Los Angeles: Rancho Los Amigos Hospital.

Mandleberg, I. A. (1975). Cognitive recovery after severe head injury. 2. Wechsler Adult Intelligence Scale during post-traumatic amnesia. *Journal of Neurology, Neurosurgery, and Psychiatry, 38,* 1127–1132.

Mandleberg, I. A., & Brooks, D. N. (1975). Cognitive recovery after severe head injury. 1. Serial testing on the Wechsler Adult Intelligence Scale. *Journal of Neurology, Neurosurgery, and Psychiatry, 38,* 1121–1126.

Mazzucchi, A., Cattelani, R., Missale, G., Gugliotta, M., Brianti, R., & Parma, M. (1992). Head injured subjects aged over 50 years: Correlations between variables of trauma and neuropsychological follow-up. *Journal of Neurology, 239,* 256–260.

McKinlay, W. W., Brooks, D. N., & Bond, M. R. (1983). Post-concussional symptoms, financial compensation and outcome of severe blunt head injury. *Journal of Neurology, Neurosurgery, and Psychiatry, 46,* 1084–1091.

McLean, A., Temkin, N. R., Dikmen, S., & Wyler, A. R. (1983). The behavioral sequelae of head injury. *Journal of Clinical Neuropsychology, 5,* 361–376.

Meyers, C. A., Levin, H. S., & Eisenberg, H. M. (1983). Early versus late lateral ventricular enlargement following closed head injury. *Journal of Neurology, Neurosurgery, and Psychiatry, 46,* 1092–1097.

Miller, J. D., Pentland, B., & Berrol, S. (1990). Early evaluation and management. In M. Rosenthal, M. R. Bond, E. R. Griffith, & J. D. Miller (Eds.), *Rehabilitation of the adult and child with traumatic brain injury* (2nd ed.) (pp. 21–51). Philadelphia: F. A. Davis.

Miller, L. (1993). *Psychotherapy of the brain-injured patient: Reclaiming the shattered self.* New York: Norton.

Narayan, R. K., Gokaslan, Z. L., Bontke, C. F., & Berrol, S. (1990). Neurologic sequelae of head injury. In M. Rosenthal, M. R. Bond, E. R. Griffith, & J. D. Miller (Eds.), *Rehabilitation of the adult and child with traumatic brain injury* (2nd ed.) (pp. 94–106). Philadelphia: F. A. Davis.

Novack, T. A., Daniel, M. S., & Long, C. J. (1984). Factors related to emotional adjustment following head injury. *International Journal of Clinical Neuropsychology, 6,* 139–142.

Oddy, M., Humphrey, M., & Uttley, D. (1978). Stresses upon the relatives of head-injured patients. *British Journal of Psychiatry, 133,* 507–513.

O'Hara, C. (1988). Emotional adjustment following minor head injury. *Cognitive Rehabilitation, 6*(2), 26–33.

O'Shaughnessy, E. J., Fowler, R. S., & Reid, V. (1984). Sequelae of mild closed head injuries. *Journal of Family Practice, 18,* 391–394.

Paniak, C. E., Shore, D. L., & Rourke, B. P. (1989). Recovery of memory after severe closed head injury: Dissociations in recovery of memory parameters and predictors of outcome. *Journal of Clinical and Experimental Psychology, 11,* 631–644.

Parker, R. S. (1990). *Traumatic brain injury and neuropsychological impairment: Sensorimotor, cognitive, emotional, and adaptive problems of children and adults.* New York: Springer-Verlag.

Peck, E. A., & Mitchell, S. A. (1990). Normative data for 538 head injury patients across seven time periods after injury. Presented at the 1990 International Neuropsychological Society Meeting in Orlando, Fl.

Povlishock, J. T., & Coburn, T. H. (1989). Morphopathological change associated with mild head injury. In H. S. Levin, H. M. Eisenberg, & A. L. Benton (Eds.), *Mild head injury* (pp. 37–53). New York: Oxford University Press.

Prigatano, G. P. (1985). *Neuropsychological rehabilitation after brain injury.* Baltimore: Johns Hopkins University Press.

Prigatano, G. P. (1987). Personality and psychosocial consequences after brain injury. In M. J. Meier, A. L. Benton, & L. Diller (Eds.), *Neuropsychological rehabilitation* (pp. 355–378). Edinburgh: Churchill Livingstone.

Prigatano, G. P. (1991). Disturbances of self-awareness of deficit after traumatic brain injury. In G. P. Prigatano & D. L. Schacter (Eds.), *Awareness after brain injury: Clinical and theoretical issues* (pp. 111–126). New York: Oxford University Press.

Richardson, J. T. E. (1990). *Clinical and neuropsychological aspects of closed head injury.* London: Taylor & Francis.

Rimel, R. W., & Jane, J. A. (1983). Characteristics of head injury patients. In M. Rosenthal, E. R. Griffith, M. R. Bond, & J. D. Miller (Eds.), *Rehabilitation of the head injured adult* (pp. 9–21). Philadelphia: F. A. Davis.

Rimel, R. W., Giordani, B., Barth, J. T., Boll, T. J., & Jane, J. A. (1981). Disability caused by minor head injury. *Neurosurgery, 9,* 221–228.

Rimel, R. W., Jane, J. A., & Bond, M. R. (1990). Characteristics of the head injured patient. In M. Rosenthal, M. R. Bond, E. R. Griffith, & J. D. Miller (Eds.), *Rehabilitation of the adult and child with traumatic brain injury* (2nd ed.) (pp. 8–16). Philadelphia: F. A. Davis.

Ruff, R. M., Evans, R., & Marshall, L. M. (1986). Impaired verbal and figural fluency after head injury. *Archives of Clinical Neuropsychology, 1,* 87–101.

Ruff, R. M., Cullum, C. M., & Luerssen, T. G. (1989a). Brain imaging and neuropsychological outcome in traumatic brain injury. In E. D. Bigler, R. A. Yeo, & E. Turkenheimer (Eds.), *Neuropsychological function and brain imaging* (pp. 161–183). New York: Plenum Press.

Ruff, R. M., Levin, H. S., Mattis, S., High, W. M., Marshall, L. F., Eisenberg, H. M., & Tabaddor, K. (1989b). Recovery of memory after mild head injury: A three-center study. In H. S. Levin, H. M. Eisenberg, & A. L. Benton (Eds.), *Mild head injury.* New York: Oxford University Press.

Russell, D., & Sharratt, A. (1992). *Academic recovery after head injury.* Springfield, IL: Charles C. Thomas.

Russell, W. R. (1932). Cerebral involvement in head injury. *Brain, 55,* 549–603.

Russell, W. R., & Nathan, P. W. (1946). Traumatic amnesia. *Brain, 69,* 280–300.

Rutherford, W. H. (1989). Postconcussion symptoms: Relationship to acute neurological indices, individual differences, and circumstances of injury. In H. S. Levin, H. M. Eisenberg, & A. L. Benton (Eds.), *Mild head injury* (pp. 217–228). New York: Oxford University Press.

Rutherford, W. H., Merrett, J. D., & McDonald, J. R. (1977). Sequelae of concussion caused by minor head injuries. *Lancet, 1,* 1–4.

Rutherford, W. H., Merrett, J. D., & McDonald, J. R. (1979). Symptoms at one year following concussion from minor head injuries. *Injury, 10,* 225–230.

Sbordone, R. J., Kral, M., Gerard, M., & Katz, J. (1984). Evidence of a "command performance syndrome" in the significant others of the victims of severe traumatic head injury. *International Journal of Clinical Neuropsychology, 6,* 183–185.

Sloan, S., Benjamin, L., & Hawkins, W. (1989). Group treatment of memory problems following closed head injury. In V. Anderson, M. Bailey, J. Ponsford, P. Snow, & M. Mealings (Eds.), *Theory and function: Bridging the gap.* Melbourne: Australian Society for the Study of Brain Impairment.

Spanbock, P. (1987). Understanding head injury from the families' perspective. *Cognitive Rehabilitation, 5*(2), 12–14.

Stambrook, M., Moore, A. D., & Peters, L. C. (1990). Social behavior and adjustment to moderate and severe traumatic brain injury: Comparison to normative and psychiatric samples. *Cognitive Rehabilitation, 8,* 26–30.

Stuss, D. T. (1987). Contribution of frontal lobe injury to cognitive impairment after closed head injury: Methods of assessment and recent findings. In H. S. Levin, J. Grafman, & H. M. Eisenberg (Eds.), *Neurobehavioral recovery from head injury* (pp. 166–177). New York: Oxford University Press.

Stuss, D. T., Ely, P., Hugenholtz, H., Richard, M. T., Larochell, S., Poirier, C. A., & Bell, I. (1985). Subtle neuropsychological deficits in patients with good recovery after closed head injury. *Neurosurgery, 17,* 41–47.

Stuss, D. T., Stethem, L. L., Hugenholtz, H., & Richard, M. T. (1989). Traumatic brain injury: A comparison of three clinical tests, and analysis of recovery. *The Clinical Neuropsychologist, 3,* 145–156.

Teasdale, G., & Jennett, B. (1974). Assessment of coma and impaired consciousness: A practical scale. *Lancet, 2,* 81–84.

Thomsen, I. V. (1974). The patient with severe head injury and his family. *Scandinavian Journal of Rehabilitation Medicine, 6,* 180–183.

Van Dongen, K. J., & Braakman, R. (1980). Late computed tomography in survivors of severe head injury. *Neurosurgery, 7,* 14–22.

Van Zomeron, A. H. (1981). *Reaction time and attention after closed head injury.* Lisse: SWETS.

Wechsler, D. A. (1987). *Wechsler Memory Scale—Revised.* New York: Psychological Corporation.

Wrightson, P., & Gronwall, D. (1981). Time off work and symptoms after minor head injury. *Injury, 12,* 445–454.

Zappala, G., & Trexler, L. E. (1992). Quantitative and qualitative aspects of memory performance after minor head injury. *Archives of Clinical Neuropsychology, 7,* 145–154.

Stroke

DESCRIPTION

Stroke or *cerebrovascular accident* (CVA) is a rapid, nonconvulsive, focal neurological deficit resulting from an infarct or hemorrhage in the cerebral vasculature (R. D. Adams & Victor, 1989; Reitan & Wolfson, 1985).

Cerebral aneurysm: Saccular or berry aneurysms are formed by the dilation of a cerebral artery and take the form of small, thin-walled blisters protruding from the arteries of the circle of Willis (90–95%) or its major branches. They tend to form at bifurcations (R. D. Adams & Victor, 1989; Reitan & Wolfson, 1985). *Subarachnoid hemorrhage* often results from a ruptured aneurysm (Hinton, 1991). *Arteriovenous malformation* is an abnormal formation of arteries and veins. *Multi-infarct dementia* is defined as dementia due to multiple infarcts. *Vascular dementia* is dementia resulting from cerebrovascular disease.

INCIDENCE AND RISK FACTORS

Stroke

Incidence

Incidence rates for men and women were 103/100,000 for Rochester, Minnesota (1975–1979). The incidence of stroke has shown a progressive decline in the United States. The period of 1975–1979 compared with 1945–1949 exhibited a 54% decline (Garraway *et al.*, 1983).

Mortality

Mortality rates for stroke in the United States have declined since 1915 (Wolf *et al.*, 1986).

Age

The incidence and prevalence of stroke increase with age.

Gender

The incidence of cerebral infarction is 1.3 times higher in men than in women (Wolf, 1990).

Ethnicity

Stroke mortality is higher among blacks. Stroke is common in Japanese, with an increasing south-to-north gradient.

Hypertension

Hypertension is the predominant risk factor for stroke. Regardless of age or gender, hypertensive individuals have 3 times the rate of atherosclerotic brain infarction of normotensive individuals (Kannel *et al.*, 1970).

Impaired Cardiac Function

Cardiac abnormalities such as congestive heart disease, cardiac failure, left ventricular atrophy, heart enlargement, and chronic atrial fibrillation increase stroke risk (Wolf, 1990).

Additional Risk Factors

Diabetes mellitus, obesity, inappropriate fibrinogen, increased hematocrit, family history of stroke, increased serum lipids, cigarette and alcohol use, oral contraceptive use, and physical inactivity increase risk for stroke (Wolf, 1990).

Cerebral Aneurysm

Prevalence

The prevalence in the United States is as high as 2000/100,000 (Sahs & Adams, 1984).

Age

The incidence is highest between the ages of 40 and 60 (Locksley, 1966).

Gender

The incidence for males is greater than for females before 40. Overall, the ratio is 3:2 females to males.

Arteriovenous Malformations

Incidence

AVMs make up approximately 1–2% of strokes (Gross *et al.,* 1984; Perret, 1975). The risks of hemorrhage have been estimated to be from 1% to 4% per annum.

Age

Hemorrhagic AVMs are more common during the 2nd through the 5th decades of life (Brown *et al.,* 1991).

Gender

They are equally frequent in males and females (R. D. Adams and Victor, 1989).

Vascular Dementia

Schoenberg (1988) reported that in a carefully designed study of Copiah County, Mississippi, the prevalence ratio for vascular dementia was 134/100,000.

ETIOLOGY AND PATHOLOGY

Stroke

Stroke can result from multiple causes and is divided into two categories: (1) ischemic stroke and (2) hemorrhagic stroke. Ischemic strokes are neurological insults that result from lack of circulation of blood due to primary thrombotic occlusion or embolic occlusion of an artery (R. D. Adams & Victor, 1989). Although there are many possible causes of thrombosis, one of the most common is arteriosclerosis. In atherosclerosis, deposits or plaques of cholesterol, lipoid material, and lipophages are formed within the intima of arteries (Reitan & Wolfson, 1985). Such a deposit is common at the bifurcation of the carotid artery. Embolic occlusion of a vessel occurs as a result of foreign material lodging in the vessel. The most common source of emboli is cardiac disorder.

Hemorrhagic stroke is commonly the result of a ruptured aneurysm or arteriovenous malformation. It may occur intracerebrally, in the subarachnoid space, intraventricularly, or subdurally.

Cerebral Aneurysm

It has been suggested that berry aneurysms may result from developmental defects in the media and elastica. It has also been suggested that they are the result of focal destruction of the internal elastic membrane due to hemodynamic forces at the apices of bifurcations (R. D. Adams & Victor, 1989). Subarachnoid hemorrhage may arise from the rupture of berry aneurysms (usually greater than 1 cm). The rupture of the aneurysm results in a discharge of blood under high pressure into the surrounding brain tissue (Reitan & Wolfson, 1985). Steinman and Bigler (1986) found all their seven patients to have sustained bilateral mesial frontal infarctions.

Arteriovenous Malformations

AVMs have been attributed to fetal abnormalities beginning approximately 3 weeks after conception (Stein & Wolpert, 1980). At this stage in development, primitive vessels divide into arteries and veins. Fistulas are formed that are supplied by hypertrophied arteries and are drained by enlarged veins. The walls of these vessels may become thin and may eventually rupture. "Cerebral steal" may occur when shunting of blood through the AVM deprives the surrounding tissue of normal supply (Mohr et al., 1989). This process may result in focal or generalized cognitive impairment.

Multi-infarct Dementia

The most common etiology of multi-infarct dementia is lacunar infarcts, followed by multiple bilateral cerebral embolization (Meyer et al., 1988a).

MEDICAL ASSESSMENT

In all forms of stroke, the primary feature is the temporal profile of neurological events. The neurological deficit develops abruptly, in a matter of seconds or at most a few days. There is then an arrest and regression in all but fatal strokes. The neurological deficit suggests both the location and the size of the lesion.

Middle cerebral artery occlusion may result in contralateral hemiplegia and hemianesthesia, contralateral homonymous hemianopia with impairment of conjugate gaze contralateral to the lesion, aphasia with language-dominant hemisphere involvement, or apractagnosia, asomatognosia, and anosognosia with nondominant hemisphere involvement (R. D. Adams & Victor, 1989; Hinton, 1991).

Carotid artery occlusion may be silent due to collateral circulation. If collaterals are compromised, deficits may be similar to those that result from middle cerebral artery occlusion. Carotid artery disease is found in 50% of patients with transient unilateral loss of vision. Oculoplethysmography, Doppler ultrasonography, phonoangiography, and digital intravenous angiography may be used to assess the degree of stenosis in the carotid artery (R. D. Adams & Victor, 1989; Hinton, 1991).

Anterior cerebral artery occlusion may result in paralysis of the contralateral foot and leg, grasp reflex, gegenhalten rigidity, abulia, gait disorder, perseveration, and urinary incontinence (R. D. Adams & Victor, 1989; Hinton, 1991).

Posterior cerebral artery occlusion may result in contralateral homonymous hemianopia or upper quadrantanopia, memory loss, dyslexia without dysgraphia, color anomia, mild contralateral hemiparesis and hemisensory loss, and ipsilateral third-nerve palsy (R. D. Adams & Victor, 1989; Hinton, 1991).

Vertebrobasilar artery occlusion may produce quadriplegia, bilateral conjugate horizontal gaze palsies, coma, or "locked in" syndrome. If disease occurs only in branches, symptoms may include ipsilateral ataxia, contralateral hemiplegia with sensory loss, internuclear ophthalmoplegia, nystagmus, vertigo, nausea, vomiting, deafness, tinnitus, palatal myoclonus, and oscillopsia (R. D. Adams & Victor, 1989; Hinton, 1991).

CT scanning is superior to MRI in distinguishing hemorrhage from infarction (Hinton, 1991). CT scan is reliable in the detection of hemorrhages that are 1–1.5 cm or more in diameter (R. D. Adams & Victor, 1989). MRI is useful for demonstrating brainstem hemorrhages and residual hemorrhages and small embolic infarctions (Ford *et al.*, 1989). The EEG is usually slower over an area of infarction (Hinton, 1991).

Cerebral Aneurysm and Subarachnoid Hemorrhage

According to R. D. Adams and Victor (1989), "the clinical sequence of sudden violent headache, collapse, relative preservation of consciousness, and a paucity of lateralizing signs in the face of massive subarachnoid hemorrhage is diagnostic of a ruptured saccular aneurysm" (p. 670). The onset of a ruptured aneurysm and subarachnoid hemorrhage is often rapid. A sudden, severe headache is experienced by 60% of victims. There may be a severe stiff neck. Twenty percent go rapidly into coma. Twenty percent have a variety of symptoms including seizures, vomiting, pain in neck, back, or limbs, and focal paralyses. Fifty percent have a delay of 6–12 hr before stupor or coma is produced (Hinton, 1991; Reitan & Wolfson, 1985). "About one-half of the men and perhaps two-thirds of the women have warning signs before the sudden and usually severe onset of subarachnoid hemorrhage due to a ruptured berry aneurysm" (Reitan & Wolfson, 1985, p. 201). The rupture of the aneurysm usually occurs when the patient is active rather than passive (R. D. Adams & Victor, 1989).

CT scan will detect blood within the brain, ventricular system, or subarachnoid spaces. The cerebrospinal fluid (CSF) is grossly bloody and exhibits increased pressure. Carotid and vertebral angiography demonstrates aneurysm in 85% of patients so diagnosed on clinical grounds (R. D. Adams & Victor, 1989).

Arteriovenous Malformations

About 50% of patients will present with a cerebral or subarachnoid hemorrhage, 30% with a seizure, and 20% with a headache. Focal neurological deficit is noted in 10% of patients (R. D. Adams and Victor, 1989). Unilateral headache and migraine is a common symptom and may precede rupture. Headache location may not correlate with the location of the AVM (Mohr *et al.*, 1989).

AVMs will often present on CT scan with a hyperdense appearance (Mohr *et al.*, 1989). A diagnosis can be made in 85–95% of cases (LeBlanc *et al.*, 1979). Angiography often demonstrates tortuous feeding arteries and draining veins embracing a blotch representing the fistula (Mohr *et al.*, 1989). Serial angiography plays an important role in preparing the patient for therapy.

Multi-infarct Dementia

Diagnosis of multi-infarct dementia involves medical history, neurological examination, and psychiatric interview with psychometric testing (Loeb, 1988). Blood chemistries, examination of CSF, EEG, CT, and MRI will assist in identifying etiologies of tumor, vascular malformation, cerebral hematoma, infections, metabolic, toxic, drug, and vitamin deficiencies, and normal pressure hydrocephalus. Alzheimer's disease may be distinguished from multi-infarct dementia as follows:

Alzheimer's disease is associated with a family history of similar disorders, insidious onset with slow progression, primitive reflexes, normal CSF, normal or diffuse slowing on EEG, normal or atrophy on CT or MRI, and bilateral temporoparietal deficits on SPECT (Loeb, 1988).

Multi-infarct dementia is associated with a history of stroke, sudden onset, focal symptoms and signs, pseudobulbar signs, signs of blood–brain barrier damage, focal slow waves on the EEG, abnormal somatosensory evoked potentials, low-density areas on CT, bright lesions on T2-weighted images, and focal flow deficits on SPECT (Loeb, 1988).

Loeb (1988) defined *possible vascular dementia* as dementia with onset of cognitive impairments around the age of 60–70 years, history of stroke, abrupt onset of cognitive impairments, and focal neurological signs and symptoms. *Probable vascular dementia* requires, in addition to the criteria for possible vascular dementia, confirmation of dementia by neuropsychological testing, low-density areas on CT scan, Modified Ischemic Score of 5–10, and laboratory studies. *Definite vascular dementia* requires, in addition, positive CSF tests for blood–brain barrier damage, focal EEG abnormalities, abnormal somatosensory evoked potentials, and deep white-matter infarctions.

The Hachinsky Ischemic Score (Hachinsky *et al.*, 1975), which assigns weights to clinical criteria for multi-infarct dementia, has been found to yield mixed results when used to differentially diagnose multi-infarct dementia vs. Alzheimer's disease (Fischer *et al.*, 1991; Meyer *et al.*, 1988b).

NEUROPSYCHOLOGICAL ASSESSMENT

The neurobehavioral consequences of stroke can include alterations in any behaviors that are regulated by the brain. The entire repertoire of higher-level human behavior (and any subset of that repertoire) may be affected (Bleiberg, 1986). Due to the multiplicity of cognitive and behavioral impairments that may result from stroke, it is impossible to delineate them completely. Impairments in cognitive–emotional functioning following only the most common strokes will be described.

Neuropsychological deficits in stroke tend to be overlooked or underestimated. Conditions such as hemiplegia capture the attention of clinicians and obscure full appreciation of disorders of higher cognitive function. Neuropsychological evaluation may delineate concurrent, more subtle deficits and strengths in cognitive functioning essential for management and rehabilitation (Finlayson, 1990; Walsh, 1991). Neuropsychological test performance may also predict outcome (Novack *et al.*, 1987).

The relationship of test performance to locus of brain damage has often been studied with groups of stroke patients. Information concerning the relationship of loci of stroke to particular tests may therefore often be found under the *Localization* subheadings of the chapters in Part III.

Left hemisphere stroke typically results in impairments in language. Impairment may be noted in the WAIS-R verbal subtests, WMS-R verbal subtests, RAVLT, CVLT, BNT, COWAT, and BDAE. Right hemisphere stroke may result in left hemispatial neglect and visuospatial and visuoconstructional functioning. WAIS-R performance tests, HVOT, JLO, LBT, VFDT, ROCFT:C&M. Sensory and motor function is likely to be impaired contralateral to the stroke (Hom, 1991; Hom & Reitan, 1990; Orsini *et al.*, 1988). The practitioner should be cautious in applying these rules of thumb. They will not apply if the patient's right hemisphere is dominant for language (see Chapter 7). The individual test descriptions should be referred to for more detailed localization information.

The Barthel Index (Mahoney & Barthel, 1965) has been used as a functional outcome measure for stroke.

Catastrophic reaction is a profound depression following stroke characterized by restlessness, hyperemotionality, sudden bursts of tears, irritation, and displacement of anxiety onto extraneous events (Robinson & Forrester, 1987; Robinson & Starkstein, 1990). Catastrophic reaction has been found to be associated with left hemisphere damage (Gainotti, 1972).

Indifference reaction is characterized by lack of interest, indifference toward failures, and explicit denial or lack of awareness of physical or mental impairments. These symptoms may be accompanied by self-reports of anxiety, slowness, and worrying. This reaction is associated with left neglect and right hemisphere lesions (Robinson & Forrester, 1987; Starkstein & Robinson, 1992). *Major depression* is associated with left frontal damage and has a natural course of about 1 year without treatment (Robinson & Forrester, 1987). *Dysthymic disorder* is associated with right or left posterior lesions and has been found to improve in only 30% of patients over 2-year follow-up (Robinson & Forrester, 1987). Depression appears to be more prevalent in the first 2 years following a stroke. Tricyclic antidepressant medications (e.g., nortriptyline) have been used successfully in treating poststroke depression (Robinson & Forrester, 1987). Depression is associated with delayed recovery (Parikh *et al.,* 1990). *Mania* may be associated with right brain damage (Cummings & Mendez, 1984).

Caution should be observed in interpreting the MMPI-2 for patients with cerebrovascular disease (Gass, 1992). Neurologic complaints may inflate scores on Scales 1, 2, 3, and 8.

Cerebral Aneurysm and Subarachnoid Hemorrhage

A ruptured communicating artery aneurysm may produce an amnestic confabulatory state similar to that of Korsakoff's syndrome (Bornstein, 1986). Lindquist and Norlen (1966) found 17 of 35 patients to have postoperative Korsakoff's syndrome, characterized by amnesia, disorientation, confabulation, and a lack of concern over deficit. Takaku *et al.* (1979) found a 14% incidence of psychological symptoms including disorientation, amnesia, and Korsakoff's syndrome for patients with anterior communicating artery aneurysms. These symptoms may persist in a small percentage of patients.

Steinman and Bigler (1986) found WAIS IQs to be generally within the normal range. WMS scores were generally impaired relative to WAIS IQs. Performance was impaired on the CT. Behavioral assessment suggested impairment in learned social behavior (diminution of initiative, impaired judgment, increased social dependency) and inability to learn (mental slowness, rigidity of thought, reduced learning capacity). The Maudsley Mentation Test has been developed for the monitoring of mental status after aneurysmal subarachnoid hemorrhage (Strong *et al.,* 1992).

Arteriovenous Malformations

Waltimo and Putkonen (1974) found no relationship between performance on the WAIS, Visual Retention test, Token Test and size, laterality, or symptoms of AVMs. Brown *et al.* (1989) found that neuropsychological measures (WAIS-R, WMS, FTT, GS, Tactile Finger Recognition, Fingertip Number Writing, and testing for visual imperception) were not sensitive to laterality of AVMs.

Multi-infarct Dementia

Performance on batteries of neuropsychological tests may not differ significantly from that of patients with Alzheimer's disease. Loring *et al.* (1986) found few differences in performance on the Satz–Mogel short form of the WAIS, SRT, CPT, SR, and several other tests. Significant differences were found only for FSIQ, VIQ, and PC. Brinkman *et al.* (1986) found no differences for the WAIS and WMS.

Some differences in language functioning have been reported. Naming impairments may be less severe than those found in Alzheimer's patients (Powell *et al.,* 1988).

Delusions (50%) and depression (25%) may occur (Cummings & Mahler, 1991).

MEDICAL TREATMENT

Ischemic Stroke

Anticoagulants such as coumarin agents, heparin, or antiplatelet agent (aspirin) may be prescribed (Hinton, 1991). Nortriptyline has been found to be effective in the treatment of poststroke depression (Lipsey *et al.,* 1984).

Cerebral Aneurysm and Subarachnoid Hemorrhage

Medical management may include strict bed rest in a darkened room, fluid administration to maintain normal circulating volume and venous pressure, elastic stockings, stool softeners, anticonvulsant medication, and if necessary, antihypertensive drugs (R. D. Adams & Victor, 1989). Surgery may involve evacuating an intracerebral clot or placing a ventriculoatrial shunt. It is commonly performed to prevent recurrence of hemorrhage. Procedures may include clipping or ligating the neck of the aneurysm, wrapping or tamponade of the aneurysmal sac, or trapping the aneurysm. Surgery may be contraindicated if the patient is stuporous or comatose—grade IV or V (Hunt & Hess, 1968). Patients whose conditions improve to the point where they can be operated on tend to fare better than those treated conservatively. Studies have suggested that patients may benefit from surgical treatment of aneurysms greater than 7 mm in diameter (R. D. Adams & Victor, 1989).

Arteriovenous Malformations

AVM are treated by radiotherapy, embolization, and surgery (Brown *et al.,* 1991).

PSYCHOSOCIAL THERAPIES

G. F. Adams and Hurwitz (1963) found that rehabilitation "failed" in approximately 50% of a sample of stroke patients due to neuropsychological deficits. Barriers to recovery were denial of illness, hemiparetic neglect, spatial disturbance, body image disturbance, motor perseveration, memory deficit, and inattentiveness. Kinsella and Ford (1980) found cognitive deficits, especially unilateral spatial neglect, to be a barrier to recovery.

Cognitive Rehabilitation: A variety of processes are involved in the recovery of function after stroke. These include: (1) selective regeneration of neural elements, (2) structural substitution, and (3) behavioral substitution (Meier & Strauman, 1991).

Techniques applicable to the remediation of cognitive deficits in stroke (e.g., aphasia, neglect, and visuospatial impairments) may be found in Chapter 35. Techniques have been reviewed by Tupper (1991).

Evans and Bishop (1990) have reported that care-giver education stabilizes aspects of family function. Counseling may help sustain treatment benefits and improve long-term patient adjustment (Evans *et al.,* 1988).

Numerous self-help books are available. These include *Stroke: A Guide for Patient and Family* (Frye-Pierson & Toole, 1987), *What Every Family Should Know About Strokes* (Hess & Bahr, 1981), and *The Road Ahead: A Stroke Recovery Guide* (National Stroke Association, 1988). An informative first-person account of a stroke has been written by Sten Lindgren (1992). Pamphlets are available from the American Heart Association. A referral might be made to the local "stroke club." The address of the National Stroke Association is 1420 Ogden Street, Denver, CO 80218.

PROGNOSIS

Ischemic Stroke

Of stroke survivors, 70–80% will have a mild or no functional deficit, 20% will be moderately disabled (ambulatory but dependent in some ADLs), and fewer than 10% will be severely disabled (Brandstater, 1990).

Cerebral Aneurysm and Subarachnoid Hemorrhage

Thirty percent die within 24 hr of the hemorrhage and an additional 20% during the first week (Reitan & Wolfson, 1985). McKissock *et al.* (1965) found the patient's state of consciousness at the time of arteriography to be the best index of prognosis. Of patients coming to angiography, 17% were stuporous or comatose. After 6 months, 8% died from the original hemorrhage and 59% had a recurrence, with 40% mortality.

Arteriovenous Malformations

In one longitudinal study of a group of patients managed without surgery, hemorrhage occurred in 42% and seizures in 18%. At 20 years after diagnosis, 29% had died and 27% had a neurologically related handicap (Crawford *et al.*, 1986). In 90% of cases, bleeding stops and the patient survives. Rebleeding occurs at a rate of 6% in the first year after hemorrhage and 2–3% thereafter (R. D. Adams and Victor, 1989).

REFERENCES

Adams, G. F., & Hurwitz, L. J. (1963). Mental barriers to recovery from stroke. *Lancet, 2,* 533–537.

Adams, R. D., & Victor, M. (1989). *Principles of neurology* (4th ed.). New York: McGraw-Hill.

Bleiberg, J. (1986). Psychological and neuropsychological factors in stroke management. In P. E. Kaplan & L. J. Cerullo (Eds.), *Stroke rehabilitation* (pp. 197–232). Boston: Butterworths.

Bornstein, R. A. (1986). Neuropsychological aspects of cerebrovascular disease and its treatment. In G. Goldstein & R. E. Tarter (Eds.), *Advances in clinical neuropsychology* (pp. 55–94). New York: Plenum Press.

Brandstater, M. E. (1990). An overview of stroke rehabilitation. *Stroke, 21*(Supplement II), II-40–II-42.

Brinkman, S. D., Largen, J. W., Cushman, L., Braun, P. R., & Block, R. (1986). Clinical validators: Alzheimer's disease and multi-infarct dementia. In L. W. Poon (Ed.), *Handbook for clinical memory assessment of older adults* (pp. 307–313). Washington, DC: American Psychological Association.

Brown, G. G., Spicer, K. B., Robertson, W. M., Baird, A. D., & Malik, G. (1989). Neuropsychological signs of lateralized arteriovenous malformations: Comparison with ischemic stroke. *The Clinical Neuropsychologist, 3,* 340–352.

Brown, G. G., Spicer, K. B., & Malik, G. (1991). Neurobehavioral correlates of arteriovenous malformations and cerebral aneurysms. In R. A. Bornstein & G. G. Brown (Eds.), *Neurobehavioral aspects of cerebrovascular disease* (pp. 202–223). New York: Oxford University Press.

Crawford, P. M., West, C. R., Chadwick, D. W., & Shaw, M. D. M. (1986). Arteriovenous malformations of the brain: Natural history in unoperated patients. *Journal of Neurology, Neurosurgery, and Psychiatry, 49,* 1–10.

Cummings, J. L., & Mahler, M. E. (1991). Cerebrovascular dementia. In R. A. Bornstein & G. G. Brown (Eds.), *Neurobehavioral aspects of cerebrovascular disease* (pp. 131–149). New York: Oxford University Press.

Cummings, J. L., & Mendez, M. F. (1984). Secondary mania with focal cerebrovascular lesions. *American Journal of Psychiatry, 141,* 1084–1087.

Evans, R. L., & Bishop, D. S. (1990). Psychosocial outcomes in stroke survivors: Implications for research. *Stroke, 21*(Supplement II), II-48–II-49.

Evans, R. L., Matlock, A., Bishop, D. S., Stranahan, S., & Pederson, C. (1988). Family intervention after stroke: Does counseling or education help? *Stroke, 19,* 1243–1249.

Finlayson, M. A. J. (1990). Neuropsychological assessment and treatment of stroke patients: An overview. *Stroke, 21*(Supplement II), II-14–II-15.

Fischer, P., Jellinger, K., Gatterer, G., & Danielczyk, W. (1991). Prospective neuropathological validation of Hachinski's Ischaemic Score in dementias. *Journal of Neurology, Neurosurgery, and Psychiatry, 54,* 580–583.

Ford, C. S., Buonanno, F. S., & Kistler, J. P. (1989). Magnetic resonance imaging in cerebrovascular disease. In J. F. Toole (Ed.), *Handbook of clinical neurology,* Volume 10 *(54): Vascular diseases, Part II* (pp. 81–103). Amsterdam: Elsevier.

Frye-Pierson, J., & Toole, J. F. (1987). *Stroke: A guide for patient and family.* New York: Raven Press.

Gainotti, G. (1972). Emotional behavior and hemispheric side of lesion. *Cortex, 8,* 41–55.

Garraway, W. M., Whisnant, J. P., & Drury, I. (1983). The changing pattern of survival following stroke. *Stroke, 14,* 699–703.

Gass, C. S. (1992). MMPI-2 interpretation of patients with cerebrovascular disease: A correction factor. *Archives of Clinical Neuropsychology, 7,* 17–27.

Gross, C. R., Kase, C. S., Mohr, J. P., Cunningham, S. C., & Baker, W. E. (1984). Stroke in south Alabama: Incidence and diagnostic features—a population based study. *Stroke, 15,* 249–255.

Hachinski, V. C., Iliff, L. D., Zilhka, L., Du Boulay, G. H., McAllister, V. L., Marshall, J., Russell, R. W. R., & Symon, L. (1975). Cerebral blood flow in dementia. *Archives of Neurology, 32,* 632–637.

Hess, L. J., & Bahr, R. E. (1981). *What every family should know about strokes.* New York: Appleton-Century-Crofts.

Hinton, R. C. (1991). Stroke. In M. A. Samuels (Ed.), *Manual of neurology: Diagnosis and therapy* (4th ed.) (pp. 197–212). Boston: Little, Brown.

Hom, J. (1991). Halstead–Reitan Battery in the neuropsychological investigation of stroke. In R. A. Bornstein & G. G. Brown (Eds.), *Neurobehavioral aspects of cerebrovascular disease* (pp. 163–181). New York: Oxford University Press.

Hom, J., & Reitan, R. M. (1990). Generalized cognitive function in stroke. *Journal of Clinical and Experimental Neuropsychology, 12,* 644–654.

Hunt, W. E., and Hess, R. M. (1968). Surgical risk as related to time of intervention in the repair of intracranial aneurysms. *Journal of Neurosurgery, 28,* 14–20.

Kannel, W. B., Wolf, P. A., Verter, J., & McNamara, P. M. (1970). Epidemiologic assessment of the role of blood pressure in stroke: The Framingham study. *JAMA, 214,* 301–310.

Kinsella, G., & Ford, B. (1980). Acute recovery patterns in stroke patients: Neuropsychological factors. *Medical Journal of Australia, 2,* 663–666.

LeBlanc, R., Ethier, R., & Little, J. R. (1979). Computerized tomography findings in arteriovenous malformations of the brain. *Journal of Neurosurgery, 51,* 765–772.

Lindgren, S. (1992). A self-report of sensory deficit after posterior right brain infarction. *Neuropsychology, 6,* 271–285.

Lindquist, G., & Norlen, G. (1966). Korsakoff's syndrome after operation on ruptured aneurysm of the communicating artery. *Acta Psychiatrica Scandinavica, 42,* 24–34.

Lipsey, J. R., Robinson, R. G., Pearlson, G. D., Rao, K., & Price, T. R. (1984). Nortriptyline treatment of post-stroke depression: A double-blind study. *Lancet, 1,* 297–300.

Locksley, H. B. (1966). Report on the Cooperative Study of Intracranial Aneurysms and Subarachnoid Hemorrhage. *Journal of Neurosurgery, 25,* 321–239.

Loeb, C. (1988). Clinical criteria for diagnosis and classification of vascular and multi-infarct dementia. In J. S. Meyer, H. Lechner, J. Marshall, & J. F. Toole (Eds.), *Vascular and multi-infarct dementia* (pp. 13–22). Mount Kisco, NY: Futura Publishing.

Loring, D. W., Meador, K. J., Mahurin, R. K., & Largen, J. W. (1986). Neuropsychological performance in dementia of the Alzheimer type and multi-infarct dementia. *Archives of Clinical Neuropsychology, 1,* 335–340.

Mahoney, F. I., & Barthel, D. W. (1965). Functional evaluation: Barthel Index. *Maryland State Medical Journal, 14,* 61–65.

McKissock, W., Richardson, A., & Walsh, L. S. (1965). Anterior communicating aneurysms: A trial of conservative and surgical treatment. *Lancet, 1,* 873–876.

Meier, M. J., & Strauman, S. E. (1991). Neuropsychological recovery after cerebral infarction. In R. A. Bornstein & G. G. Brown (Eds.), *Neurobehavioral aspects of cerebrovascular disease* (pp. 271–296). New York: Oxford University Press.

Meyer, J. S., McClintic, K., Sims, P., Rogers, R. L., & Mortel, K. F. (1988a). Etiology, prevention, and treatment of vascular and multi-infarct dementia. In J. S. Meyer, H. Lechner, J. Marshall, & J. F. Toole (Eds.), *Vascular and multi-infarct dementia* (pp. 129–147). Mount Kisco, NY: Futura Publishing.

Meyer, J. S., Rogers, R. L., Judd, B. W., Mortel, K. F., & Sims, P. (1988b). Cognition and cerebral blood flow fluctuate together in multi-infarct dementia. *Stroke, 19,* 163–169.

Mohr, J. P., Stein, B. M., & Hilal, S. K. (1989). Arteriovenous malformations. In J. F. Toole (Ed.), *Handbook of clinical neurology,* Volume 10(54): *Vascular diseases, Part II* (pp. 361–393). Amsterdam: Elsevier.

National Stroke Association (1988). *The road ahead: A stroke recovery guide.* Denver: National Stroke Association.

Novack, T. A., Haban, G., Graham, K., & Satterfield, W. T. (1987). Prediction of stroke rehabilitation outcome from psychologic screening. *Archives of Physical Medicine, 68,* 729–735.

Orsini, D. L., Van Gorp, W. G., & Boone, K. B. (1988). *The neuropsychology casebook.* New York: Springer-Verlag.

Parikh, R. M., Robinson, R. G., Lipsey, J. R., Starkstein, S. E., Federoff, J. P., & Price, T. R. (1990). The impact of poststroke depression on recovery in activities of daily living over a 2-year followup. *Archives of Neurology, 47,* 785–789.

Perret, G. (1975). The epidemiology and clinical course of arteriovenous malformations. In H. W. Pia, J. R. W. Gleave, E. Grote, and J. Zierski (Eds.), *Cerebral angiomas: Advances in diagnosis and therapy* (pp. 21–26). New York: Springer-Verlag.

Powell, A., Cummings, J. L., Hill, M. A., & Benson, D. F. (1988). Speech and language alterations in multi-infarct dementia. *Neurology, 38,* 717–719.

Reitan, R. M., & Wolfson, D. (1985). *Neuroanatomy and neuropathology: A clinical guide for neuropsychologists.* Tucson: Neuropsychology Press.

Robinson, R. G., & Forrester, A. W. (1987). Neuropsychiatric aspects of cerebrovascular disease. In R. E. Hales & S. C. Yudolfsky (Eds.), *The American Psychiatric Press textbook of neuropsychiatry* (pp. 191–208). Washington, DC: American Psychiatric Press.

Robinson, R. G., & Starkstein, S. E. (1990). Current research in affective disorders following stroke. *Journal of Neuropsychiatry and Clinical Neurosciences, 2,* 1–14.

Sahs, A. L., & Adams, H. P. (1984). Aneurysmal subarachnoid hemorrhage. *Seminars in Neurology, 4,* 271–296.

Schoenberg, B. S. (1988). Epidemiology of vascular and multi-infarct dementia. In J. S. Meyer, H. Lechner, J. Marshall, & J. F. Toole (Eds.), *Vascular and multi-infarct dementia* (pp. 47–59). Mount Kisco, NY: Futura Publishing.

Starkstein, S. E., & Robinson, R. G. (1992). Neuropsychiatric aspects of cerebral vascular disorders. In S. C. Yudofsky & R. E. Hayes (Eds.), *Textbook of neuropsychiatry* (2nd ed.) (pp. 449–472). Washington, DC: American Psychiatric Press.

Stein, B. M., & Wolpert, S. M. (1980). Arteriovenous malformations of the brain. I. Current concepts and treatment. *Archives of Neurology, 37,* 1–5.

Steinman, D. R., & Bigler, E. D. (1986). Neuropsychological sequelae of ruptured anterior communicating artery aneurysm. *International Journal of Clinical Neuropsychology, 8,* 135–140.

Strong, A. J., Wyke, M. A., Daum, I., Darkins, A. W., & Volans, A. P. (1992). The Maudsley Mentation Test: A method for extended monitoring of mental status after aneurysmal subarachnoid hemorrhage. *Neurosurgery, 31,* 886–890.

Takaku, A., Tanaka, S., Mori, T., & Suzuki, J. (1979). Postoperative complications in 1,000 cases of intracranial aneurysms. *Surgical Neurology, 12,* 137–144.

Tupper, D. E. (1991). Rehabilitation of cognitive and neuropsychological deficit following stroke. In R. A. Bornstein & G. G. Brown (Eds.), *Neurobehavioral aspects of cerebrovascular disease* (pp. 337–358). New York: Oxford University Press.

Walsh, K. W. (1991). *Understanding brain damage: A primer of neuropsychological evaluation.* Edinburgh: Churchill-Livingston.

Waltimo, O., & Putkonen, A. (1974). Intellectual performance of patients with intracranial arteriovenous malformations. *Brain, 97,* 511–520.

Wolf, P. A. (1990). An overview of the epidemiology of stroke. *Stroke, 21*(Supplement II), II-4–II-6.

Wolf, P. A., Kannel, W. B., & McGee, D. L. (1986). Epidemiology of strokes in North America. In H. J. M. Barnett, B. M. Stein, J. P. Mohr, & F. M. Yatsu (Eds.), *Stroke: Pathophysiology, diagnosis, and management,* Volume 1 (pp. 19–29). New York: Churchill-Livingston.

Epilepsy

DESCRIPTION

Seizures

Seizures may be defined as paroxysmal events of cerebral origin (Dodrill, 1981) or as "the clinical manifestation of an abnormal and excessive discharge of a set of neurons of the brain" (Hauser *et al.*, 1991, p. 429). *Generalized seizures* involve the entire brain and are bilaterally symmetrical and without focal onset. *Partial seizures* are of focal onset. Consciousness is not impaired in *simple seizures,* but is impaired in *complex seizures. Idiopathic seizures,* in contrast to *symptomatic seizures,* occur in the absence of historical insult to the brain (Hauser *et al.*, 1991). If a seizure lasts 30 min or more, the patient is said to be in *status epilepticus* (Uthman & Wilder, 1989). The classification schemata for seizures are further elaborated in three papers by the Commission on Classification and Terminology of the International League Against Epilepsy (1981, 1985, 1989).

Epilepsy

In epilepsy, the patient experiences recurrent seizures (Fernandez & Samuels, 1991).

Tonic–Clonic (Grand Mal) Seizures

The seizure may be preceded by subjective phenomena heralding its approach (the prodrome). In the tonic phase (10–20 sec), there is a sudden contraction of the muscles. There may be a cry as the respiratory muscles contract and the patient falls to the ground. The tongue may be bitten, and the patient may involuntarily urinate. In the clonic phase (usually less than 1 min), there is a mild generalized tremor that becomes coarser and evolves into violent muscular contractions. The patient is apneic until the end of the clonic phase, when a deep respiration occurs and all the muscles relax. The patient may remain unconscious for a period of time and awake with soreness and a headache (Adams & Victor, 1989).

Absence (Petit Mal) Seizures

Absence seizures are characterized by sudden onset, interruption of ongoing activities, a blank stare, and a brief (2- to 30-sec) loss of consciousness and may be associated with 3/sec minor motor activity (e.g., facial twitching) and with 3/sec generalized spikes and slow waves seen on the EEG. There is no aura or postictal state (Adams & Victor, 1989; Commission on Classification and Terminology of the International League Against Epilepsy, 1981; Fernandez & Samuels, 1991).

Simple Partial Seizures

Simple partial seizures begin locally in part of the brain and involve no impairment in consciousness. They may involve elementary motor, sensory, or autonomic symptoms. Jacksonian motor seizures, for example, may begin with the tonic contraction of the hand, face, or foot on one side of the body. This transforms to clonic movements that "march" to other muscles on the same side of the body (Adams & Victor, 1989).

Complex Partial Seizures

In a complex partial seizure, the aura or subjective experience heralding the seizure may be a complex hallucination or perceptual illusion. Experiences of deja vu, jamais vu, depersonalization, abdominal sensations, or feelings of fear and anxiety may occur. Consciousness is impaired but not lost, and automatisms, such as lipsmacking, fumbling of hands, or walking in a daze, may occur (Adams & Victor, 1989).

Reflex Epilepsy

In reflex epilepsy, seizures are regularly elicited by a specific stimulus (Tassinari et al., 1991). Stimuli may be flashes of light, patterns, eye closure, reading, and even eating. Cases of self-induced seizures have been documented.

Pseudoepileptic Seizures

Pseudoepileptic seizures are paroxysmal episodes of behavior that resemble seizures but lack characteristic epileptic clinical and electrographic features and have no identifiable physiological cause (Wilkus et al., 1984).

INCIDENCE, PREVALENCE, AND RISK FACTORS

Epilepsy

Incidence

Studies report an incidence of 20–50/100,000 (Zielinski, 1988).

Prevalence

The prevalence rate of epilepsy has been found to be between 4 and 10/1000 (Zielinski, 1988). A prevalence of 6.8/1000 was found for Rochester, Minnesota (Hauser et al., 1991). In this study, more than 60% of all active prevalence cases were partial epilepsy. Seventy-five percent were classified as idiopathic.

Age

The incidence decreases after the first decade until 60 and above, when it may increase (Zielinski, 1988). Hauser *et al.* (1991) found that more than 50% were diagnosed in the first 20 years of life.

Gender

Males tend to have a higher incidence than females (Zielinski, 1988).

Genetics

The risk for epilepsy in offspring has been reported to be in the range of 2–4%, while the population base rate is 1–2% (Anderson & Hauser, 1988). The risk is higher if: (1) the parent had idiopathic epilepsy, (2) the affected parent is the mother, (3) the epilepsy developed at a younger age, and (4) the affected parent has an affected parent or sibling.

Generalized Tonic–Clonic Seizures

Anderson & Hauser (1988) estimate a risk level of 5% when a sibling has absence seizures or generalized tonic–clonic seizures and a generalized spike and wave EEG. The addition of further factors such as having had a parent with idiopathic epilepsy may increase the estimate.

Absence Seizures

Age

The onset is usually between 4 and 8 years (Fernandez & Samuels, 1991).

Gender

The ratio of girls to boys is approximately 2:1 (Wallace, 1988).

Genetics

See *Generalized Tonic–Clonic Seizures* above.

Partial Seizures

The risk of seizures has been reported to be 3% for epilepsy and 5% for any nonfebrile seizure (by the age of 40) for siblings of individuals with partial seizures (Anderson & Hauser, 1988). An exception is siblings of individuals with benign childhood epilepsy with centrotemporal spikes, for whom the risk is 15%.

Pseudoepileptic Seizures

Pseudoepileptic seizures have been reported to account for 8–20% of cases that were evaluated for drug-resistant epilepsy (Ramani, 1986).

ETIOLOGY AND PATHOLOGY

Anything that insults the brain can cause seizures. The etiology and pathology of epilepsy are complex and multifaceted. In cases of idiopathic (primary) epilepsy, the brain has been grossly and microscopically normal. Many secondary epilepsies involve definable pathologies such as neuronal loss, gliosis, vascular malformations, and tumors (Adams & Victor, 1989).

Absence Seizures

Absence seizures have been described in patients with mesial frontal lesions, diencephalic lesions, and diffuse neuronal disease. However, they generally are not preceded by an identifiable neurological lesion (Dreifuss, 1991).

MEDICAL ASSESSMENT

Diagnosis occurs on three levels (Porter, 1989). Etiological diagnosis pertains to the cause of the seizures. Seizure diagnosis is the seizure type. Epilepsy syndrome diagnosis identifies the cluster of signs and symptoms. The medical history is essential to diagnosis. It should include a description of possible prodromal or precipitating factors and the seizure itself. History should also include birth history, patient's mother's perinatal history, and family history. A general physical examination and review of systems are of value in detecting systemic mechanisms of significance. Routine laboratory studies include a blood count, urinalysis, serum chemistry, and electrolytes (Stevenson & King, 1987). The EEG is essential for determining the form of the seizure discharge and its locus. EEG abnormality is associated with epilepsy in approximately 90% of cases (Stevenson & King, 1987). Special activation and recording procedures may be required to elicit abnormalities: hyperventilation, photic stimulation, sleep recording, and drug activation.

MRI is preferred to CT to evaluate the brain in patients with symptomatic epilepsy (Riela & Penry, 1991; Sperling, 1990). Neoplastic lesions may be detected when CT scans are unremarkable. An increase in signal intensity in T2-weighted images in mesial temporal regions has been reported in refractory partial epilepsy (Sperling, 1990).

PET studies, in partial epilepsy, have found focal, cortical hypometabolism (Sperling, 1990). Interictal cerebral hypoperfusion and ictal and immediate postictal hyperfusion in patients with partial epilepsy have been found with SPECT.

Absence Seizures

Absence seizures are identified by their clinical presentation and EEG as specified in the preceding description. Hyperventilation or photic stimulation is sometimes used to precipitate the EEG abnormality. Since the patient is often unaware of the attacks, a history must be obtained from a family member or other observer (Fernandez & Samuels, 1991). In absence status epilepticus, the patient may appear confused or stuporous and the EEG shows continuous spike and wave activity (Dreifuss, 1991).

Pseudoepileptic Seizures

Mulder (1991) has provided an extensive list of historical and behavioral criteria for the differential diagnosis of pseudoepileptic seizures. Although clinical observation during a seizure provides the essential information in distinguishing true seizures from pseudoepileptic seizures, EEG recordings can enhance diagnostic accuracy (Scott, 1982). No spikes or other rhythmical seizure elements are usually seen. Rarely, interseizure forms such as localized sharp waves and complexes may continue during the attack. Clusters of muscle activity appear more random and less rhythmic than those seen in true seizures. In the postattack period, alpha activity returns immediately and in abundance if the eyes remain shut. The addition of videotape recording to the patient's monitoring can assist in diagnosing pseudoepileptic seizures (Feldman *et al.*, 1982).

NEUROPSYCHOLOGICAL ASSESSMENT

Epilepsy

A rationale for neuropsychological testing in epilepsy has been presented by Dodrill (1988, 1991). Pertinent areas in neuropsychological evaluation of epilepsy include assessment of underlying brain disturbance, immediate and long-term effects of the epileptic attacks, and effects of antiepileptic medications on mental abilities. A neuropsychological assessment is especially important for patients who are experiencing adjustment difficulties or for whom assessment of strengths and weaknesses would assist treatment, educational, and vocational planning. Dodrill (1991) has suggested that the expense of comprehensive neuropsychological evaluations may be offset by their value in assisting patients' vocational planning.

Klove and Matthews (1974) have noted that there is little evidence to suggest specific types or patterns of cognitive impairment unique to epilepsy. The neuropsychological correlates of seizure history have been summarized by Dodrill and Matthews (1992).

Dodrill (1978, 1981) has constructed a neuropsychological battery for the evaluation of patients with epilepsy. Measures accepted for the battery were those that maximally distinguished epileptic from nonepileptic individuals. These included measures from the CT, TPT (Total Time, Memory, Localization), SR, FTT, TMTB, AST (Errors and Constructional Dyspraxia), Sensory–Perceptual Examination, Name Writing, Seashore Tonal Memory, Stroop (Part I, Part II), and WMS—Russell Revision (LM and VR). The number of tests outside normal limits was also found to be a significant measure. Dodrill has provided cutoff scores for each of the measures.

Although WAIS IQs and subtest scores correlated significantly with tests in a version of the HRNB, Kupke and Lewis (1985) concluded that the WAIS could usefully be added to the battery for interpretation of VIQ–PIQ differences and subtest profile interpretation. A factor analysis of the HRNB (including the WAIS) yielded five factors labeled: (1) Verbal Comprehension, (2) Motor Skills, (3) Perceptual Organization, (4) Selective Attention, and (5) Abstract Reasoning (Fowler *et al.*, 1987). Patients with left-sided foci obtained the lowest residual scores on Verbal Comprehension and Abstract Reasoning. Patients with right-sided foci obtained the lowest residual scores on Perceptual Organization.

Intracarotid Sodium Amytal Testing

Amytal testing has been commonly used to determine the side of speech representation and memory prior to neurosurgery for epilepsy (Milner, 1974). Clinical neuropsychologists often play a crucial role in assessing cognition during this procedure. The Wada technique of intracarotid injection of sodium Amytal (amobarbital) is performed first on either the right or the left side and then on the other side. At the Montreal Neurological Institute, sodium

Amytal is injected into the carotid artery of one side while the patient slowly counts aloud. The drug inactivates one hemisphere, producing a contralateral hemiplegia, hemianopia, and partial hemiplegia. When the hemisphere dominant for speech is injected, the patient may be mute for about 2 min and then make dysphasic errors—misnaming of common objects and errors in repeating well-known series. When the nondominant hemisphere is injected, speech is rarely interrupted more than a few seconds, and no mistakes are made in naming or serial repetition. A mild, bilateral dysphasia is seen in patients with a bilateral representation of speech (Milner, 1974).

A variety of techniques are used in the evaluation of memory functioning. In the Oregon Comprehensive Epilepsy Program, baseline recognition memory is assessed using objects, words, and pictures prior to administration (Walker *et al.*, 1987). Assessment is also performed during administration and after the effects of the drug have dissipated.

A three-part repetitive task modeled after a technique used by Carl Dodrill has been used at the University of Rochester Medical Center (P. G. Como, personal communication, Dec. 27, 1991). The patient is asked to name an object, read a short sentence, and recall the object most recently shown. The object-naming task is used to assess laterality of language function, the reading task is a distracter, and the recall task is used to assess immediate memory. The tasks are practiced repeatedly prior to the Amytal injection. Memory and new learning are also evaluated by presenting one object, one word, two pictured objects, and a nursery rhyme while the patient is under Amytal and obtaining recall and recognition afterward (Montreal procedure). Finally, the patient is interviewed for accuracy of recall of five major events that occurred during the procedure: speech blockage, hemiparesis, and errors in naming, reading, and recall.

In the Wada procedure developed at the Medical College of Georgia, language tasks include overlearned verbal sequences, comprehension, confrontation naming, and repetition (Loring *et al.*, 1992a,b). Language ratings are summed and a laterality ratio is computed. Stimuli to be remembered are presented at two times during the procedure. Eight common objects are presented to assess early item memory. When language functioning has minimally resumed, additional memory items are presented. After the effects of medication have worn off, recognition memory is assessed.

Attention

DSym (Wechsler–Bellevue Intelligence Scale) has been found to be impaired in patients with posttraumatic epilepsy (Dikmen & Reitan, 1978).

Memory

Dodrill (1978) found epileptic patients to be impaired on VR-WMS (cutoff < 11) and LM-WMS (cutoff < 19).

Intelligence

VIQ, PIQ, and FSIQ have been found to be impaired in patients with epilepsy with and without known etiology (Klove and Matthews, 1974). VIQ, PIQ, FSIQ, Information, and Comprehension (Wechsler–Bellevue Intelligence Scale) have been found to be impaired in patients with posttraumatic epilepsy (Dikmen & Reitan, 1978).

Speech/Language

Dodrill (1978) found epileptic patients to be impaired on the SR (cutoff < 26), but unimpaired on the SSPT, the Seashore Tonal Memory Test (cutoff < 22), and the AST (cutoff > 2). The SR has been found to be impaired in patients with epilepsy with and without known etiology; however, the SSPT was unimpaired (Klove & Matthews, 1974). Similarities (Wechsler–Bellevue Intelligence Scale) has been found to be impaired in patients with posttraumatic epilepsy (Dikmen & Reitan, 1978).

Arithmetic

Arithmetic (Wechsler–Bellevue Intelligence Scale) has been found to be impaired in patients with posttraumatic epilepsy (Dikmen & Reitan, 1978).

Visuospatial Functioning

Dodrill (1978) found epileptic patients to be impaired on Constructional Dyspraxia. Performance has been reported to be impaired on the TMTA in patients with epilepsy with and without known etiology (Klove & Matthews, 1974). Block Design (Wechsler–Bellevue Intelligence Scale) has been found to be impaired in patients with posttraumatic epilepsy (Dikmen & Reitan, 1978).

Sensory Functioning

Dodrill (1978) found epileptic patients to be impaired on TPT Total Time (cutoff > 16.2), Memory (cutoff < 8), and Localization (cutoff < 4). The RKSPE also exhibited impairment (cutoff > 6). TPT mean time per block, Memory, and Localization have been found to be impaired in patients with epilepsy with and without known etiology (Klove & Mathews, 1974). TPT Total Time has been found to be impaired in patients with posttraumatic epilepsy (Dikmen & Reitan, 1978).

Motor Functioning

Dodrill (1978) found epileptic patients to be impaired on the FTT (cutoff males < 101 taps/5 trials of 10 sec each; females < 92) and Name Writing Total (cutoff < 0.85 letter/sec). Klove and Matthews (1974) reported that FTT performance was not impaired in patients with epilepsy with and without known etiology relative to controls.

Executive Functioning

Dodrill (1978) found epileptic patients to be impaired on the TMTB (cutoff > 81) and the Halstead CT (cutoff > 53). Stroop performance was impaired (Part I cutoff > 93 sec; Part II cutoff > 150 sec). The TMTB and CT have been found to be impaired in patients with epilepsy with and without known etiology (Klove & Matthews, 1974). The CT has been found to be impaired in patients with posttraumatic epilepsy (Dikmen & Reitan, 1978).

General Indices of Impairment

Dodrill (1978) found epileptic patients to be impaired on the Halstead Impairment Index. A cutoff of >6 tests outside the cutoff limits classified 83% of controls and 79% of epileptics correctly (Dodrill, 1978). The Halstead Impairment Index was found to exhibit impairment in patients with epilepsy with and without known etiology (Klove & Matthews, 1974).

LNNB

Berg and Golden (1981) reported a hit rate of 77.3% for idiopathic epilepsy and 88.9% for symptomatic epilepsy. Post hoc *t*-tests revealed that the control group differed from both epilepsy groups on all but the Left and Right Hemisphere and Tactile Scales. Hermann and Melyn (1985) obtained a hit rate of 47% for idiopathic epilepsy and 30% for symptomatic epilepsy using a criterion for classification of "brain damaged" of two or more scales (exclusive of Writing, Arithmetic, Right and Left Hemisphere Scales) elevated above the critical value. They explain the difference between their results and those of Berg and Golden on the basis of methodological differences such as the greater percentage of patients with primary generalized epilepsy in the Berg and Golden sample. In Hermann and Melyn's sample, the Intellectual Processes Scale was most commonly in the impaired range, followed by the Tactile, Visual, Receptive Speech, Reading, and Memory Scales.

Personality

Dodrill *et al.* (1980) have developed an inventory specifically to assess psychosocial functioning in people with epilepsy. The Washington Psychosocial Seizure Inventory (WPSI) is a self-report inventory composed of 132 items. The WPSI assesses Family Background, Emotional Adjustment (problems of depression, tension, anxiety, oversensitivity, and generalized dissatisfaction with life), Interpersonal Adjustment (comfort in social situations, having a sufficient number of social contacts), Vocational Adjustment, Financial Status (feeling of financial security), Adjustment to Seizures (resentment about condition, ill at ease because of the possibility of attacks), Medicine and Medical Management, (reactions to attending physician, acceptance of medications), and Overall Psychosocial Functioning. The Inventory also contains three validity scales: (1) No. Blank, (2) Lie (to assess obvious tendencies to make one's self look overly good), and (3) Rare Items (items endorsed by no more than 15% of patients). A profile is produced that predicts professionals' ratings of adjustment significance and may assist in identifying areas that represent greatest adjustment difficulties. A similar inventory (Adolescent Psychosocial Seizure Inventory) has been developed for adolescents (Batzel *et al.*, 1991).

Sonnen (1991) has suggested that fear of seizures may be more responsible than social stigma for the social and vocational withdrawal seen in epilepsy patients. A substantial percentage of patients are afraid that they might die with their next seizure. Depression is one of the more common psychological problems for adults with epilepsy (Hermann *et al.*, 1992).

Pseudoepileptic Seizures

Wilkus *et al.* (1984) found no differences between a group of patients diagnosed pseudo-epileptic by EEG and closed-circuit TV monitoring and epileptic patients on any of the subtests of the WAIS or any of 16 measures from Dodrill's Neuropsychological Battery for

Epilepsy. For both groups, approximately one half of the tests were outside normal limits. In contrast to this finding, Sackellares *et al.* (1985) reported that pseudoepileptic patients had significantly higher mean WAIS IQ scores and scores on the TPT, CT, SRT, and SSPT than patients with epileptic seizures.

Pseudoepileptic patients exhibited an MMPI with Hs and Hy elevated and higher than D. A set of rules was devised using the MMPI. A patient was classified as having pseudoepileptic attacks if: (1) Hs or Hy is 70 or higher and one of two highest points (with the exception of the Mf and Si Scales), (2) Hs or Hy is 80 or higher (even though not among the two highest points), or (3) Hs and Hy are both higher than 59 and both are at least 10 points higher than D. Wilkus *et al.* (1984) found that 80–90% of a cross-validation sample were correctly classified. They advised caution in the application of these rules. Henrichs *et al.* (1988) reported a hit rate of 89% for calling not pseudoepileptic seizure and 41% for calling pseudoepileptic seizure. They concluded that the rules may be of value in ruling out the probability of pseudoepileptic seizures; however, inferring pseudoepileptic seizure is likely to be correct less than 50% of the time.

MEDICAL THERAPY

Medical treatment may involve: (1) removal of precipitating factors, (2) establishing and maintaining appropriate physical and mental hygiene, (3) antiepileptic medication, and (4) surgical excision of epileptic foci (Adams & Victor, 1989). Removal of precipitating factors may entail treatment of hyponatremia and hypocalcemia.

According to Adams and Victor (1989, p. 266), "approximately 75 percent of patients with convulsive seizures can have their attacks controlled completely or reduced in frequency and severity by the use of antiepileptic drugs." The most commonly used drugs for the control of tonic–clonic seizures and simple or complex partial seizures are phenobarbital (Luminal), phenytoin (Dilantin), carbamazepine (Tegretol), and primidone (Mysoline). See Chapter 49 for toxic effects and effects on cognition. Ethosuximide (Zarontin) and valproic acid (Depakene and Depakote) have been used to control absence seizures (Dreifuss, 1991).

A temporal lobectomy is sometimes performed as a treatment for refactory, disabling complex partial seizure disorders (Robinson & Saykin, 1992). This surgery may result in a variety of cognitive and psychosocial sequelae (Bladin, 1992).

PSYCHOSOCIAL THERAPIES

Behavioral therapy may be effective in treating epilepsy, especially reflex epilepsy (Forster, 1977; Tarlow, 1989). Forster has described several behavioral methods for treating reflex epilepsy: (1) avoidance of the stimulus; (2) repeated presentation of an altered stimulus (a nonepiletogenic stimulus similar to the epiletogenic stimulus); (3) repeated stimulations in the postictal refractory state; (4) vigilance inhibition — signaling of the occurrence of events related to seizure production (e.g., a particular letter in reading epilepsy), which may block the occurrence of the seizures; and (5) avoidance conditioning (Forster, 1977). Operant procedures have been used to decrease seizure frequency by providing social reinforcement during seizure-free periods and withdrawing reinforcement during seizures (Cautela & Flannery, 1973). Daniels (1975) used operant and covert conditioning techniques to treat seizure disorders. Relaxation (Wells *et al.,* 1978) and EEG biofeedback (Lantz & Sterman, 1992) have also been used in the treatment of seizure disorders.

Counseling may address issues such as perception of disability relative to work, fears about injury, or embarrassment as the result of a seizure. The therapist, in consultation with the physician, may need to counsel the patient on risk factors. According to Sonnen (1991), a number of risk factors have been exaggerated in importance. Contrary to popular belief, people with epilepsy are less likely to have an accident than other people. There is a small subgroup of people with epilepsy who are more accident-prone: people with a secondary type of epilepsy with tonic–clonic seizures. Each case must be evaluated individually. With higher-risk patients, greater restrictions may need to be applied. Sonnen (1991) has suggested the use of medical identification bracelets, contact lenses, and a pillow that allows air to pass, for some patients. Although 99% of patients live in houses without special provisions, in problem cases, modifications may be made to protect the patient in case of sudden falls, a "do not disturb" card may be used instead of a lock on the bathroom, and shields may be used on the stove and hot appliances. Sonnen (1991) has listed a number of recommendations regarding swimming. Tub baths present an unrecognized danger because the legs are raised during a generalized tonic–clonic seizure and the body may slide downward, forcing the head under. Showers may be preferable. "Most people with epilepsy can use public transport on their own" (Sonnen, 1991). Contrary to public expectations, people with epilepsy have a normal or lower than normal accident rate at work. Employers often fear that employing people with epilepsy may result in emotional stress for other employees, dangerous behavior that jeopardizes the company, significantly increased absenteeism, disability, and expensive claims, and low productivity. Research has not confirmed these fears. Education of employees can help them accept epileptic seizures (Sonnen, 1991).

Sonnen (1991, p. 756) has stated that "because epilepsy is a chronic condition restrictions will have lifelong consequences. A certain degree of carelessness can become a virtue." Risk-taking can be allowed for leisure and pleasure, which are as important as school and work. Risks can be communicated by comparing them to risks of similar magnitude so that they may be more readily understood and the patient can make an informed decision about which risks to accept.

Living Well with Epilepsy (Gumnit, 1990) or *Epilepsy Explained* (Laidlaw & Laidlaw, 1980) can provide useful information to patients and their families. A referral to the local chapter of the Epilepsy Foundation may also be helpful.

The unemployment rate for people with epilepsy has been reported to be 13–23% (Epilepsy Foundation of America, 1975). Early assessment and intervention may be helpful to individuals who are at greatest risk of being chronically unemployed. Risk factors include early age of onset, additional disabilities, associated neuropsychological impairment, long-term, complex, anticonvulsant regimen, male gender. and dysfunctional parenting styles (Fraser, 1991). Early intervention programs may include outreach to physicians concerning the needs of youngsters with epilepsy, provision of independent living skills training, and development of school-to-work transition programs. Adults may benefit from vocational evaluation, individual counseling, and participation in a job-finding club. Participation in such a club can build self-esteem and facilitate comfort with disclosure of the seizure condition. Driving is restricted in most countries after a seizure disorder has been diagnosed (Parsonage, 1991). The length of restriction varies from 6 months to 5 years.

Absence seizures, especially when frequent, may disrupt attention, thinking, and learning and impact negatively on educational performance. Intervention and support may be required at school and home.

PROGNOSIS

There is a 60–80% chance of a recurrence following a first seizure. The second seizure follows within a month in one third of cases and within a year in four fifths (Elwes &

Reynolds, 1991). Annegers *et al.* (1979) found that 20 years after diagnosis of epilepsy, 70% of patients were in 5-year remission. Fifty percent of patients were seizure-free and had successfully withdrawn from medication. Negative prognostic factors include partial seizures, a positive family history of epilepsy, a high pretreatment seizure frequency, and an associated neurological, social, or psychiatric handicap (Elwes & Reynolds, 1991).

Absence Seizures

Sato *et al.* (1983) found 78% of patients to be seizure-free after 6–8 years. Factors suggestive of a good prognosis are no other seizure type present, onset between 4 and 8 years of age, prompt response to treatment with a single drug, classic EEG pattern, and normal intelligence (Dreifuss, 1991; Fernandez & Samuels, 1991).

Pseudoepileptic Seizures

Lempert and Schmidt (1990) found that two thirds of a group of patients continued to have pseudoepileptic seizures at 2 years. Krumholz and Niedermeyer (1983) found 10 of 34 patients to continue to have pseudoepileptic seizures after 5 years.

REFERENCES

Adams, R. D., & Victor, M. (1989). *Principles of neurology* (4th ed.). New York: McGraw-Hill.

Anderson, V. E., & Hauser, W. A. (1988). Genetics. In J. Laidlaw, A. Richens, & J. Oxley (Eds.), *A textbook of epilepsy* (pp. 49–77). Edinburgh: Churchill-Livingston.

Annegers, J. F., Hauser, W. A., & Elveback, L. R. (1979). Remission of seizures and relapse in patients with epilepsy. *Epilepsia, 20,* 729–737.

Batzel, L. W., Dodrill, C. B., Dubinsky, B. L., Ziegler, R. G., Connolly, J. E., Freeman, R. D., Farwell, J. R., & Vining, E. P. G. (1991). An objective method for the assessment of psychosocial problems in adolescents with epilepsy. *Epilepsia, 32,* 202–211.

Berg, R. A., & Golden, C. J. (1981). Identification of neuropsychological deficits in epilepsy using the Luria–Nebraska Neuropsychological Battery. *Journal of Consulting and Clinical Psychology, 49,* 745–747.

Bladin, P. F. (1992). Psychosocial difficulties and outcome after temporal lobectomy. *Epilepsia, 33,* 898–907.

Cautela, J., & Flannery, R. (1973). Seizures: Controlling the uncontrollable. *Journal of Rehabilitation, 39,* 34–39.

Commission on Classification and Terminology of the International League Against Epilepsy (1981). Proposal for revised clinical and electroencephalographic classification of epileptic seizures. *Epilepsia, 22,* 489–501.

Commission on Classification and Terminology of the International League Against Epilepsy (1985). Proposal for classification of epilepsies and epileptic syndromes. *Epilepsia, 26,* 268–278.

Commission on Classification and Terminology of the International League Against Epilepsy (1989). Proposal for revised classification of epilepsies and epileptic syndromes. *Epilepsia, 30,* 389–399.

Daniels, L. (1975). Treatment of grand mal epilepsy by covert and operant conditioning techniques: A case study. *Psychosomatics, 16,* 65–67.

Dikmen, S., & Reitan, R. M. (1978). Neuropsychological performance in posttraumatic epilepsy. *Epilepsia, 19,* 177–183.

Dodrill, C. B. (1978). A neuropsychological battery for epilepsy. *Epilepsia, 19,* 611–623.

Dodrill, C. B. (1981). Neuropsychology of epilepsy. In S. B. Filskov & T. J. Boll (Eds.), *Handbook of clinical neuropsychology* (pp. 366–395). New York: Wiley.

Dodrill, C. B. (1988). Neuropsychology. In J. Laidlaw, A. Richens, & J. Oxley (Eds.), *A textbook of epilepsy* (pp. 406–420). Edinburgh: Churchill-Livingston.

Dodrill, C. B. (1991). Neuropsychology. In M. Dam & L. Gram (Eds.), *Comprehensive epileptology* (pp. 473–484). New York: Raven Press.

Dodrill, C. B., & Matthews, C. G. (1992). The role of neuropsychology in the assessment and treatment of persons with epilepsy. *American Psychologist, 47,* 1139–1142.

Dodrill, C. B., Batzel, L. W., Queisser, H. R., & Temkin, N. R. (1980). An objective method for the assessment of psychological and social problems among epileptics. *Epilepsia, 21,* 123–135.

Dreifuss, F. E. (1991). Absence epilepsies. In M. Dam & L. Gram (Eds.), *Comprehensive epileptology* (pp. 145–153). New York: Raven Press.

Elwes, R. D. C., & Reynolds, E. H. (1991). The early prognosis of epilepsy. In M. Dam & L. Gram (Eds.), *Comprehensive epileptology* (pp. 715–727). New York: Raven Press.

Epilepsy Foundation of America (1975). *Basic statistics on the epilepsies.* Philadelphia: F. A. Davis.

Feldman, R. G., Paul, N. L., & Cummins-Ducharme, J. (1982). Videotape recording in epilepsy and pseudoseizures. In T. L. Riley & A. Roy (Eds.), *Pseudoseizures* (pp. 122–131). Baltimore: Williams & Wilkins.

Fernandez, R. J., & Samuels, M. A. (1991). Epilepsy. In M. A. Samuels (Ed.), *Manual of neurology: Diagnosis and therapy* (pp. 82–118). Little, Brown.

Forster, F. M. (1977). *Reflex epilepsy, behavioral therapy and conditional reflexes.* Springfield, IL: Charles C. Thomas.

Fowler, P. C., Richards, H. C., Berent, S., & Boll, T. J. (1987). Epilepsy, neuropsychological deficits, and EEG lateralization. *Archives of Clinical Neuropsychology, 2,* 81–92.

Fraser, R. T. (1991). Vocational rehabilitation. In M. Dam & L. Gram (Eds.), *Comprehensive epileptology* (pp. 729–742). New York: Raven Press.

Gumnit, R. J. (1990). *Living well with epilepsy.* New York: Demos.

Hauser, W. A., Annegers, J. F., & Kurland, L. T. (1991). Prevalence of epilepsy in Rochester, Minnesota: 1940–1980. *Epilepsia, 32,* 429–445.

Henrichs, T. F., Tucker, D. M., Farha, J., & Novelly, R. A. (1988). MMPI indices in the identification of patients evidencing pseudoseizures. *Epilepsia, 29,* 184–187.

Hermann, B. P., & Melyn, M. (1985). Identification of neuropsychological deficits in epilepsy using the Luria–Nebraska Neuropsychological Battery: A replication attempt. *Journal of Clinical and Experimental Psychology, 7,* 305–313.

Hermann, B. P., Whitman, S., & Anton, M. (1992). A multietiological model of psychological and social dysfunction in epilepsy. In T. L. Bennett (Ed.), *The neuropsychology of epilepsy* (pp. 39–57). New York: Plenum Press.

Klove, H., & Matthews, C. G. (1974). Neuropsychological studies of patients with epilepsy. In R. M. Reitan & L. A. Davison (Eds.), *Clinical neuropsychology: Current status and applications* (pp. 237–265). Washington, DC: Winston.

Krumholz, A., & Niedermeyer, E. (1983). Psychogenic seizures: A clinical study with follow up data. *Neurology,* 498–502.

Kupke, T., & Lewis, R. (1985). WAIS and neuropsychological tests: Common and unique variance within an epileptic population. *Journal of Clinical and Experimental Neuropsychology, 7,* 353–366.

Laidlaw, M. V., & Laidlaw, J. (1980). *Epilepsy explained.* Edinburgh: Churchill-Livingston.

Lantz, D., & Sterman, M. B. (1992). Neuropsychological prediction and outcome measures in relation to EEG feedback training for the treatment of epilepsy. In T. L. Bennett (Ed.), *The neuropsychology of epilepsy* (pp. 213–231). New York: Plenum Press.

Lempert, T., & Schmidt, D. (1990). Natural history and outcome of psychogenic seizures: A clinical study in 50 patients. *Journal of Neurology, 237,* 35–38.

Loring, D. W., Meador, K. J., & Lee, G. P. (1992a). Criteria and validity issues in Wada assessment. In T. L. Bennett (Ed.), *The neuropsychology of epilepsy* (pp. 233–245). New York: Plenum Press.

Loring, D. W., Meador, K. J., Lee, G. P., & King, D. W. (1992b). *Amobarbital effects and lateralized brain function: The Wada test.* New York: Springer-Verlag.

Milner, B. (1974). Hemispheric specialization: Scope and limits. In F. O. Schmitt & F. G. Worden (Eds.), *The neurosciences: Third study program* (pp. 75–89). Cambridge, MA: MIT Press.

Mulder, O. G. (1991). Management of pseudo-epileptic seizures. In M. Dam & L. Gram (Eds.), *Comprehensive epileptology* (pp. 495–504). New York: Raven Press.

Parsonage, M. (1991). Drivers' licenses. In M. Dam & L. Gram (Eds.), *Comprehensive epileptology* (pp. 743–752). New York: Raven Press.

Porter, R. J. (1989). *Epilepsy: 100 elementary principles.* London: W. B. Saunders.

Ramani, V. (1986). Intensive monitoring of psychogenic seizures, aggression and dyscontrol syndromes. In R. J. Gumnit (Ed.), *Advances in neurology,* Volume 46, *Intensive neurodiagnostic monitoring* (pp. 203–217). New York: Raven Press.

Riela, A. R., & Penry, J. K. (1991). Magnetic resonance imaging. In M. Dam & L. Gram (Eds.), *Comprehensive epileptology* (pp. 359–374). New York: Raven Press.

Robinson, L. J., & Saykin, A. J. (1992). Psychological and psychosocial outcome of anterior temporal lobectomy. In T. L. Bennett (Ed.), *The neuropsychology of epilepsy* (pp. 181–197). New York: Plenum Press.

Sackellares, J. C., Giordoni, B., Berent, S., Seidenberg, M., Dreifuss, F., Vanderzaut, C. W., & Boll, T. J. (1985). Patients with pseudoseizures: intellectual and cognitive performance. *Neurology, 35,* 116–119.

Sato, S., Dreifuss, F. E., & Penry, J. K. (1983). Long term follow up of absence seizures. *Neurology, 33,* 1590–1595.

Scott, D. F. (1982). The use of EEG in pseudoseizures. In T. L. Riley & A. Roy (Eds.), *Pseudoseizures* (pp. 113–121). Baltimore: Williams & Wilkins.

Sonnen, A. E. H. (1991). How to live with epilepsy. In M. Dam & L. Gram (Eds.), *Comprehensive epileptology* (pp. 753–767). New York: Raven Press.

Sperling, M. R. (1990). Neuroimaging in epilepsy: Contribution of MRI, PET and SPECT. *Seminars in Neurology, 10,* 349–356.

Stevenson, J. M., & King, J. H. (1987). Neuropsychiatric aspects of epilepsy and epileptic seizures. In R. E. Hales & S. C. Yudolfsky (Eds.), *The American Psychiatric Press textbook of neuropsychiatry.* Washington, DC: American Psychiatric Press.

Tarlow, G. (1989). *Clinical handbook of behavior therapy: Adult medical disorders.* Cambridge, MA: Brookline Books.

Tassinari, C. A., Rubboli, G., & Michelucci, R. (1991). Reflex epilepsy. In M. Dam & L. Gram (Eds.), *Comprehensive epileptology* (pp. 233–246). New York: Raven Press.

Uthman, B. M., & Wilder, B. J. (1989). Emergency management of seizures: An overview. *Epilepsia, 30*(Supplement 2), S33–S37.

Walker, J. A., Stanulis, R. G., & Laxer, K. D. (1987). What stages of memory do the temporal lobes serve? A sodium amytal perspective. In J. Engle, G. A. Ojemann, H. O. Luders, & P. D. Williamson (Eds.), *Fundamentals of human brain function* (pp. 111–117). New York: Raven Press.

Wallace, S. J. (1988). Seizures in children. In J. Laidlaw, A. Richens, & J. Oxley (Eds.), *A textbook of epilepsy* (pp. 78–143). Edinburgh: Churchill-Livingston.

Wells, K., Turner, S., Bellack, A., & Hersen, M. (1978). Effects of cue-controlled relaxation on psychomotor seizures: An experimental analysis. *Behavior Research and Therapy, 16,* 51–53.

Wilkus, R. J., Dodrill, C. B., & Thompson, P. M. (1984). Intensive EEG monitoring and psychological studies of patients with pseudoepileptic seizures. *Epilepsia, 25,* 100–107.

Zielinski, J. J. (1988). Epidemiology. In J. Laidlaw, A. Richens, & J. Oxley (Eds.), *A textbook of epilepsy* (pp. 21–48). Edinburgh: Churchill-Livingston.

Alzheimer's Disease

DESCRIPTION

Alzheimer's disease is a progressive degenerative neurological disorder characterized by an insidious onset, a slow, progressive course, and decline in memory and language functioning (Group for the Advancement of Psychiatry, 1988).

INCIDENCE, PREVALENCE, AND RISK FACTORS

Incidence

The incidence has been estimated as 123 cases/100,000 from a study of Rochester, Minnesota (Schoenberg et al., 1987).

Age

In a study of a geographically defined, urban, working-class community in East Boston, Massachusetts, the prevalence rate was 3.0% for individuals 65–74 years of age, 18.7% for individuals 75–84, and 47.2% for those over 85 (Evans et al., 1989).

Gender

Age-adjusted prevalence rates for women are higher than for men (Jorm et al., 1987).

Family History

First-degree relatives of patients with Alzheimer's disease have increased incidence of dementia (Henderson, 1990).

ETIOLOGY AND PATHOLOGY

Neurofibrillary tangles and neuritic plaques may be found in the hippocampus and adjacent structures and in the neocortex (Price, 1986). The primary neurochemical deficiency in Alzheimer's disease is an impairment in cholinergic transmission (Coyle et al., 1983).

Although there are a variety of theories of Alzheimer's disease (vascular, viral, autoimmune, toxic, and genetic), none has been validated (Group for the Advancement of Psychiatry, 1988).

MEDICAL ASSESSMENT

There is no known peripheral biochemical marker for Alzheimer's disease (Katzman, 1986). A definitive diagnosis of Alzheimer's disease can be made only on the basis of a cerebral biopsy or an autopsy. In clinical practice, diagnosis must therefore be made on the basis of history, behavioral and intellectual impairments, and laboratory tests to rule out treatable dementias and other possible disorders. Laboratory tests commonly include CT scan, chest film, comprehensive biochemical screening, determination of vitamin B_{12} level, thyroid-function tests, a serological test for syphilis, and possibly an examination of CSF (Katzman, 1986). Recommendations for medical evaluation may be found in the NIH Consensus Development Conference Statement (NIH Consensus Development Panel, 1987). Although a CT scan cannot definitively diagnose Alzheimer's disease, it can assist in ruling out other possible etiologies such as stroke (A. L. Powell & Benson, 1990). Patients with advanced Alzheimer's disease may exhibit enlarged lateral or third ventricles, or both, and widened sulci (Naugle & Bigler, 1989). Early in the disease, changes may not be detectable. MacInnes et al. (1990) found that radiologists using subjective ratings of CT scans diagnosed only 20% of patients with dementia correctly. PET (Friedland et al., 1989) and SPECT (Schmitt et al., 1992) may reveal temporoparietal cortical hypometabolism. Evoked potentials (P300) may be delayed (Goodwin et al., 1978). P300 may be more sensitive under mnemonic demand (de Toledo-Morell et al., 1991).

Criteria have been established for the diagnosis of probable Alzheimer's disease (McKhann et al., 1984). They include: (1) dementia established by clinical diagnosis, documented by mental status testing, and confirmed by neuropsychological tests; (2) deficits in two or more areas of cognition; (3) progressive worsening of memory and other cognitive functions; (4) no disturbance of consciousness; (5) onset between the ages of 40 and 90; and (6) "absence of systemic disorders or other brain diseases that in and of themselves could account for the progressive deficits in memory and cognition" (McKhann et al., 1984, p. 940). Further elaborations of the criteria may be found in the article by McKhann et al. (1984).

The progression of Alzheimer's disease has been conceptualized as having three stages (Cummings & Benson, 1983; Group for the Advancement of Psychiatry, 1988). In Stage I (mild, 1–3 years), new learning and recent memory may be impaired, but the patient is oriented as to time, date, and location. There may be a mild deficit in remote memory. Topographic disorientation (lost in unfamiliar places) and impaired visuoconstructional ability may be noted. Word finding, word fluency, and anomia may be present. Activities of daily living (ADLs) are intact. The EEG and CT are normal.

In Stage II (moderate, 2–10 years), recent and remote recall, spatial orientation, and constructional ability become more severely impaired, but the patient may be able to travel to familiar locations. Word finding becomes more impaired, with limited vocabulary and sentence structure. ADLs are grossly intact, although assistance in decision-making and planning may sometimes be required. The patient may with draw from challenging situations. Denial, indifference, and apathy may be noted. The EEG may exhibit slowing, while the CT may be normal or exhibit mild ventricular and sulcal enlargement.

In Stage III (severe, 8–12 years), memory and cognition are severely deteriorated.

Assistance is required in all areas. Limb rigidity and flexion posture are present. The EEG is slow, and ventricular and sulcal enlargement is present on CT.

Initial symptoms may first appear in any of the areas of functioning commonly affected in Alzheimer's disease: (1) memory (Grady et al., 1988), (2) language (Kirshner et al., 1984), and (3) visuospatial functioning.

Huff et al. (1987b) found that aside from the mental status findings of a standardized neurological exam, the presence of release signs, olfactory deficit, impaired stereognosis, gait disorder, and abnormalities on cerebellar testing helped in differentiating patients with probable Alzheimer's disease from controls.

NEUROPSYCHOLOGICAL ASSESSMENT

Since the diagnosis of Alzheimer's disease depends partly on the determination of cognitive impairment, neuropsychological testing can make a valuable contribution to diagnosis. It is also useful for assessing intact cognitive strengths, areas of impairment, and changes over time. According to the NIH Consensus Development Conference Statement (NIH Consensus Development Panel, 1987, p. 3415).

> neuropsychological evaluation is appropriate (1) to obtain baseline information against which to measure change in cases in which diagnosis is in doubt, (2) before and after treatment, (3) in cases of exceptionally bright individuals suspected of early dementia, (4) in cases of ambiguous imaging findings that require elucidation, (5) to help distinguish dementia from depression and delirium, and (6) to provide additional information about the extent and nature of impairment following focal or multifocal brain injury.

Neuropsychological testing can assist in the early detection of Alzheimer's disease. Welsh et al. (1992) found delayed recall and confrontation naming to be most sensitive. Fluency, praxis, and recognition memory were useful in staging. Hom (1992) found that Alzheimer's disease patients differed significantly from normals ("late confusional" to "early dementia" stages) on all the HRNB tasks with the exception of simple motor and sensory tasks. The literature suggests that clinical interview and collateral history are critical in evaluating dementia (Huff et al., 1987a; Jorm & Korten, 1988; Morris et al., 1991).

Behavior Rating Scales

Numerous behavior rating scales have been developed (McDonald, 1986).

Mental Status

Ratings on the MMSE may correlate with ratings on the Global Deterioration Scale (Reisberg et al., 1986b).

Attention

DS Forward is unimpaired in the early stages (Corkin et al., 1986; Weingartner et al., 1981), but becomes increasingly impaired over time (Kaszniak et al., 1979). D Sym may exhibit impairment (Reisberg et al., 1986a). Lines et al. (1991) found no difference between controls and patients with mild Alzheimer's disease on a CPT.

Memory

Explicit memory is often severely and consistently disrupted, while acquisition of visuo-motor skills may remain intact (Carlesimo & Oscar-Berman, 1992). Brinkman *et al.* (1983) found that Alzheimer's patients performed significantly less well than controls on all subscales of the Russell revision of the WMS. Difficult pairs in the Paired-Associates subtest of the WMS may be sensitive even in cases of questionable dementia (Duchek *et al.,* 1991). A gentle temporal gradient may be noted in remote memory loss (Kopelman, 1989). The SRT has been found to be sensitive to the memory impairment associated with Alzheimer's. Masur *et al.* (1989) reported predictive values of 86% for consistent long-term storage, 89% for long-term retrieval, 91% for sum of recall, and 100% for storage estimate.

General Intelligence and Social Understanding

The WAIS IQ is likely to be diminished (Miller, 1977). Fuld (1984) has suggested that the following profile [associated with administration of an anticholinergic drug (Drachman & Leavitt, 1974)] might be associated with Alzheimer's disease. The profile is defined as follows: (1) A = (Information + Vocabulary)/2; B = (Similarities + Digit Span)/2; C = (Digit Symbol + Block Design)/2; D = Object Assembly; A > B > C ≤ D and A > D. Evidence for this contention has been mixed (Brinkman & Braun, 1984; Filley *et al.,* 1987; Logsdon *et al.,* 1989; Satz *et al.,* 1987).

Speech/Language

BDAE Visual Confrontation Naming (objects, actions, and forms), Body-Part Naming, Complex Ideational Material, and Commands may be impaired (Rosen, 1983). Using the BDAE and additional tests, Cummings *et al.* (1985) found fluent paraphasic speech and impaired auditory comprehension with relative preservation of the ability to repeat, character-istics of transcortical sensory aphasia, in Alzheimer's patients (mean MMSE = 10.50). In the late stage of Alzheimer's disease, repetition deteriorates and verbal output resembles that of Wernicke's aphasia. Moderately demented patients with probable Alzheimer's disease were impaired on the 60-item BNT (Williams *et al.,* 1989). A cutoff score of 51 correctly classified 80% of Alzheimer's patients and 86% of normal controls. Descriptive writing may exhibit letter, spelling, and content word errors (Neils *et al.,* 1989). Impairment may be noted on the Token Test (Corkin *et al.,* 1986). Nebes (1989) has written a comprehensive review of semantic memory in Alzheimer's disease.

Visuospatial Functioning

Patients with Alzheimer's disease may exhibit impairments on BD, ROCFT:C, and Ravens Colored Progressive Matricies (Freedman & Dexter, 1991; Gainotti *et al.,* 1992). Performances may be quantitatively similar to those of patients with right hemisphere brain injury. Drawing and copying may be impaired (Ober *et al.,* 1991). Performance may be impaired on the FR and the JLO (Brouwers *et al.,* 1984).

Olfaction

Olfactory deficits may be associated with Alzheimer's disease (Gilbert, 1986; S. Hart & Semple, 1990).

Motor Functioning

The FTT is usually intact (Reisberg *et al.*, 1986a).

Executive Functioning

Impairment is likely in both letter and categorical word fluency (Ober *et al.*, 1986; Rosen, 1980). Performance has been found deficient, relative to normals, on a modified WCST (R. P. Hart *et al.*, 1988). The test did not distinguish patients with mild Alzheimer's disease from patients with depression.

Personality

Passive behavioral changes are present in mild Alzheimer's disease (Rubin, 1990). Agitation increases throughout the course. Self-centered behavior is prominent during the moderate stage. Depressed mood may occur in 40–50% of patients, with depressive disorders occurring in 10–20% of patients (Wragg & Jeste, 1989). Bozzola *et al.* (1992) found 61.3% of a group of Alzheimer's disease patients to exhibit diminished initiative; 55%, relinquishment of hobbies; and 41.3%, increased rigidity. Care-givers have reported inconsistently depressed mood (46.2%), agitation (46.2%), and sleep disturbance (41.8%) in patients (Devanand *et al.*, 1992).

Distinguishing dementia from depression or pseudodementia is a common diagnostic problem. Distinguishing severe dementia from depression may be accomplished with some confidence. Patients with depression rarely score below 12 on the MMSE, and they rarely display grossly disturbed behavior such as trying to eat a pencil or putting underwear on over outerwear (Spar & La Rue, 1990). Distinguishing mild dementia from depression can be extremely difficult. The capacity of neuropsychological testing to contribute significantly to resolving this diagnostic dilemma has been questioned (Caine, 1986). Walsh (1991) has stated, to the contrary, that if careful qualitative observations are made, neuropsychological testing can be useful in the context of the patient's history. Wells (1979) has suggested that inconsistencies in the test performance may be more suggestive of depression than of dementia. Some rules of thumb for making the distinction are as follows:

Dementia is associated with an indistinct and extended onset, a slow progression (Bigler, 1988; Salzman & Gutfreund, 1986; Strub & Black, 1988). Depressed mood follows memory loss. The patient does not complain of and is unaware of his or her cognitive symptoms in the moderate to severe stages. The patient may attempt to be cooperative during testing. Everyday behavior is congruent with cognitive loss. Affect is limited. Recent memory is invariably impaired. Remote memory is relatively preserved in early stages.

Depression is associated with a distinct and brief onset with a rapid progression (Bigler, 1988; Salzman & Gutfreund, 1986; Strub & Black, 1988). Memory loss follows depressed mood. The patient complains in detail about and is aware of his or her cognitive symptoms. Poor cooperation or effort is noted during testing. Everyday behavior is incongruent with cognitive loss. Affective change is noted. Recent memory may be impaired, but inconsistencies may be noted. Gaps in remote memory may be noted.

Jones *et al.* (1992) found the TOT and the BVRT to be indicators of later-developing dementia. Lamberty and Bieliauskas (1993) reported that dementia and depression can be effectively distinguished by medical and neuropsychological evaluation. For depression, very mild impairments in cognitive functioning with greater impairments on motor and attentional tasks are expected. More substantial impairments are expected for Alzheimer's disease. For depression, "shallow" encoding of information, decreased response latency, and adequate encoding of information with serial presentation are often noted. For Alzheimer's disease, lack of ability to systematically encode information and little benefit from serial presentation of materials may be found. In depression, in contrast to dementia, delayed recall may be within normal limits. In depression, there may be reduced verbal fluency, while in dementia, a more general deficit in verbal functioning is noted.

It may also be helpful to compare the patient's profile of cognitive functioning with the profiles presented in Chapters 40 through 45, and 51. If depression is suspected, a trial of antidepressant medication is often administered (Salzman & Gutfreund, 1986; Spar & La Rue, 1990). A retest may be appropriate to determine whether there has been any change in cognitive functioning. Retests at 6 months to 1 year may be helpful for patients who are suspected of having a dementing disorder or elderly patients who are periodically depressed (Walsh, 1991).

Approximately one third of patients experience psychotic symptoms, with persecutory delusions most common. Psychotic symptoms, especially delusions, are more common in patients with a higher level of cognitive functioning.

MEDICAL TREATMENT

There is no effective medical treatment for Alzheimer's disease (Adams & Victor, 1989; Kaszniak, 1986).

PSYCHOSOCIAL THERAPIES

Individual psychotherapy may assist the patient in coping in the early stages when the patient is aware of intellectual decline (Group for the Advancement of Psychiatry, 1988). Therapy may focus on stress reduction and maximizing the patient's feelings of dignity. In the middle stages, reality orientation may improve the patient's feeling of well-being and help structure the patient's life. Behavioral programs may be useful if behavior problems arise. Cognitive rehabilitation has had very limited success. Environmental modifications such as the removal of hazards and the use of memory prostheses have been recommended (Group for the Advancement of Psychiatry, 1988). The burden of care on family members may result in depression. Family therapy involves education about the disease and practicalities of treatment.

Self-help books include *Alzheimer's: A Caregiver's Guide and Sourcebook* (Gruetzner, 1988), *Alzheimer's Disease: A Guide for Families* (L. S. Powell & Courtice, 1986), and *Alzheimer's, Stroke, and 29 Other Neurological Disorders Sourcebook* (Bair, 1993).

Referral should be made to the local chapter of the Alzheimer's Disease and Related Disorder Association. The address of the national office is: 70 East Lake Street, Suite 600, Chicago, IL 60601.

PROGNOSIS

Predictors of progression of cognitive dysfunction include aggressive behavior, sleep disturbance, history of alcohol abuse, presence of language impairment, extrapyramidal motor signs, myoclonus, psychoses, and hearing impairment (Mortimer *et al.*, 1992). Severity of memory or language deficits or both has been correlated with mortality rate (Heyman *et al.*,

1987). Psychotic symptoms during the mild stage are associated with more rapid cognitive deterioration (Rubin, 1990). The course of the disease from onset to death is approximately 5–10 years (Group for the Advancement of Psychiatry, 1988).

REFERENCES

Adams, R. D., & Victor, M. (1989). *Principles of neurology* (4th ed.). New York: McGraw-Hill.

Bair, F. E. (1993). *Alzheimer's, stroke, and 29 other neurological disorders sourcebook.* Detroit: Omnigraphics.

Bigler, E. D. (1988). *Diagnostic clinical neuropsychology.* Austin: University of Texas Press.

Bozzola, F. G., Gorelick, P. B., & Freels, S. (1992). Personality changes in Alzheimer's disease. *Archives of Neurology, 49,* 297–300.

Brinkman, S. D., & Braun, P. (1984). Classification of dementia patients by a WAIS profile related to central cholinergic deficits. *Journal of Clinical and Experimental Neuropsychology, 6,* 393–400.

Brinkman, S. D., Largen, J. W., Gerganoff, S., & Pomara, N. (1983). Russell's revised Wechsler Memory Scale in the evaluation of dementia. *Journal of Clinical Psychology, 39,* 989–993.

Brouwers, P., Cox, C., Martin, A., & Chase, T. (1984). Differential perceptual–spatial impairment in Huntington's and Alzheimer's dementias. *Archives of Neurology, 41,* 1973–1976.

Caine, E. D. (1986). The neuropsychology of depression: The pseudodementia syndrome. In I. Grant & K. M. Adams (Eds.), *Neuropsychological assessment of neuropsychiatric disorders* (pp. 221–243). New York: Oxford University Press.

Carlesimo, G. A., & Oscar-Berman, M. (1992). Memory deficits in Alzheimer's patients: A comprehensive review. *Neuropsychology Review, 3,* 119–169.

Corkin, S., Growdin, J. H., Sullivan, E. V., Nissen, M. J., & Huff, F. J. (1986). Assessing treatment effects: A neuropsychological battery. In L. W. Poon (Ed.), *Handbook for clinical memory assessment of older adults* (pp. 156–167). Washington, DC: American Psychological Association.

Coyle, J. T., Price, D. L., & DeLong, M. R. (1983). Alzheimer's disease: A disorder of cortical cholinergic innervation. *Science, 219,* 1184–1219.

Cummings, J. L., & Benson, D. F. (1983). *Dementia: A clinical approach.* Boston: Butterworths.

Cummings, J. L., Benson, D. F., Hill, M. A., & Read, S. (1985). Aphasia in dementia of the Alzheimer type. *Neurology, 35,* 394–397.

De Toledo-Morrell, L., Evers, S., Hoeppner, T. J., Morrell, F., Garron, D. C., & Fox, J. H. (1991). A "stress" test for memory dysfunction: Electrophysiologic manifestations of early Alzheimer's disease. *Archives of Neurology, 48,* 605–609.

Devanand, D. P., Miller, L., Richards, M., Marder, R., Bell, K., Mayeux, R., & Stern, Y. (1992). The Columbia University Scale for psychopathology in Alzheimer's disease. *Archives of Neurology, 49,* 371–376.

Drachman, D. A., & Leavitt, J. (1974). Human memory and the cholinergic system: A relationship to aging? *Archives of Neurology, 30,* 113–121.

Duchek, J. M., Cheney, M., Ferraro, R., & Storandt, M. (1991). Paired associate learning in senile dementia of the Alzheimer type. *Archives of Neurology, 48,* 1038–1040.

Evans, D. A., Funkenstein, H. H., Albert, M. S., Scherr, P. A., Cook, N. R., Chown, M. J., Hebert, L. E., Hennekens, C. H., & Taylor, J. O. (1989). Prevalence of Alzheimer's disease in a community population of older persons: Higher than previously reported. *JAMA, 262,* 2551–2556.

Filley, C. M., Kobayashi, J., & Heaton, R. K. (1987). Wechsler Intelligence Scale profiles, the cholinergic system, and Alzheimer's disease. *Journal of Clinical and Experimental Neuropsychology, 9,* 180–186.

Freedman, L., & Dexter, L. E. (1991). Visuospatial ability in cortical dementia. *Journal of Clinical and Experimental Neuropsychology, 13,* 677–690.

Friedland, R. P., Jagust, W. J., Huesman, R. H., Koss, E., Knittel, B., Mathis, C. A., Ober, B. A., Mazoyer, B. M., & Budinger, T. F. (1989). Regional cerebral glucose transport and utilization in Alzheimer's disease. *Neurology, 39,* 1427–1434.

Fuld, P. A. (1984). Test profile of cholinergic dysfunction and Alzheimer-type dementia. *Journal of Clinical Neuropsychology, 6,* 380–392.

Gainotti, G., Parlato, V., Monteleone, D., & Carlomagno, S. (1992). Neuropsychological markers of dementia on visual–spatial tasks: A comparison between Alzheimer's type and vascular forms of dementia. *Journal of Clinical and Experimental Neuropsychology, 14,* 239–252.

Gilbert, A. N. (1986). The neuropsychology of olfaction in Alzheimer's disease. *Neurobiology of Aging, 7,* 578–579.

Goodwin, D. C., Squires, K. C., & Starr, A. (1978). Long latency event–related components of the auditory evoked potential in dementia. *Brain, 101,* 635–648.

Grady, C. L., Haxby, J. V., Horwitz, B., Sundaram, M., Berg, G., Schapiro, M., Friedland, R. P., & Rapoport, S. I. (1988). Longitudinal study of the early neuropsychological and cerebral metabolic changes in dementia of the Alzheimer type. *Journal of Clinical and Experimental Neuropsychology, 5,* 576–596.

Group for the Advancement of Psychiatry. (1988). *The psychiatric treatment of Alzheimer's disease.* New York: Brunner/Mazel.

Gruetzner, H. (1988). *Alzheimer's: A caregiver's guide and sourcebook.* New York: Wiley.

Hart, R. P., Kwentus, J. A., Wade, J. B., & Taylor, J. R. (1988). Modified Wisconsin Sorting Test in elderly normal, depressed and demented patients. *The Clinical Neuropsychologist, 2,* 49–56.

Hart, S., & Semple, J. M. (1990). *Neuropsychology and the dementias.* London: Taylor & Francis.

Heyman, A., Wilkinson, W. E., Hurwitz, B. J., Helms, M. J., Haynes, C. S., Utley, C. M., & Gwyther, L. P. (1987). Early-onset Alzheimer's disease: Clinical predictors of institutionalization and death. *Neurology, 37,* 980–984.

Henderson, A. J. (1990). Epidemiology of dementia disorders. In R. J. Wurtman, S. Corkin, J. H. Growdin, E. Ritter-Walker (Eds.) *Advances in neurology, Volume 51, Alzheimer's disease.* New York: Raven Press.

Hom, J. (1992). General and specific cognitive dysfunctions in patients with Alzheimer's disease. *Archives of Clinical Neuropsychology, 7,* 121–133.

Huff, F. J., Becker, J. T., Belle, S. H., Nebes, R. D., Holland, A. L., & Boller, F. (1987a). Cognitive deficits and clinical diagnosis of Alzheimer's disease. *Neurology, 37,* 1119–1124.

Huff, F. J., Boller, F., Lucchelli, F., Querriera, R., Beyer, J., & Belle, S. (1987b). The neurologic examination in patients with probable Alzheimer's disease. *Archives of Neurology, 44,* 929–932.

Jorm, A. F., & Korten, A. E. (1988). Assessment of cognitive decline in the elderly by informant interview. *British Journal of Psychiatry, 152,* 209–213.

Jorm, A. F., Korten, A. E., & Henderson, A. S. (1987). The prevalence of dementia: A quantitative integration of the literature. *Acta Psychiatrica Scandinavica, 76,* 465–479.

Jones, R. D., Tranel, D., Benton, A., & Paulsen, J. (1992). Differentiating dementia from "pseudodementia" early in the clinical course: Utility of neuropsychological tests. *Neuropsychology, 6,* 13–21.

Kaszniak, A. W. (1986). The neuropsychology of dementia. In I. Grant & K. M. Adams (Eds.), *Neuropsychological assessment of neuropsychiatric disorders* (pp. 172–220). New York: Oxford University Press.

Kaszniak, A. W., Garron, D. C., & Fox, J. H. (1979). Differential effects of age and cerebral atrophy upon span of immediate recall and paired associate learning in older patients suspected of dementia. *Cortex, 15,* 285–295.

Katzman, R. (1986). Alzheimer's disease. *New England Journal of Medicine, 314,* 964–973.

Kirshner, H. S., Webb, W. G., Kelly, M. P., & Wells, C. E. (1984). Language disturbance: An initial symptom of cortical degenerations and dementia. *Archives of Neurology, 41,* 491–496.

Kopelman, M. D. (1989). Remote and autobiographical memory, temporal context memory and frontal atrophy in Korsakoff and Alzheimer patients. *Neuropsychologia, 27,* 437–460.

Lamberty, G. J., & Bieliauskas, L. A. (1993). Distinguishing between depression and dementia in the elderly: A review of neuropsychological findings. *Archives of Clinical Neuropsychology, 8,* 149–170.

Lines, C. R., Dawson, C., Preston, G. C., Reich, S., Foster, C., & Traub, M. (1991). Memory and attention in patients with senile dementia of the Alzheimer type and in normal elderly subjects. *Journal of Clinical and Experimental Neuropsychology, 13,* 691–702.

Logsdon, R. G., Teri, L., Williams, D. E., Vitiello, M. V., & Prinz, P. N. (1989). The WAIS-R profile: A diagnostic tool for Alzheimer's disease? *Journal of Clinical and Experimental Neuropsychology, 11,* 892–898.

MacInnes, W. D., Rysavy, J. A., McGill, J. E., Mahoney, P. D., Wilmot, M. D., Frick, M. P., & Elyaderani, M. K. (1990). The usefulness and limitations of CT scans in the diagnosis of Alzheimer's disease. *International Journal of Clinical Neuropsychology, 12,* 127–130.

Masur, D. M., Fuld, P. A., Blau, A. D., Thal, L. J., Levin, H. S., & Aronson, M. K. (1989). Distinguishing normal and demented elderly with the Selective Reminding Test. *Journal of Clinical and Experimental Neuropsychology, 11,* 615–630.

McDonald, R. S. (1986). Assessing treatment effects: Behavior Rating Scales. In L. W. Poon (Ed.), *Handbook for clinical memory assessment of older adults* (pp. 129–138). Washington, DC: American Psychological Association.

McKhann, G., Drachman, D., Folstein, M., Katzman, R., Price, D., & Stadlan, E. M. (1984). Clinical diagnosis of Alzheimer's disease: Report of the NINCDS–ADRDA Work Group under the auspices of the Department of Health and Human Services Task Force on Alzheimer's disease. *Neurology, 34,* 939–944.

Miller, E. (1977). *Abnormal ageing: The psychology of senile and presenile dementia.* New York: Wiley.

Morris, J. C., McKeel, D. W., Storandt, M., Rubin, E. H., Price, J. L., Grant, E. A., Ball, M. J., & Berg, L. (1991). Very mild Alzheimer's disease: Informant-based clinical psychometric, and pathologic distinction from normal aging. *Neurology, 41,* 469–478.

Mortimer, J. A., Ebbitt, B., Jun, S., & Finch, M. D. (1992). Predictors of cognitive and functional progression in patients with probable Alzheimer's disease. *Neurology, 42,* 1689–1696.

Naugle, R. I., & Bigler, E. D. (1989). Brain imaging and neuropsychological identification of dementia of the Alzheimer's type. In E. D. Bigler, R. A. Yeo, & E. Turkheimer (Eds.). *Neuropsychological function and brain imaging* (pp. 185–218). New York: Plenum Press.

Nebes, R. D. (1989). Semantic memory in Alzheimer's disease. *Psychological Bulletin, 3,* 377–394.

Neils, J., Boller, F., Gerdeman, B., & Cole, M. (1989). Descriptive writing abilities in Alzheimer's disease. *Journal of Clinical and Experimental Neuropsychology, 11,* 692–698.

NIH Consensus Development Panel (1987). Differential diagnosis of dementing diseases. *JAMA, 258,* 3411–3416.

Ober, B. A., Dronkers, N. F., Koss, E., Delis, D. C., & Friedland, R. P. (1986). Retrieval from semantic memory in Alzheimer-type dementia. *Journal of Clinical and Experimental Neuropsychology, 8,* 75–92.

Ober, B. A., Jagust, W. J., Koss, E., Delis, D. C., & Friedland, R. P. (1991). Visuoconstructive performance and regional cerebral glucose metabolism in Alzheimer's disease. *Journal of Clinical and Experimental Neuropsychology, 13,* 752–772.

Powell, A. L., & Benson, D. F. (1990). Brain imaging techniques in the diagnosis of dementia. *Neuropsychology Review, 1,* 3–19.

Powell, L. S., & Courtice, K. (1986). *Alzheimer's disease: A guide for families.* Reading, MA: Addison-Wesley.

Price, D. L. (1986). New perspectives on Alzheimer's disease. *Annual Review of Neuroscience, 9,* 489–512.

Reisberg, B., Ferris, S. H., Borenstein, J., Sinaiko, E., de Leon, M. J., & Buttinger, C. (1986a). Assessment of presenting symptoms. In L. W. Poon (Ed.), *Handbook for clinical memory assessment of older adults* (pp. 108–128). Washington, DC: American Psychological Association.

Reisberg, B., Ferris, S. H., de Leon, M. J., & Crook, T. (1986b). The Global Deterioration Scale for the assessment of primary degenerative dementia. *American Journal of Psychiatry, 139,* 1136–1139.

Rosen, W. G. (1980). Verbal fluency in aging and dementia. *Journal of Clinical Neuropsychology, 2,* 135–146.

Rosen, W. G. (1983). Neuropsychological investigation of memory, visuoconstructional, visuoperceptual, and language abilities in senile dementia of the Alzheimer type. In R. Mayeux & W. G. Rosen (Eds.), *The dementias* (pp. 65–73). New York: Raven Press.

Rubin, E. H. (1990). Psychopathology of senile dementia of the Alzheimer type. In R. J. Wurtman, S. Corkin, J. H. Growdon, & E. Ritter-Walker (Eds.), *Advances in Neurology,* Volume 51, *Alzheimer's disease.* New York: Raven Press.

Salzman, C., & Gutfreund, M. J. (1986). Clinical techniques and research strategies for studying depression and memory. In L. W. Poon (Ed.), *Handbook for clinical memory assessment of older adults* (pp. 257–267). Washington, DC: American Psychological Association.

Satz, P., Van Gorp, W. G., Soper, H. V., & Mitrushina, M. (1987). WAIS-R marker for dementia of the Alzheimer type? An empirical and statistical induction test. *Journal of Clinical and Experimental Neuropsychology, 9,* 767–774.

Schmitt, F. A., Shih, W., & DeKosky, S. T. (1992). Neuropsychological correlates of single photon emission computed tomography (SPECT) in Alzheimer's disease. *Neuropsychology, 6,* 159–171.

Schoenberg, B. S., Kokmen, E., & Okazaki, H. (1987). Alzheimer's disease and other dementing illnesses in a defined United States population: Incidence rates and clinical features. *Annals of Neurology, 22,* 724.

Spar, J. E., & La Rue, A. (1990). *A concise guide to geriatric psychiatry.* Washington, DC: American Psychiatric Press.

Strub, R. L., & Black, F. W. (1988). *Neurobehavioral disorders: A clinical approach.* Philadelphia: F. A. Davis.

Walsh, K. W. (1991). *Understanding brain damage: A primer of neuropsychological evaluation.* Edinburgh: Churchill-Livingston.

Weingartner, H., Kaye, W., Smallberg, S. A., Ebert, M. H., Gillin, J. C., & Sitaran, N. (1981). Memory failures in progressive idiopathic dementia. *Journal of Abnormal Psychology, 90,* 187–196.

Wells, C. E. (1979). Pseudodementia. *American Journal of Psychiatry, 136,* 895–900.

Welsh, K. A., Butters, N., Hughes, J. P., Mohs, R. C., & Heyman, A. (1992). Detection and staging of dementia in Alzheimer's disease. *Archives of Neurology, 49,* 448–452.

Williams, B. W., Mack, W., & Henderson, V. W. (1989). Boston Naming Test in Alzheimer's disease. *Neuropsychologia, 27,* 1073–1079.

Wragg, R. E., & Jeste, D. V. (1989). Overview of depression and psychosis in Alzheimer's disease. *American Journal of Psychiatry, 146,* 577–587.

Parkinson's Disease

DESCRIPTION

Parkinson's disease is a progressive degenerative neurological disorder characterized by resting tremor affecting primarily the distal part of the extremities, especially the hands; slowness of movement known, as "bradykinesia"; rigidity or increased muscle tone; and loss of normal postural reflexes that takes the form of involuntary flexion of the trunk, limbs, and head. Other symptoms may include cogwheel rigidity, a festinating gate, micrographia, hypophonia, and a monotonous voice (Adams & Victor, 1989).

INCIDENCE, PREVALENCE, AND RISK FACTORS

Incidence and Prevalence

The incidence for the general population is approximately 20/100,000 (Schoenberg, 1986). Prevalence ratios have ranged from 30/100,000 to 180/100,000 (Schoenberg, 1986). A similar incidence has been found for both sexes, urban and rural residences, social status, ethnicity, and occupation. Whether Parkinson's disease is equally distributed worldwide continues to be debated.

Age

The age of onset for Parkinson's disease is generally between 40 and 70 years of age, with a peak in the 60s and 70s (Adams & Victor, 1989). Approximately 1% of the population over 50 is affected.

ETIOLOGY AND PATHOLOGY

The etiology of idiopathic Parkinson's disease is unknown.

The pathology involves damage to the pigmented neuronal systems of the brainstem. The substantia nigra is affected with a loss of pigmented cells (Adams & Victor, 1989; Jellinger, 1986). Lewy bodies (eosinophilic cytoplasmic inclusions) are often found in remaining cells in the substantia nigra and the locus ceruleus (Forno, 1986). There is a loss of dopamine-containing neurons in the substantia nigra, resulting in a severe loss of striatal

271

dopamine—the primary neurochemical abnormality in Parkinson's disease (Hornykiewicz & Kish, 1986).

MEDICAL ASSESSMENT

Diagnosis involves the use of clinical signs, history, and other factors to distinguish idiopathic Parkinson's disease from progressive supranuclear palsy, Shy–Drager syndrome, and striatonigral degeneration secondary to drugs or poisons (Adams & Victor, 1989). The EEG may be normal or show nonspecific slowing. CT may be normal or show cerebral atrophy (Freedman, 1990). MRI may reveal signal hypointensity in the substantia nigra of patients with both atypical parkinsonism and Parkinson's disease (Olanow, 1992).

NEUROPSYCHOLOGICAL ASSESSMENT

Spatial orientation, ability to shift mental set, effortful memory, verbal fluency, initiation, and facial expression have been reported deficient in Parkinson's disease (Raskin et al., 1990). A subgroup of Parkinson's patients develop dementia, possibly due to concomitant Alzheimer's disease. An assessment of cognitive and emotional functioning is therefore important in defining the Parkinson's disease patient's constellation of symptoms and in recommending appropriate supports. Raskin et al. (1990) have described an extensive battery designed to assess the areas of cognitive functioning commonly impaired in Parkinson's disease.

Although cognitive impairment has been found to be associated with Parkinson's disease, Parkinson's patients have been found to be generally accurate in judgments of their disability (Brown et al., 1989).

Behavior Rating Scales

Hoehn and Yahr (1967) have developed a rating scale for patients with Parkinson's disease.

Mental Status

Cognitive impairments may not be observed on the MMSE in nondemented Parkinson's disease patients (Youngjohn et al., 1992).

Attention

Performance on DSym-WAIS (Boller et al., 1984) and (DSMT) (Taylor et al., 1986) is impaired. Motor slowing may result in slowed reaction time (Daum & Quinn, 1991). Impaired simple reaction time and choice reaction time have been reported (Jordan et al., 1992).

Memory

Impaired memory functioning is a common but not invariable finding in nondemented patients. Impairment may be noted on the SRT—Total, Long Term Recall, and Recognition (Helkala et al., 1989). The RAVLT may be impaired in nondemented patients (Taylor et al.,

1987). For patients in Hoehn and Yahr (1967) stages 1–3, performance is impaired on the subtests of the BVRT that require drawing, but not on the BVRT:G (Boller *et al.*, 1984). PA-WMS, LM-WMS (delayed), and VR-WMS (delayed) may be impaired in nondemented patients (Bowen, 1976). Performance on LM- and VR-WMS, and the ROCFT:M may be impaired even in high-functioning patients (Mohr *et al.*, 1990). Patients may be impaired on procedural learning (Saint-Cyr *et al.*, 1988). Remote dating capacity may exhibit greater impairment than remote memory for content (Sagar *et al.*, 1988).

Intelligence

The PIQ is generally lower than the VIQ (Loranger *et al.*, 1972).

Speech/Language

Seventy percent of patients with Parkinson's disease exhibit hypokinetic dysarthria: monotony of pitch and loudness, reduced stress, short phrases, and segmented rushes of speech (Levin *et al.*, 1992). Vocabulary is unimpaired in early stages (Sullivan *et al.*, 1989). The PPVT is unimpaired in patients with mild functional impairment (Bayles & Tomoeda, 1983). Studies show BNT performance to be within normal limits for nondemented patients (Matison *et al.*, 1982).

Using items derived from the BDAE and the WAB, Cummings *et al.* (1988) found impaired phrase length, grammatical complexity, speech melody, writing mechanics, writing to dictation, narrative writing, word list generation, loudness, pitch, articulation, speech rate, and overall speech intelligibility in patients without overt dementia (MMSE > 24). Comprehension, repetition, naming, reading, and automatic speech were unimpaired. Parkinson's disease patients with overt dementia were more impaired than Parkinson's patients without dementia on phrase length, speech melody, information content of spontaneous speech, phrase repetition, comprehension of written and spoken commands, naming, writing mechanics, writing to dictation, narrative writing, alphabet recitation, word list generation, loudness, pitch, articulation, speech rate, and general intelligibility. Parkinson's disease patients with dementia exhibited richer information content of spontaneous speech, better word list generation, and better naming, but more impaired writing mechanics, phrase length, speech melody, and grammatical complexity than Alzheimer's disease patients.

Visuospatial Functioning

Although some impairment of performance on visuospatial tasks is due to impaired motor functioning, impairment has also been noted on tasks with no motor component. BD, OA, and JLO may be impaired (Boller *et al.*, 1984). PA-WAIS-R may be impaired (Sullivan *et al.*, 1989). HVOT performance may be unimpaired (Boller *et al.*, 1984). However, for patients with 5–10 years' duration, performance may be impaired on the HVOT and FR (Levin *et al.*, 1992). ROCFT:C may be impaired even in high-functioning patients (Mohr *et al.*, 1990). Performance on RPM may be impaired in nondemented patients (Growdon *et al.*, 1990).

Motor Functioning

Performance is likely to be impaired on the FTT and PPT in stage 1–3 patients (Boller *et al.*, 1984).

Executive Functioning

Impairment may be noted on the WCST (Pillon *et al.*, 1986; Taylor *et al.*, 1986). In stages 1–3, on the Nelson (1976) version, patients may complete fewer categories or make significantly more perseverative errors, or both, than controls (Canavan *et al.*, 1989; Lees & Smith, 1983). In high-functioning patients, there may be no impairment (Mohr *et al.*, 1990). Halstead CT performance may be deficient (Reitan & Boll, 1971). No impairment may be noted in verbal fluency for patients in stages 1–4 (Hanley *et al.*, 1990).

LNNB

Personality

Estimates of the prevalence of depression in Parkinson's disease range from 39% to 90% (Bieliauskas *et al.*, 1986). Bieliauskas & Glantz (1989) found 70% of their sample to be depressed using the MMPI D-Scale and 67% using the Hamilton Depression Rating Scale. Depression does not appear to increase with disease progression and may be reactive rather than an integral part of the disease process (Bieliauskas & Glantz, 1989; Huber *et al.*, 1990). The Beck Depression Inventory has been found useful for assessing depression in Parkinson's disease (Levin *et al.*, 1988). Psychosis may result from increased L-Dopa (Fischer *et al.*, 1990).

MEDICAL TREATMENT

There is no effective long-term therapy. Anticholinergics such as Artane and Cogentin may be prescribed early in the course of the disease. L-Dopa, in commercial preparations such as Sinemet, may improve symptoms such as hypokinesia by supplementing depleted dopamine. Psychiatric side effects include depression or psychosis or both. Dyskinesia may also result. The patient may become so sensitive that hourly vacillations may occur from mobility to complete immobility—the on/off phenomenon. Dopaminergic agents such as amantadine and bromocriptine may supplement the effect of L-Dopa. Surgical lesioning of the globus pallidus or ventrolateral thalamus has been performed in patients with uncontrolled, severe unilateral tremor (Adams & Victor, 1989).

PSYCHOSOCIAL THERAPIES

Patients often feel embarrassed, apathetic, inadequate, and lonely (Dakof & Mendelsohn, 1986). They are less likely than their peers to be working, participating in household management, and enjoying a close circle of friends.

Although motoric symptoms may hinder the development of therapeutic rapport, the intact language ability of most Parkinson's disease patients can support psychotherapy. Involvement in medically appropriate exercise and sports activities may help the patient cope with symptoms (Dakof & Mendelsohn, 1986). A variety of sensory and rhythmic cues can be used to help the patient modify bradykinetic movement. For example, taps can be put on shoes to provide auditory feedback for walking and prevent festination. Depression is a common emotional response to Parkinson's disease. There may be an increased risk for suicide, especially in individuals who strongly value physical mobility and power. If depression is diagnosed, therapy addressing issues of lost functional capacities should be provided.

Due to the initial effectiveness of medications such as L-Dopa, patients and their families tend to become "believers" in their medication. As drugs lose their efficacy, patients may experience severe disillusionment. Counseling may be especially helpful at this time. Sexual dysfunction is common both in patients and in their partners (Brown *et al.*, 1990). In the later stages of the disease, the patient's emotional flattening, apathy, and impaired ability to relate socially may be extremely painful for the spouse and other family members, and counseling may be appropriate.

Group Therapy

Patients have problems being in public, asking for help, and accepting the illness. They may be helped by informational, therapeutic workshops (Ellgring *et al.*, 1990).

The self-help book *Parkinson's Disease: A Guide for Patient and Family* (Duvoisin, 1984) may be useful for the patient and family members. A referral may be made to the local Parkinson's disease self-help group and to the United Parkinson Foundation, 220 South State Street, Chicago, IL 60604.

PROGNOSIS

The duration of illness varies with age of onset. Hoehn and Yahr (1967) found that for patients with age of onset greater than 50, the mean duration was 8 years, with a range of 1–30. A longer mean duration was found for younger patients. Prevalence figures for Parkinsonian dementia range from 3% to 50%. More recent studies have suggested percentages in the higher end of the range (Lees & Smith, 1983).

Patients who develop dementia tend to be older, to develop the disease later, and to exhibit more hypokinesis and arteriosclerosis. General disturbance of EEG, low HVA level in CSF, less response to L-Dopa, and pretreatment cognitive decline were also associated with a greater likelihood of developing dementia (Portin & Rinne, 1986).

REFERENCES

Adams, R. D., & Victor, M. (1989). *Principles of neurology.* New York: McGraw-Hill.

Bayles, K., & Tomoeda, C. (1983). Confrontation naming impairment in dementia. *Brain and Language, 19,* 98–114.

Bieliauskas, L. A., & Glantz, R. H. (1989). Depression type in Parkinson disease. *Journal of Clinical and Experimental Neuropsychology, 11,* 597–604.

Bieliauskas, L. A., Klawans, H. L., & Glantz, R. H. (1986). Depression and cognitive changes in Parkinson's disease: A review. In M. D. Yahr & K. J. Bergmann (Eds.), *Advances in neurology,* Volume 45, *Parkinson's disease* (pp. 437–438). New York: Raven Press.

Boller, F., Passafiume, D., Keefe, N. C., Rogers, K., Morrow, L., & Kim, Y. (1984). Visuospatial impairment in Parkinson's disease: Role of perceptual and motor factors. *Archives of Neurology, 41,* 485–490.

Bowen, F. (1976). Behavioral alterations in patients with basal ganglia lesions. In M. Yahr (Ed.), *The basal ganglia.* New York: Raven Press.

Brown, R. G., MacCarthy, B., Jahanshahi, M., & Marsden, C. D. (1989). Accuracy of self-reported disability in patients with parkinsonism. *Archives of Neurology, 46,* 955–959.

Brown, R. G., Jahanshahi, M., Quinn, N., & Marsden, C. D. (1990). Sexual function in patients with Parkinson's disease and their partners. *Journal of Neurology, Neurosurgery, and Psychiatry, 53,* 480–486.

Canavan, A. G. M., Passingham, R. E., Marsden, C. D., Quinn, N., Wyke, M., & Polkey, C. E. (1989). The performance on learning tasks of patients in the early stages of Parkinson's disease. *Neuropsychologia, 27,* 141–156.

Cummings, J. L., Darkins, A., Mendez, M., Hill, M. A., & Benson, D. F. (1988). Alzheimer's disease and Parkinson's disease: Comparison of speech and language alterations. *Neurology, 38*, 680–684.

Dakof, G. A., & Mendelsohn, G. A. (1986). Parkinson's disease: The psychological aspects of a chronic illness. *Psychological Bulletin, 99*, 375–387.

Daum, I., & Quinn, N. (1991). Reaction times and visual spatial processing in Parkinson's disease. *Journal of Clinical and Experimental Neuropsychology, 13*, 972–982.

Duvoisin, R. C. (1984). *Parkinson's disease: A guide for patient and family* (2nd ed.). New York: Raven Press.

Ellgring, H., Seiler, S., Nagel, U., Perleth, B., Gasser, T., & Oertel, W. H. (1990). Psychosocial problems of Parkinson's patients: Approaches to assessment and treatment. In M. B. Streifler, A. D. Korczyn, E. Melamed, & M. B. H. Youdin (Eds.), *Advances in Neurology,* Volume 53, *Parkinson's disease: Anatomy, pathology, and therapy* (pp. 349–353) New York: Raven Press.

Fischer, P., Danielczyk, W., Simanyi, M., & Streifler, M. B. (1990). Dopaminergic psychosis in advanced Parkinson's disease. In M. B. Streifler, A. D. Korczyn, E. Melamed, & M. B. H. Youdin (Eds.), *Advances in Neurology,* Volume 53, *Parkinson's disease: Anatomy, pathology, and therapy* (pp. 391–397) New York: Raven Press.

Forno, L. S. (1986). The Lewy body in Parkinson's disease. In M. D. Yahr & K. J. Bergmann (Eds.), *Advances in neurology,* Volume 45, *Parkinson's disease* (pp. 35–43). New York: Raven Press.

Freedman, M. (1990). Parkinson's disease. In J. L. Cummings (Ed.), *Subcortical dementia* (pp. 108–122). New York: Oxford University Press.

Growdon, J. H., Corkin, S., & Rosen, T. J. (1990). Distinctive aspects of cognitive dysfunction in Parkinson's disease. In M. B. Streifler, A. D. Korczyn, E. Melamed, & M. B. H. Youdin (Eds.), *Advances in Neurology,* Volume 53, *Parkinson's disease: Anatomy, pathology, and therapy* (pp. 365–376) New York: Raven Press.

Hanley, J. R., Dewick, H. C., Davies, A. D. M., Playfer, J., & Turnbull, C. (1990). Verbal fluency in Parkinson's disease. *Neuropsychologia, 28*, 737–741.

Helkala, E., Laulumaa, V., Soininen, H., & Riekkinen, P. J. (1989). Different error pattern of episodic and semantic memory in Alzheimer's disease and Parkinson's disease with dementia. *Neuropsychologia, 27*, 1241–1248.

Hoehn, M. M., & Yahr, M. D. (1967). Parkinsonism: Onset, progression, and mortality. *Neurology, 17*, 427–442.

Hornykiewicz, O., & Kish, S. J. (1986). Biochemical pathophysiology of Parkinson's disease. In M. D. Yahr & K. J. Bergmann (Eds.), *Advances in neurology,* Volume 45, *Parkinson's disease* (pp. 19–34). New York: Raven Press.

Huber, S. J., Freidenberg, D. L., Paulson, G. W., Shuttleworth, E. C., & Christy, J. A. (1990). The pattern of depressive symptoms varies with progression of Parkinson's disease. *Journal of Neurology, Neurosurgery, and Psychiatry, 53*, 275–278.

Jellinger, K. (1986). Overview of morphological changes in Parkinson's disease. In M. D. Yahr & K. J. Bergmann (Eds.), *Advances in neurology,* Volume 45, *Parkinson's disease* (pp. 1–18). New York: Raven Press.

Jordan, N., Sagar, H. J., & Cooper, J. A. (1992). Cognitive components of reaction time in Parkinson's disease. *Journal of Neurology, Neurosurgery, and Psychiatry, 55*, 658–664.

Lees, A. J., & Smith, E. (1983). Cognitive deficits in the early stages of Parkinson's disease. *Brain, 106*, 257–270.

Levin, B. E., Llabre, M. M., & Weiner, W. J. (1988). Parkinson's disease and depression: Psychometric properties of the Beck Depression Inventory. *Journal of Neurology, Neurosurgery, and Psychiatry, 51*, 1401–1404.

Levin, B. E., Tomer, R., & Rey, G. J. (1992). Cognitive impairments in Parkinson's disease. In J. M. Cedarbaum & S. T. Gancher (Eds.), *Parkinson's disease* (pp. 471–485). Philadelphia: W. B. Saunders.

Loranger, A., Goodell, H., McDowell, F., Lee, J., & Sweet, R. (1972). Intellectual impairment in Parkinson's syndrome. *Brain, 95*, 405–412.

Matison, R., Mayeux, R., Rosen, J., & Fahn, S. (1982). "Tip-of-the-tongue" phenomenon in Parkinson's disease. *Neurology, 32*, 567–570.

Mohr, E., Juncos, J., Cox, C., Litvan, I., Fedio, P., & Chase, T. N. (1990). Selective deficits in cognition and memory in high-functioning Parkinsonian patients. *Journal of Neurology, Neurosurgery, and Psychiatry, 53*, 603–606.

Nelson, H. E. (1976). A modified card sorting test sensitive to frontal deficits. *Cortex, 12*, 313–324.

Olanow, C. W. (1992). Magnetic resonance imaging in parkinsonism. In J. M. Cedarbaum & S. T. Gancher (Eds.), *Parkinson's disease* (pp. 405–420). Philadelphia: W. B. Saunders.

Pillon, B., Dubois, B., Lhermitte, F., & Agid, Y. (1986). Heterogeneity of cognitive impairment in supranuclear palsy, Parkinson's disease, and Alzheimer's disease. *Neurology, 36,* 1179–1185.

Portin, R., & Rinne, U. K. (1986). Predictive factors for cognitive deterioration and dementia in Parkinson's disease. In M. D. Yahr & K. J. Bergmann (Eds.), *Advances in neurology,* Volume 45, *Parkinson's disease* (pp. 413–416). New York: Raven Press.

Raskin, S. A., Borod, J. C., & Tweedy, J. (1990). Neuropsychological aspects of Parkinson's disease. *Neuropsychology Review, 1,* 185–221.

Reitan, R. M., & Boll, T. J. (1971). Intellectual and cognitive functions in Parkinson's disease. *Journal of Consulting and Clinical Psychology, 37,* 364–369.

Sagar, H. J., Cohen, N. J., Sullivan, E. V., Corkin, S., & Growdon, J. H. (1988). Remote memory function in Alzheimer's disease and Parkinson's disease. *Brain, 111,* 185–206.

Saint-Cyr, J. A., Taylor, A. E., & Lang, A. E. (1988). Procedural learning and neostriatal dysfunction in man. *Brain, 110,* 35–51.

Schoenberg, B. S. (1986). Descriptive epidemiology of Parkinson's disease: Disease distribution and hypothesis formulation. In M. D. Yahr & K. J. Bergmann (Eds.), *Advances in neurology,* Volume 45, *Parkinson's disease* (pp. 277–283). New York: Raven Press.

Sullivan, E. V., Sagar, H. J., Gabrieli, J. D. E., Corkin, S., & Growdon, J. H. (1989). Different cognitive profiles on standard behavioral tests in Parkinson's disease and Alzheimer's disease. *Journal of Clinical and Experimental Neuropsychology, 11,* 799–820.

Taylor, A. E., Saint-Cyr, J. A., & Lang, A. E. (1986). Frontal lobe dysfunction in Parkinson's disease: The cortical focus of neostriatal outflow. *Brain, 109,* 845–883.

Taylor, A. E., Saint-Cyr, J. A., & Lang, A. E. (1987). Parkinson's disease: Cognitive changes in relation to treatment response. *Brain, 110,* 35–51.

Youngjohn, J. R., Beck, J., Jogerst, G., & Caine, C. (1992). Neuropsychological impairment, depression, and Parkinson's disease. *Neuropsychology, 6,* 149–158.

Multiple Sclerosis

DESCRIPTION

Multiple sclerosis (MS) is a neurological disease involving a fluctuating or progressive clinical course and multiple lesions in the white matter of the CNS.

INCIDENCE AND RISK FACTORS

Age

The onset in two thirds of cases is between 20 and 40 years of age; 95% of cases occur between 10 and 50 (Adams & Victor, 1989).

Gender

The ratio of females to males is 1.7:1.0.

Geographic Location

Residence in higher latitudes during adolescence is associated with greater risk. The prevalence is 1/100,000 in equatorial regions, 6–14/100,000 in the southern United States and Europe, and 30–80/100,000 in the northern United States and Europe (Kurtze *et al.*, 1979).

Family

Having a first-degree relative with MS is associated with 5–15 times greater risk (Adams & Victor, 1989).

ETIOLOGY AND PATHOLOGY

The disease is characterized by demyelinating plaques. Plaques occur throughout the white matter of the CNS and are common in the periventricular white matter (Raine, 1990). The etiology is unknown.

MEDICAL ASSESSMENT

Symptoms are variable but may include motor weakness, paresthesias, visual impairment, nystagmus, dysarthria, intention tremor, ataxia, impairment of deep sensation, bladder dysfunction, and paraparesis. There is no single specific diagnostic test for MS. Diagnosis involves the following: (1) On objective neurological examination, there is a dysfunction of the CNS reflecting white matter involvement. (2) Examination or history suggests involvement of more than one part of the CNS. (3) Symptoms are either relapsing and remitting or chronically progressive. (4) The patient is 10–50 years old. (5) Symptoms cannot be explained by another disease process (W. B. Matthews, 1985; Peyser & Poser, 1986; Sibley, 1990).

Other diagnostic evidence may include: (1) CT scans may detect the presence of scattered lesions, but are unable to detect many plaques. (2) MRI is more sensitive to the plaques formed in MS and is the neuroimaging technique of choice (Hier, 1991; Willoughby & Paty, 1990). However, demyelination as visualized on MRI may have only modest correlations with neuropsychological impairment (Huber et al., 1992). (3) The EEG may show nonspecific changes in the form of slow waves. (4) Evoked-potential studies may confirm the existence of lesions. (5) The finding of CSF oligoclonal immunoglobin G may help confirm diagnosis (Hier, 1991). (6) The hot bath test may aid diagnosis by exacerbating symptoms (Hier, 1991).

NEUROPSYCHOLOGICAL ASSESSMENT

Neuropsychological evaluation may be diagnostically useful in identifying a second CNS lesion in a person presenting with the first symptoms of a demyelinating disorder (Peyser & Poser, 1986). It may also be useful in providing a cognitive profile of the patient for use in long-term management and treatment. Franklin et al. (1990) have provided a list of indications for neuropsychological assessment. The indications include: (1) patient complaints of cognitive impairments affecting functioning at work or home; (2) employer reports of reduced work capacity; (3) vocational counseling; (4) patient complaints of cognitive difficulties that may interfere with successful completion of a rehabilitation program; (5) baseline prior to immunosuppressive therapy; (6) patient with relapsing–remitting disease and very little neurological impairment reports cognitive impairments; (7) patient reports subtle or fluctuating cognitive deficits that may have functional consequences; and (8) "patient has an unexplained or treatment-resistant bipolar or other affective disorder which may have resulted from MS lesions" (Franklin et al., 1990, p. 169). Indications for counseling before deciding on testing and contradictions for testing are also listed.

A variety of cognitive impairments have been found in patients with MS, and there is considerable interpatient variability in the severity of cognitive deficits. There is no unique profile of cognitive deficits associated with MS that distinguishes it from other neurological disorders. Care must be taken to dissociate cognitive impairments from impairments due to motor dysfunction.

Cognitive impairment in MS may involve impaired speed of information-processing independent of motor involvement (Rao et al., 1989b), intact span memory but impaired long-term memory (Rao, 1986), generally intact language (Fennell & Smith, 1990), and impairments in concept formation, abstract reasoning, behavioral fluency, planning, and organizational skills (Fennell & Smith, 1990).

Cognitive impairment is related to the type and stage of MS. Heaton et al. (1985) found minimal impairment in relapsing–remitting MS but impairment on all HRNB cognitive test measures in chronic–progressive MS. According to White (1990), in the early stages, patients may show deficits of tasks such as the PASAT and WCST. In moderate stages, patients may exhibit impaired anterograde memory and visuospatial functioning with intact language. In later stages, a more global impairment of cognitive functioning may occur, and deficits may be noted in naming, general language, visuospatial skills, and memory.

Behavioral Rating Scales

Kurtzke (1955, 1983) has developed a disability rating scale [Expanded Disability Status Scale (EDSS)] for patients with MS.

Metal Status

The MMSE has been found to be relatively insensitive to cognitive impairment in MS. Rao *et al.* (1991) found the MMSE to exhibit a specificity of 98% and a sensitivity of 23%. A Brief Cognitive Battery consisting of the SRT, the Spatial Recall Test (Barbizet & Cany, 1968), the PASAT, and the COWAT attained a sensitivity of 68% and a specificity of 85% using a criterion of two or more tests impaired (Rao *et al.*, 1991).

Attention

Studies of DS have been mixed (White, 1990). DS Backward may be impaired (Rao *et al.*, 1991). The PASAT may be impaired (Litvan *et al.*, 1988; Rao *et al.*, 1991).

Memory

Recognition memory is often unimpaired. Recall for supraspan lists and delayed recall for both verbal and visual materials may be impaired (Rao, 1986; Rao *et al.*, 1989a). SRT performance is likely to be compromised (Rao *et al.*, 1991). Fischer (1988) reported impairment on all the Indexes of the WMS-R: 20% of the patients exhibited global impairment, 56% had intact attention but milder deficits in learning and long term memory, and 24% were intact. Minden *et al.* (1990) found memory impairment to be related to lower socioeconomic status, chronic progressive type, and use of antianxiety medication. It was not significantly related to severity of disability, duration of symptoms, or depression.

Intelligence

Information and Comprehension are often found to be intact (Heaton *et al.*, 1985; White, 1990), but have been reported to be significantly impaired compared to normals (Rao *et al.*, 1991).

Speech/Language

Verbal abilities are generally intact (Goldstein & Shelly, 1974; White, 1990). However, in some studies, Vocabulary (Ivnik, 1978), the COWAT (Rao *et al.*, 1991), and the TWF (Heaton *et al.*, 1985) have been reported to be impaired.

Arithmetic

A-WAIS (Heaton *et al.*, 1985) and A-WAIS-R (Rao *et al.*, 1991) have been found to be impaired.

Visuospatial Functioning

Impairments may be seen on tests of visuospatial functioning, but it has been difficult to dissociate perceptual and motor components. For chronic–progressive patients, impairment has been noted on all the WAIS Performance tests (Heaton *et al.*, 1985), but for relapsing–remitting patients, only OA was impaired. Rao *et al.* (1991) found RPM, JLO, FR, and the VFDT but not the HVOT to be impaired.

Sensory Functioning

Findings are variable but are more likely in chronic–progressive MS (Heaton *et al.*, 1985). TPT Time may be impaired (C. G. Matthews *et al.*, 1970).

Motor Functioning

Motor functioning is almost invariably impaired. Decrements in performance are likely on the FTT (C. G. Matthews *et al.*, 1970; Goldstein & Shelly, 1974; Heaton *et al.*, 1985), GP (Goldstein & Shelly, 1974; Heaton *et al.*, 1985), and GS (Heaton *et al.*, 1985).

Executive Functioning

Performance on tests of executive functioning and conceptual reasoning such as the WCST (Heaton *et al.*, 1985) and the CT (Heaton *et al.*, 1985; Rao *et al.*, 1991) may be impaired.

LNNB

The Motor Functions Scale may be elevated (Moses & Maruish, 1988).

Personality

Depression is a common concomitant to MS. Shiffer and Babigian (1984) found that during a 13-year period, 62% of MS patients received a depressive spectrum diagnosis. Shiffer (1990) found the lifetime risk for bipolar disorder of patients with MS to be twice that of populations free of neurological disease. Elevations on scales 1, 2, 3, and 8 of the MMPI may be due to sensitivities of these scales to physical symptoms associated with MS (Marsh *et al.*, 1982; Meyerink *et al.*, 1988). Adjustment for items directly sensitive to the neurological disorder may be needed to obtain an accurate profile of the patient's emotional functioning. Euphoria is sometimes present, especially in patients who exhibit significantly impaired cognitive functioning and more extensive brain involvement (Rabins, 1990). Psychosis is rare (Hier, 1991).

MEDICAL TREATMENT

There is no cure for multiple sclerosis. Treatment is directed at relieving symptoms and assisting the patient in coping with the illness. ACTH and prednisone may speed recovery from acute relapses, but may induce cognitive–affective side effects (see Chapter 49). Diazepam (Valium) and baclofen may be prescribed for spasticity. A variety of procedures treat complications such as bladder, bowel, and sexual dysfunction (Adams & Victor, 1989; Hier, 1991).

PSYCHOSOCIAL THERAPIES

Patients with MS may experience depression, anxiety, grief about losses, and lowered self-esteem. Harrower (1990) has described the experiences of "marginality," uncertainty, and loss of control with which the patient must cope.

Individual Psychotherapy

As the disease varies, the patient's need for psychological support is likely to vary. Patients can often benefit from ongoing intermittent therapy responsive to changes in the patient's status in contrast with brief, short-term therapy. Therapy may be especially helpful in assisting the patient in overcoming grief and depression in response to the losses inflicted by MS. The patient may experience a partial loss of control as total loss of control (Minden, 1992). The patient may benefit from the facilitation of healthy grieving, support, and increased awareness of available options. Therapy may also help the patient resolve preexisting problems that MS has exacerbated.

Patients may be referred to *Multiple Sclerosis: A Guide for Patients and Their Families* (Scheinberg & Holland, 1987). The patient and family should be informed of the National Multiple Sclerosis Society, 205 East 42nd Street, New York, NY 10017, and the local MS group.

Cognitive Rehabilitation

The patient may benefit from training in the use of notebooks or computer databases to record appointments and daily activities, if motor functioning permits. Well-established recording behaviors should assist the individual during periods when memory is compromised, if writing or typing skills are intact or appropriate adaptive aides are provided. Formal study of cognitive rehabilitation with MS patients is just beginning (LaRocca, 1990).

Family Therapy

Family or marital therapy may assist the family in coping with problems such as overinvolvement in the patient's disability, feelings of loss if the patient's functioning is severely compromised, and feelings of being "used."

Group Therapy

A group setting can be effective in providing information and an understanding that the patient is not "alone" (Crawford & McIvor, 1985). An ongoing therapy group can help patients "troubleshoot" their mutual problems and provide insight into their feelings about and methods of coping with their disabilities.

PROGNOSIS

The duration and course of multiple sclerosis is extremely variable. A 60-year study of 174 patients revealed that 74% of patients with MS survived 25 years, compared to 86% in the general population. After 25 years, one third of surviving patients were still working, and two thirds were still ambulatory (Percy *et al.*, 1971).

REFERENCES

Adams, R. D., & Victor, M. (1989). *Principles of neurology* (4th ed.). New York: McGraw-Hill.

Barbizet, J., & Cany, E. (1968). Clinical and psychometrical study of a patient with memory disturbances. *International Journal of Neurology, 7,* 44–54.

Beatty, P. A., & Gange, J. J. (1977). Neuropsychological aspects of multiple sclerosis. *Journal of Nervous and Mental Disease, 164,* 42–50.

Crawford, J. D., & McIvor, G. P. (1985). Group psychotherapy: Benefits in multiple sclerosis. *Archives of Physical Medicine and Rehabilitation, 66,* 810–813.

Fennell, E. B., & Smith, M. C. (1990). Neuropsychological assessment. In S. M. Rao (Ed.), *Neurobehavioral aspects of multiple sclerosis* (pp. 63–81). New York: Oxford University Press.

Fischer, J. S. (1988). Using the Wechsler Memory Scale—Revised to detect and characterize memory deficits in multiple sclerosis. *The Clinical Neuropsychologist, 2,* 149–172.

Franklin, G. M., Nelson, L. M., Heaton, R. K., & Filley, C. M. (1990). Clinical perspectives in the identification of cognitive impairment. In S. M. Rao (Ed.), *Neurobehavioral aspects of multiple sclerosis* (pp. 161–174). New York: Oxford University Press.

Goldstein, G., & Shelly, C. H. (1974). Neuropsychological diagnosis of multiple sclerosis in a neuropsychiatric setting. *Journal of Nervous and Mental Disease, 158,* 280–289.

Harrower, M. (1990). Introduction. In S. M. Rao (Ed.), *Neurobehavioral aspects of multiple sclerosis* (pp. 177–179). New York: Oxford University Press.

Heaton, R. K., Nelson, L. M., Thompson, D. S., Burks, J. S., & Franklin, G. M. (1985). Neuropsychological findings in relapsing–remitting and chronic–progressive multiple sclerosis. *Journal of Consulting and Clinical Psychology, 53,* 103–110.

Hier, D. B. (1991). Demyelinating diseases. In M. A. Samuels (Ed.), *Manual of neurology: Diagnosis and therapy* (4th ed.) (pp. 266–275). Boston: Little, Brown.

Huber, S. J., Bornstein, R. A., Rammohan, K. W., Christy, J. A., Chakeres, D. W., & McGhee, R. B. (1992). Magnetic resonance imaging correlates of neuropsychological impairment in multiple sclerosis. *Journal of Neuropsychiatry and Clinical Neurosciences, 4,* 152–158.

Ivnik, R. J. (1978). Neuropsychological test performance as a function of the duration of MS-related symptomatology. *Journal of Clinical Psychiatry, 39,* 304–307.

Kurtzke, J. F. (1955). A scale for evaluating disability in multiple sclerosis. *Neurology, 11,* 686–694.

Kurtzke, J. F. (1983). Rating neurologic impairment in multiple sclerosis: An expanded disability status scale (EDSS). *Neurology, 33,* 1444–1452.

Kurtzke, J. F., Beebe, G. W., & Norman, J. E. (1979). Epidemiology of multiple sclerosis in US veterans. I. Race, sex, and geographic distribution. *Neurology, 29,* 1228–1235.

LaRocca, N. G. (1990). A rehabilitation perspective. In S. M. Rao (Ed.), *Neurobehavioral aspects of multiple sclerosis* (pp. 215–229). New York: Oxford University Press.

Litvan, I., Grafman, J., Vendrell, P., & Martinez, J. M. (1988). Slowed information processing in multiple sclerosis. *Archives of Neurology, 45,* 281–285.

Marsh, G. G., Hirsch, S. H., & Leung, G. (1982). Use and misuse of the MMPI in multiple sclerosis. *Psychological Reports, 51,* 1127–1134.

Matthews, C. G., Cleeland, C. S., & Hooper, C. L. (1970). Neuropsychological patterns in multiple sclerosis. *Diseases of the Nervous System, 31,* 161–170.

Matthews, W. B. (Ed.). (1985). *McAlpine's multiple sclerosis.* Edinburgh: Churchill-Livingston.

Meyerink, L. H., Reitan, R. M., & Selz, M. (1988). The validity of the MMPI with multiple sclerosis patients. *Journal of Clinical Psychology, 44,* 764–769.

Minden, S. L. (1992). Psychotherapy for people with multiple sclerosis. *Journal of Neuropsychiatry and Clinical Neurosciences, 4,* 198–213.

Minden, S. L., Moes, E. J., Orav, J., Kaplan, E., & Reich, P. (1990). Memory impairment in multiple sclerosis. *Journal of Clinical and Experimental Neuropsychology, 12,* 566–586.

Moses, J. A., & Maruish, M. E. (1988). A critical review of the Luria–Nebraska Neuropsychological Battery literature: Specific neurologic syndromes. *International Journal of Clinical Neuropsychology, 10,* 178–188.

Percy, A. K., Nobrega, F. T., Okazaki, H., Galattre, E., & Kurland, L. T. (1971). Multiple sclerosis in Rochester, Minnesota: A 60-year appraisal. *Archives of Neurology, 25,* 105–111.

Peyser, J. M., & Poser, C. M. (1986). Neuropsychological correlates of multiple sclerosis. In S. B. Filskov & T. J. Boll (Eds.), *Handbook of clinical neuropsychology,* Volume 2 (pp. 364–397). New York: Wiley.

Rabins, P. V. (1990). Euphoria in multiple sclerosis. In S. M. Rao (Ed.), *Neurobehavioral aspects of multiple sclerosis* (pp. 180–185). New York: Oxford University Press.

Raine, C. S. (1990). Neuropathology. In S. M. Rao (Ed.), *Neurobehavioral aspects of multiple sclerosis* (pp. 15–36). New York: Oxford University Press.

Rao, S. M. (1986). Neuropsychology of multiple sclerosis: A critical review. *Journal of Clinical and Experimental Neuropsychology, 8,* 503–542.

Rao, S. M., Leo, G. J., & St. Aubin-Faubert, P. (1989a). On the nature of memory disturbance in multiple sclerosis. *Journal of Clinical and Experimental Neuropsychology, 11,* 699–712.

Rao, S. M., St. Aubin-Faubert, P., & Leo, G. J. (1989b). Information processing speed in patients with multiple sclerosis. *Journal of Clinical and Experimental Neuropsychology, 11,* 471–477.

Rao, S. M., Leo, G. J., Bernardin, L., & Unverzagt, F. (1991). Cognitive dysfunction in multiple sclerosis. I. Frequency, patterns, and prediction. *Neurology, 41,* 685–691.

Scheinberg, L. C., & Holland, N. J. (Eds.) (1987). *Multiple sclerosis: A guide for patients and their families.* New York: Raven Press.

Shiffer, R. B. (1990). Disturbances of affect. In S. M. Rao (Ed.), *Neurobehavioral aspects of multiple sclerosis* (pp. 186–195). New York: Oxford University Press.

Shiffer, R. B., & Babigian, H. M. (1984). Behavioral disorders in multiple sclerosis, temporal lobe epilepsy, and amyotrophic lateral sclerosis: An epidemiologic study. *Archives of Neurology, 41,* 1067–1069.

Sibley, W. A. (1990). The diagnosis and course of multiple sclerosis. In S. M. Rao (Ed.), *Neurobehavioral aspects of multiple sclerosis* (pp. 5–14). New York: Oxford University Press.

White, R. F. (1990). Emotional and cognitive correlates of multiple sclerosis. *Journal of Neuropsychiatry, 2,* 422–428.

Willoughby, E. W., & Paty, D. W. (1990). Brain imaging in multiple sclerosis. In S. M. Rao (Ed.), *Neurobehavioral aspects of multiple sclerosis* (pp. 37–62). New York: Oxford University Press.

Huntington's Disease

DESCRIPTION

Huntington's disease is an inherited, autosomal dominant, degenerative neurological disorder characterized by dyskinesia (e.g., chorea and other motor abnormalities), nonaphasic dementia, and disorders of mood such as depression (Folstein, 1989; Folstein *et al.,* 1990).

PREVALENCE, INCIDENCE, AND RISK FACTORS

Prevalence

Estimates of prevalence in Caucasian populations range from 4.1 to 7.5 cases/100,000. Huntington's disease has also been found in other racial groups (Narabayashi, 1973; Wright *et al.,* 1981).

Age

The average age of onset is between 36 and 45 years (Folstein, 1989).

ETIOLOGY AND PATHOLOGY

Atrophy and neuronal loss occur in the striatum. Loss is noted primarily in the caudate, putamen, and pallidum. Loss may be noted in the cortex and other areas in the corticosubcortical circuit. It has been hypothesized that the Huntington's disease gene results in an excessive stimulation and destruction of striatal neurons (Folstein, 1989).

MEDICAL ASSESSMENT

Chorea is quick, unintended movements of the body. It peaks at about 10 years after onset, but may diminish in patients who survive 15 years, with the patient left in a state of akinetic mutism. Chorea is increased by stressful tasks such as counting backward by 7s and decreased by voluntary movements such as writing and walking. Motor restlessness, dystonia, tremor, and myoclonic jerks may also be noted. Cognitive dysfunction has been found to be correlated with caudate atrophy (Starkstein *et al.*, 1988).

NEUROPSYCHOLOGICAL ASSESSMENT

Premorbid performance on the WAIS has not been found to be a useful predictor of illness (Josiassen, *et al.*, 1982; Strauss & Brandt, 1986). Bamford and Caine (1986) have reviewed the literature. A comparison of test results from studies of Huntington's disease vs. other dementing disorders has been compiled by Brown and Marsden (1988).

Behavioral Rating Scales

A scale for assessing functional disability has been developed (Shoulson, 1981; Shoulson & Fahn, 1979).

Mental Status Testing

SSS is impaired first. Recall of three words is affected early. The more difficult orientation items and copying a pentagon may be impaired later in the course. Repetition of three words, naming simple objects, reading, and easy orientation items are preserved even at moderate levels of dementia (Folstein, 1989).

Attention

DS-WAIS and DSym-WAIS have been found to be impaired early (Fedio *et al.*, 1979; Josiassen *et al.*, 1982).

Memory

The ROCFT:M (Fedio *et al.*, 1979), SRT (Fisher *et al.*, 1983), and ACT (Bamford & Caine, 1986) may be impaired. Delayed recall is impaired (Wilson *et al.*, 1987). Recognition has been found to be less impaired than recall (Butters *et al.*, 1986; Moss *et al.*, 1986). Recently diagnosed patients with Huntington's disease may exhibit impairment on tests of remote memory (Albert *et al.*, 1981).

General Intelligence and Social Understanding

FSIQ decreases slowly over the course of the illness. I-WAIS and C-WAIS may be relatively spared (Caine *et al.*, 1978; Josiassen *et al.*, 1982). PA-WAIS is impaired early (Caine *et al.*, 1978; Josiassen *et al.*, 1982).

Speech/Language

Speech may be dysrhythmic and slow with a loss of volume at the ends of phrases (Ramig, 1986). V-WAIS and S-WAIS are often spared (Caine *et al.*, 1978; Josiassen *et al.*, 1982). PPVT may be intact (Fisher *et al.*, 1983). Verbal fluency as assessed on the COWAT is impaired, while confrontation naming as assessed on the BNT is unimpaired (Butters *et al.*, 1978).

Arithmetic

A-WAIS has been found to be impaired early (Fedio *et al.,* 1979; Josiassen *et al.,* 1982).

Visuospatial Functioning

BD-WAIS and OA-WAIS may be impaired early (Folstein, 1989). The ROCFT:C may be impaired; however, deficits in visuospatial functioning not attributable to impaired motor functioning have been reported (Fedio *et al.,* 1979).

Executive Functioning

Performance on tasks requiring shifts of set may be impaired. Performance on TMTB is impaired (Starkstein *et al.,* 1988). The WCST and PMT may be impaired (Fisher *et al.,* 1983; Folstein, 1989).

LNNB

Moses *et al.* (1981) found impaired memory and visuospatial abilities on the LNNB in recently diagnosed patients.

Personality

Disorders of affect, especially depression, may occur prior to the onset of motor symptoms. Data suggest that the depression is not simply reactive (Folstein, 1989). Apathy, irritability, impaired self-perception, anxiety, and inappropriate hypersexuality or hyposexuality may accompany the disease progression. Fedio *et al.* (1979) found MMPI elevations on Scales 8, 2, and 7; however, no statistically significant difference between Huntington's disease patients and other groups of brain-injured patients and no unique profile have been reported (Boll *et al.,* 1974; Norton, 1975).

MEDICAL TREATMENT

There is no medical treatment that can cure or delay the onset or slow the course of Huntington's disease.

PSYCHOSOCIAL THERAPIES

Genetic counseling may be appropriate for individuals who may be carriers (Folstein, 1989).

Psychotherapy and family therapy may assist the patient and family in coping with the disease (Folstein, 1989).

PROGNOSIS

Death occurs an average of 16 years after onset (Conneally, 1984).

REFERENCES

Albert, M. S., Butters, N., & Brandt, J. (1981). Development of remote memory loss in patients with Huntington's disease. *Journal of Clinical Neuropsychology, 3,* 1–12.

Bamford, K. A., & Caine, E. D. (1986). The neuropsychology of Huntington's disease: Problems of clinical–pathological correlation in progressive brain illness. In G. Goldstein & R. E. Tarter (Eds.), *Advances in clinical neuropsychology,* Volume 3 (pp. 181–212). New York: Plenum Press.

Boll, T., Heaton, R., & Reitan, R. (1974). Neuropsychological and emotional correlates of Huntington's disease. *Journal of Nervous and Mental Disease, 158,* 61–69.

Brown, R. G., & Marsden, C. D. (1988). "Subcortical dementia": The neuropsychological evidence. *Neuroscience, 25,* 363–387.

Butters, N., Sax, D., Montgomery, K., & Tarlow, S. (1978). Comparison of the neuropsychological deficits associated with early and advanced Huntington's disease. *Archives of Neurology, 35,* 585–589.

Butters, N., Wolfe, J., & Granholm, E. (1986). An assessment of verbal recall, recognition, and fluency abilities in patients with Huntington's disease. *Cortex, 22,* 11–32.

Caine, E. D., Hunt, R. D., Weingartner, H., & Ebert, M. H. (1978). Huntington's dementia: Clinical and neuropsychological features. *Archives of General Psychology, 35,* 377–384.

Conneally, P. M. (1984). Huntington's disease: Genetics and epidemiology. *American Journal of Human Genetics, 36,* 506–526.

Fedio, P., Cox, C. S., Neophytides, A., Canal-Frederick, G., & Chase, T. N. (1979). Neuropsychological profile of Huntington's disease: Patients and those at risk. *Advances in neurology,* Volume 23 (pp. 239–255). New York: Raven Press.

Fisher, J. M., Kennedy, J. L., Caine, E. D., & Shoulson, I. (1983). Dementia in Huntington disease: A cross-sectional analysis of intellectual decline. In R. Mayeux & W. G. Rosen (Eds.), *The dementias* (pp. 229–238). New York: Raven Press.

Folstein, S. E. (1989). *Huntington's disease: A disorder of families.* Baltimore: Johns Hopkins University Press.

Folstein, S. E., Brandt, J., & Folstein, M. F. (1990). Huntington's disease. In J. L. Cummings (Ed.), *Subcortical dementia* (pp. 87–107). New York: Oxford University Press.

Josiassen, R. C., Curry, L., Roemer, R. A., DeBease, C., & Mancall, E. L. (1982). Patterns of intellectual deficit in Huntington's disease. *Journal of Clinical Neuropsychology, 4,* 173–183.

Moses, J. A., Golden, C. J., Berger, P. A., & Wisniewski, A. M. (1981). Neuropsychological deficits in early, middle, and late stages of Huntington's disease as measured by the Luria-Nebraska Neuropsychological Battery. *International Journal of Neuroscience, 14,* 95–100.

Moss, M. B., Albert, M. S., Butters, N., & Payne, M. (1986). Differential patterns of memory loss among patients with Alzheimer's disease, Huntington's disease, and alcoholic Korsakoff's syndrome. *Archives of Neurology, 43,* 239–246.

Narabayashi, H. (1973). Huntington's chorea in Japan: Review of the literature. *Advances in Neurology, 1,* 253–259.

Norton, J. (1975). Patterns of neuropsychological test performance in Huntington's disease. *Journal of Nervous and Mental Disease, 161,* 276–279.

Ramig, L. A. (1986). Acoustic analyses of phonation in patients with Huntington's disease: Preliminary report. *Annals of Otology, Rhinology, and Laryngology, 95,* 288–293.

Shoulson, I. (1981). Huntington's disease: Functional capacities in patients treated with neuroleptic and antidepressant drugs. *Neurology, 31,* 1333–1335.

Shoulson, I., & Fahn, S. (1979). Huntington's disease: Clinical care and evaluation. *Neurology, 29,* 1–3.

Starkstein, S. E., Brandt, J., Folstein, S., Strauss, M., Berthier, M. L., Pearlson, G. D., Wong, D., McDonnell, A., & Folstein, M. (1988). Neuropsychologic and neuroradiologic correlates in Huntington's disease. *Journal of Neurology, Neurosurgery, and Psychiatry, 51,* 1259–1263.

Strauss, M. E., & Brandt, J. (1986). Attempt at preclinical identification of Huntington's disease using the WAIS. *Journal of Clinical and Experimental Neuropsychology, 8,* 210–218.

Wilson, R. S., Como, P. G., Garron, D. C., Klawans, H. L., Barr, A., & Klawans, D. (1987). Memory failure in Huntington's disease. *Journal of Clinical and Experimental Neuropsychology, 9,* 147–154.

Wright, H. H., Still, C. N., & Abramson, R. K. (1981). Huntington's disease in black kindreds in South Carolina. *Archives in Neurology, 38,* 412–414.

Progressive Supranuclear Palsy

DESCRIPTION

Progressive supranuclear palsy (Steele–Richardson–Olszewski syndrome) is a degenerative neurological disorder characterized by disturbance of gait with frequent falls, disorders of articulation, vertical gaze paralysis, problems in looking down while eating, horizontal gaze paralysis, limb rigidity, face or limb bradykinesia, hyperreflexia, pseudobulbar palsy, and neck rigidity (Lees, 1990; Maher & Lees, 1986; Steele *et al.,* 1964).

INCIDENCE, PREVALENCE, AND RISK FACTORS

Prevalence

Prevalence has been reported to be 1.39/100,000 (Lees, 1990). It has been estimated that 4–12% of patients diagnosed as having Parkinson's disease may have progressive supranuclear palsy (Lees, 1990).

Age

The median age of onset is approximately 65 years (Maher & Lees, 1986).

ETIOLOGY AND PATHOLOGY

The cause of progressive supranuclear palsy is unknown (Adams & Victor, 1989). Areas of damage include: (1) the pallidosubthalamic complex, (2) the zona compacta of the substantia nigra, and (3) the superior colliculus, periaqueductal gray matter, and pretectal areas. Most areas of the cerebral neocortex, with the possible exception of the frontal lobe, are undamaged. Dopamine levels have been found to be decreased in both the caudate nucleus and putamen (Lees, 1990).

MEDICAL ASSESSMENT

Diagnosis involves the use of clinical signs, history, and other factors to distinguish progressive supranuclear palsy from other disorders. CT may reveal atrophy of the midbrain tegmentum, superior colliculus, and pons and mild atrophy in the prefrontal and temporal regions (Mascucci *et al.*, 1985).

NEUROPSYCHOLOGICAL ASSESSMENT

Cognitive impairment in progressive supranuclear palsy has been found primarily in areas requiring processing of visual information, especially on tasks requiring visual searching or scanning ability (Kimura *et al.*, 1981). Impairment may also be found on "frontal" tasks, but language functioning is generally intact (Maher *et al.*, 1985). If dementia occurs, it is usually in the later stages of the disease.

Orientation

O-WMS is unimpaired (Pillon *et al.*, 1986).

Attention

DS-WAIS (Pillon *et al.*, 1986; Maher *et al.*, 1985) and DSym-WAIS may be impaired (Fisk *et al.*, 1982; Kimura *et al.*, 1981).

Memory

Impairments may be noted in LM-WMS, PA-WMS, and VR-WMS (Pillon *et al.*, 1986).

General Intelligence

PIQ (Fisk *et al.*, 1982) and PA-WAIS may be impaired (Maher *et al.*, 1985).

Speech/Language

S-WAIS is likely to be unimpaired (Pillon *et al.*, 1986; Maher *et al.*, 1985).

Arithmetic

A-WAIS may be impaired (Pillon *et al.*, 1986; Maher *et al.*, 1985).

Visuospatial Functioning

RPM may be impaired (Pillon *et al.*, 1986). PC-WAIS has been found in some studies to be unimpaired (Fisk *et al.*, 1982; Kimura *et al.*, 1981) and in others to be impaired (Maher *et al.*, 1985). BD-WAIS may also be impaired (Maher *et al.*, 1985).

Executive Functioning

WCST may be impaired (Pillon *et al.,* 1986). Impaired verbal fluency may be noted on the COWAT (Milberg & Albert, 1989).

MEDICAL TREATMENT

L-Dopa, dopamine agonists, anticholinergics, methysergide, and amitriptyline are not consistently effective in providing symptomatic relief (Adams & Victor, 1989; Maher & Lees, 1986).

PROGNOSIS

Median survival from onset is 6 years. Neither age at onset nor presence of dysphasia or cognitive impairment is related to prognosis (Maher & Lees, 1986).

REFERENCES

Adams, R. D., & Victor, M. (1989). *Principles of neurology* (4th ed.). New York: McGraw-Hill.

Fisk, J. D., Goodale, M. A., Burkhart, G., & Barnett, H. J. M. (1982). Progressive supranuclear palsy: The relationship between ocular motor dysfunction and psychological test performance. *Neurology, 32,* 698–705.

Kimura, D., Barnett, H. J. M., & Burkhart, G. (1981). The psychological test pattern in progressive supranuclear palsy. *Neuropsychologia, 19,* 301–306.

Lees, A. J. (1990). Progressive supranuclear palsy (Steele–Richardson–Olszewski Syndrome). In J. L. Cummings (Ed.), *Subcortical dementia.* New York: Oxford University Press.

Maher, E. R., & Lees, A. J. (1986). The clinical features and natural history of the Steele–Richardson–Olszewski syndrome (progressive supranuclear palsy). *Neurology, 36,* 1005–1008.

Maher, E. R., Smith, E. M., & Lees, A. J. (1985). Cognitive deficits in the Steele–Richardson–Olszewski syndrome (progressive supranuclear palsy). *Journal of Neurology, Neurosurgery, and Psychiatry, 48,* 1234–1239.

Masucci, E. F., Borts, F. T., Smirniotopoulos, J. G., & Kurtzke, J. F. (1985). Thin section CT of midbrain abnormalities in progressive supranuclear patsy. *American Journal of Neuroradiology, 6,* 767–772.

Milberg, W., & Albert, M. (1989). Cognitive differences between patients with progressive supranuclear palsy and Alzheimer's disease. *Journal of Clinical and Experimental Neuropsychology, 11,* 605–614.

Pillon, B., Dubois, B., L'Hermitte, F., & Agid, Y. (1986). Heterogeneity of intellectual impairment in progressive supranuclear palsy, Parkinson's disease and Alzheimer's disease. *Neurology, 36,* 1179–1185.

Steele, J. C., Richardson, J. C., & Olszewski, J. (1964). Progressive supranuclear palsy: A heterogeneous degeneration involving the brain stem, basal ganglia and cerebellum with vertical gaze and pseudobulbar palsy, nuchal dystonia and dementia. *Archives of Neurology, 10,* 333–358.

Human Immunodeficiency Virus

DESCRIPTION

Human Immunodeficiency Virus-1

Human immunodeficiency virus-1 (HIV-1) is a ribonucleic acid virus in the family Retroviridae and subfamily Lentivirinae. HIV has been shown to be the causative agent in AIDS (Fultz, 1989). HIV-2, which may produce similar symptoms, is less common than HIV-1 and is less well studied (Ewing, 1990).

Acquired Immunodeficiency Syndrome

The Centers for Disease Control (CDC) surveillance case definition of acquired immunodeficiency syndrome (AIDS) is complex. A patient is diagnosed with AIDS if one or more specific opportunistic infections or neoplasms are diagnosed in the absence of a known cause of immunodeficiency other than HIV. AIDS may be diagnosed if the patient is known to be HIV-positive and if there is HIV encephalopathy, HIV wasting syndrome, or a variety of manifestations of opportunistic infections or neoplasms (Centers for Disease Control, 1987; Ewing, 1990; Robertson & Hall, 1992).

Persistent Generalized Lymphadenopathy

Persistent generalized lymphadenopathy (PGL) is defined as palpable lymphadenopathy for more than 3 months at two or more extrainguinal sites in the absence of a condition that could explain findings other than HIV (Centers for Disease Control, 1986).

AIDS-Related Complex

AIDS-related complex (ARC) has a variety of definitions. The term has generally been applied to patients who have constitutional signs such as weight loss, fevers, night sweats, or infections that do not define the patient as having AIDS (Yarchoan & Pluda, 1988).

AIDS Dementia Complex

The three-part nomenclature has been justified as follows: (1) "AIDS" emphasizes the comparability of the syndrome to other AIDS-defining systemic sequelae of HIV-1; (2)

"dementia" suggests the intellectual decline that is the usual presenting symptom; and (3) "complex" refers to the collection of cognitive, motor, and behavioral symptoms that make up the syndrome (Sidtis & Price, 1990). AIDS dementia complex (ADC) has been described as a subacute or chronic progressive CNS disorder characterized by cognitive, motor, and behavioral dysfunction. It has been claimed to be a subcortical dementia with diffuse cognitive deficit, psychomotor slowing, motor impairment, and behavioral apathy (Price *et al.*, 1988). For research purposes, the neurological manifestations of HIV-1 have been labeled "HIV-1-associated cognitive/motor complex" (Working Group of the American Academy of Neurology AIDS Task Force, 1991, p. 779). This is further broken down into "HIV-1-associated dementia complex" and "HIV-1-associated myelopathy" (severe manifestations) and "HIV-1-associated minor cognitive/motor disorder" (mild manifestations) (Working Group of the American Academy of Neurology AIDS Task Force, 1991, p. 779).

INCIDENCE, PREVALENCE, AND RISK FACTORS

HIV-1

Sexual Risk Factors

Numerous male homosexual partners and frequent receptive anal intercourse have been identified as risk factors for HIV infection (Geodert & Blattner, 1988). A high HIV antibody prevalence has been found among prostitutes in some locations. Contact with female prostitutes has been one of the primary modes of transmission into the heterosexual community.

Parenteral Drug Abuse

Frequency of drug injection and sharing of needles have been identified as risk factors (Geodert & Blattner, 1988).

Transfusion

Prior to HIV screening of donated blood in the spring of 1985, there was a significant risk of transmission of HIV. Hemophiliacs and other patients in routine need of blood or blood products were at the greatest risk. Screening of blood and of donors has significantly lowered the risk (Geodert & Blattner, 1988).

Geography

The prevalence and incidence of HIV vary greatly with geographic location and with the population studied. These rates are changing rapidly, and the practitioner is advised to acquire the latest statistics available for his or her locality. As of June 30, 1988, 100,410 cases of AIDS from 138 countries had been reported to the World Health Organization. The United States had the most cases, followed by France, Brazil, and West Germany. In 1988, it was estimated that 5–10 million people were affected with HIV-1 worldwide (Mann & Chin, 1988). As of February 1992, 202,843 AIDS cases had been reported in the United States (Steger, 1993).

ADC

It has been estimated that 70–90% of AIDS patients develop neuropsychological impairment (Navia, 1990). ADC can develop as the initial clinical manifestation of HIV-1 infection (Navia & Price, 1987).

ETIOLOGY AND PATHOLOGY

HIV-1

HIV integrates into host DNA, is tropic and lytic for CD4 T-helper cells, and latently infects cells of monocyte lineage that migrate throughout the body (Fultz, 1989). T-helper cells perform recognition and induction functions involved in the immune response to foreign stimuli. HIV gradually depletes T-helper cells, this depletion resulting in a progressive loss of immune responsiveness. The patient becomes increasingly susceptible to opportunistic infections and malignancies (McDougal et al., 1989). Opportunistic infections may include *Pneumocystis carinii* pneumonia, cerebral toxoplasmosis (a common cause of encephalitis), *Cryptococcus neoformans* (a common cause of meningitis), cryptosporidiosis, cytomegalovirus (which may cause retinitis and colitis), and *Mycobacterium avium–intracellulare* (Libman & Witzburg, 1993). Neoplastic diseases such as Karposi's sarcoma may occur. Non-Hodgkin's lymphoma and Hodgkin's disease may be found in AIDS.

Transmission is primarily by intimate sexual contact, intravenous drug abuse with sharing of blood-contaminated needles, and transfusion of contaminated blood. Transmission has not been shown to occur by casual contact with infected persons in the home or hospital, the shared communion cup, mosquitoes, or hepatitis vaccination (Ewing, 1990).

ADC

ADC is caused by direct brain infection by HIV-1 (Navia, 1990). Histological examination has revealed damage in central white and deep gray matter regions, in the basal ganglia and thalamus. A diffuse pallor of the centrum semiovale, usually associated with reactive astrocytosis, is often found (Navia, 1990).

MEDICAL ASSESSMENT

HIV-1

Infection with HIV is followed in 2–3 weeks by acute onset of fever and malaise, sore throat, rash, myalgia, lymphadenopathy, retroorbital pain, meningitis, encephalitis, and neuropathy. The symptoms resolve in 1–4 weeks. The appearance of antibodies specific to HIV proteins (seroconversion) generally occurs about 2 months after infection, although longer periods have been reported. Serological tests include enzyme-linked immunosorbent assay (ELISA) and Western blot (WB) (Ewing, 1990). Since HIV depletes T-helper cells, which in turn compromises immunoresponsiveness, clinical severity parallels T-helper-cell depletion (McDougal et al., 1989). The diagnosis of HIV infection is best accomplished by serological testing (Chaisson & Volberding, 1990).

HIV infection may result in numerous symptoms due to the complexity of the action of the virus and its effect on the immune system. The CDC classification system may be summarized as follows:

Group I. Acute infection
Group II. Asymptomatic infection
Group III. Persistent generalized lymphadenopathy
Group IV. Other diseases
        Subgroup A. Constitutional disease
        Subgroup B. Neurological disease
        Subgroup C. Secondary infectious diseases
        Subgroup D. Secondary cancers
        Subgroup E. Other conditions

AIDS is not likely to occur in the first 2 years after seroconversion. In homosexual men, cumulative AIDS incidence is 30% by 7–8 years after seroconversion (Goedert & Blattner, 1988).

MRI is generally more sensitive than CT in detecting intracranial lesions in AIDS due to its sensitivity to white-matter lesions (Olsen & Cohen, 1988). CT scan may reveal focal lesions that appear as low-intensity, ring-enhancing lesions or atrophy (De La Paz & Enzmann, 1988). MRI may demonstrate high-T2-signal-intensity lesions.

ADC

Early symptoms may include cognitive slowness, impaired attention and concentration, forgetfulness, confusion, clumsiness, impaired fine motor ability, tremor, loss of balance, leg weakness, reduced spontaneity, apathy, and social withdrawal. Early signs include psychomotor slowing, impaired word reversal and serial subtraction, blunted affect, organic psychosis, impaired rapid movements, sustention tremor, hyperreflexia, limb paresis, and impaired tandem gait (Navia, 1990). Care must be taken in making a diagnosis due to the possibility of misinterpreting complaints such as forgetfulness, difficulty in attention and concentration, slowing of cognitive functions, and loss of interest in everyday activities secondary to reactive depression (Fernandez & Levy, 1990).

Diffuse cerebral atrophy, sometimes associated with ventricular dilation, may be found. MRI and occasionally CT may reveal a patchy or diffuse attenuation of white matter (Navia, 1990).

NEUROPSYCHOLOGICAL ASSESSMENT

A comprehensive neurobehavioral assessment, including a neuropsychological evaluation, is essential to avoid potential misdiagnosis and potential mismanagement when a patient is infected with HIV. Such an assessment can assist in distinguishing between organic and psychosocial factors. The test results can provide a determination of level of impairment in cognitive areas that might be affected by HIV and secondary diseases. Specifically, they can provide information about the patient's ability to comprehend and comply with his or her treatment and may be useful. Issues of competency may be addressed in the context of return to work or solo living. If a baseline is obtained early in the course of the disorder, cognitive changes can be monitored over time and therapeutic recommendations regarding clinical management can be made. The tests may be used to detect early prodromal cognitive changes associated with delirium. Selection of neuropsychological instruments must be based in part on the patient's endurance and ability to respond. Lengthy batteries may not be appropriate (Fernandez & Levy, 1990).

Research on the effect of HIV on the neuropsychological functioning of HIV-positive individuals has focused on three subgroups: (1) asymptomatic HIV-positive individuals, (2) patients with ARC, and (3) patients with AIDS (Kaemingk & Kaszniak, 1989). Research on asymptomatic HIV has been mixed. Some earlier studies (Grant et al., 1987; Silberstein et al., 1987) of HIV+, asymptomatic individuals tended to find some impairment on neuropsychological tests; other studies have found no impairment (Franzblau et al., 1991; Kokkevi et al., 1991; Martin et al., 1993; Selnes et al., 1990). HIV-related cognitive changes tend to occur with the onset of constitutional symptoms or AIDS-defining illnesses (E. N. Miller et al., 1990).

Bornstein et al. (1992) noted mild but persistent behavioral impairment in a group of HIV-positive individuals. Impairments were noted on the GP and SRT. Levin et al. (1992) found impairments in word fluency and arithmetic.

A history of head injury may exacerbate neuropsychological deficits in HIV-positive patients (Marder et al., 1992). However, a history of minor head injury may not correlate with neuropsychological impairment (Bornstein et al., 1992, 1993).

ARC and PGL

Individuals who were asymptomatic, except for lymphadenopathy or T4 counts less than 700, were found to be impaired on tests of verbal memory (LM-WMS Delayed Recall, SRT-Retrieval, Storage, and Consistent Retrieval) and speed of information-processing of certain types of information [Posner Letter Matching Task (Posner & Mitchell, 1967) and figural visual search speed]. Impairment was also noted on the MMSE relative to HIV-negative individuals, although performance was not in the clinically impaired range. No impairment was noted on the BNT, V-WAIS-R, COWAT, DS-WAIS-R, continuous paired-associate learning, VR-WMS, BD-WAIS-R, mental rotation, simple reaction time, or two-choice reaction time (Wilkie et al., 1990).

Saykin et al. (1987) found impairment in language (naming and fluency), attention, visual and auditory information-processing, psychomotor function, and memory in patients with PGL. Impairment was noted on I-WAIS-R, COWAT, BNT, animal naming, LM-WMS (Immediate), TMTA, TMTB, SCWT Color, SCWT Interference, FTT nondominant hand, and CVLT Tuesday List. Impairment was also noted on two impairment indices devised by Saykin et al. (1987) and based on all 28 tests administered. Impairment was not suggested on the Halstead Impairment Index. No impairment, relative to controls, was noted on the Halstead CT, TPT, V-WAIS-R, BD-WAIS-R, LM-WMS (Delayed), VMS-WMS, DS-WAIS-R, SSPT, SRT, SR, DSym-WAIS-R, SCWT Word, finger sequencing or touching, FTT dominant hand, CVLT (all measures except the Tuesday list), or graphesthesia.

AIDS

Studies have found significant variability in the specific domains of cognitive functioning that are impaired in HIV-1 infection. Saykin et al. (1987) reported impairment in the area of verbal abilities. Grant et al. (1987) reported neither language impairments nor psychomotor slowing, but impaired CT performance. Van Gorp et al. (1989) found a pattern of deficits in nonverbal memory and timed psychomotor tasks with relatively preserved attention/concentration and language skills. Skoraszewski et al. (1991) found AIDS subjects impaired on all tests administered. Impairment was noted in psychomotor slowing, decreased attention and fine motor control, abstraction, memory, and verbal spontaniety.

Mental Status

The MMSE was found not to be impaired by Van Gorp *et al.* (1989).

Impairment Ratings

On a measure termed "global judgment," 87% of AIDS patients were found to be impaired vs. 9% of HIV-negative controls (Grant *et al.*, 1987).

Attention

Performance on the PASAT, DS-WAIS-R (Grant *et al.*, 1987; Skoraszewski *et al.*, 1991), and DSym-WAIS-R (Skoraszewski *et al.*, 1991; Van Gorp *et al.*, 1989) has been noted to be impaired.

Intelligence

VIQ, PIQ, and FSIQ may be impaired (Van Gorp *et al.*, 1989). Performance on S-WAIS-R (Van Gorp *et al.*, 1989) and Shipley IQ Estimate (Skoraszewski *et al.*, 1991) may exhibit impairment.

Memory

Performance on LM-WMS (Grant *et al.*, 1987; Skoraszewski *et al.*, 1991), VR-WMS (Handelsman *et al.*, 1992; Skoraszewski *et al.*, 1991; Van Gorp *et al.*, 1989), ROCFT:M (Van Gorp *et al.*, 1989), and RAVLT Delayed Recognition (Van Gorp *et al.*, 1989) may exhibit impairment.

Speech/Language

COWAT may exhibit impairment (Skoraszewski *et al.*, 1991). V-WAIS-R may decline (Handelsman *et al.*, 1992).

Visuospatial Functioning

Performance on BD-WAIS-R, PC-WAIS-R (Van Gorp *et al.*, 1989), and the TMTA (Skoraszewski *et al.*, 1991; Van Gorp *et al.*, 1989) may be impaired.

Motor Functioning

Impaired FTT performance may be noted (Handelsman *et al.*, 1992; Skoraszewski *et al.*, 1991).

Executive Functioning

Performance on the CT (Grant *et al.*, 1987) and TMTB (Handelsman *et al.*, 1992; Skoraszewski *et al.*, 1991; Van Gorp *et al.*, 1989) may exhibit impairment.

LNNB

Ayers *et al.* (1987) found symptomatic HIV-positive patients to be more impaired than HIV-negative patients on the LNNB. Infected groups had greater impairment on the Motor-C1, Tactile-C3, Receptive Speech-C4, Expressive Speech-C6, Reading-C8, and Memory-C10.

Personality

Patients with ARC and AIDS have been found to be significantly higher than HIV-negative individuals on the MMPI Hypochondriasis (Hs), Depression (D), Hysteria (Hy), and Schizophrenia (Sc) scales (Ayers *et al.*, 1987). PGL patients were higher than controls only on the Hs Scale (Saykin *et al.*, 1987). No difference between groups was noted on the Zung Self-Rating Depression Scale.

Individuals who have been diagnosed with HIV infection may experience fear for the future course of the disease and fear about the potential reactions of others. The patient may exhibit shock and denial when first diagnosed. If this reaction occurs, reassurance and health information may be only partly assimilated. The patient may exhibit withdrawal, aggression, and cognitive correlates of shock, such as distractibility, poor short-term memory, and disorientation (D. Miller, 1990).

Anxiety is commonly experienced by HIV-infected individuals. Anxiety may manifest as diarrhea, nausea, sweating, tremor, visual disturbances, dizziness, skin rashes, and lethargy, which may be misinterpreted by the patient as directly resulting from HIV infection. Panic attacks may occur. D. Miller (1990) has provided a list of 14 sources of anxiety in HIV-positive individuals.

Depression may occur in response to expectations about the inevitability of disease progression, loss of control, and self-blame and guilt about being exposed to HIV or having exposed others. Withdrawal is often a prominent sign of depression in those recently diagnosed as HIV-positive and may interfere with the process of acceptance and the learning of adaptive responses. Patients should be evaluated for suicidality. Depressed mood does not account for the cognitive sequelae of HIV (Grant *et al.*, 1993; Hinkin *et al.*, 1992).

Obsessive rumination may develop as a preoccupation with checking the body for emerging signs of the disease and involuntary dwelling on images or thoughts of HIV. Patients may resort to alcohol or drug use or participate in high-risk activities as a means of coping.

D. Miller (1990) has developed an outline for formal psychosocial examination of patients with HIV infection.

MEDICAL TREATMENT

There is no cure for HIV infection. Zidovudine or azidothymidine (AZT), an antiretroviral drug, has been found to decrease the number of life-threatening illnesses and to prolong survival (Masur, 1990). Appropriate treatment is to be provided for infections such as *Pneumocystis* pneumonia, herpes simplex, varicella-zoster, cytomegalovirus, *Cryptococcus neo-*

formans, and numerous other infections to which the immunocompromised HIV-positive patient may be susceptible.

Anxiety may be treated with small doses of short- to intermediate-acting benzodiazepines. In severely medically ill or demented patients, very small dosages of opiates may be preferred (Busch & Maxwell, 1990).

Tricyclic antidepressants may be prescribed, although patients with AIDS may be highly sensitive to anticholinergic side effects of medication (Busch & Maxwell, 1990). The use of psychostimulants such as methylphenidate or dextroamphetamine has been advocated for severely CNS-compromised, depressed HIV patients (Busch & Maxwell, 1990; Fernandez & Levy, 1990).

Symptoms of psychotic severity may occur during an acute medical episode or as a side effect of medication. Very low doses of high-potency neuroleptic medications may be helpful in controlling psychotic symptoms and severe agitation (Busch & Maxwell, 1990). An increased incidence of extrapyramidal side effects has been reported.

PSYCHOSOCIAL THERAPIES

Counseling is important at many stages of the testing, diagnosis, and illness. It should be available before and after HIV antibody testing and for those who are HIV-positive and asymptomatic, have ARC, or have AIDS. If ADC is suspected, counseling may focus on management of the implications of this condition for the patient, close friends, and family (R. Miller & Bor, 1988). Intervention may include: (1) allowing the patient to ventilate and be heard; (2) providing the patient with information about the disease process, treatment options, healthful behaviors, psychosocial coping strategies, and community resources; (3) psychotherapeutic support for the patient and significant others; and (4) referral to community services. D. Miller (1990) has developed a flow chart for psychosocial support in the context of HIV testing. *AIDS: A Guide to Clinical Counselling* (R. Miller & Bor, 1988) contains detailed examples of counseling sessions with HIV-positive patients and information useful for counseling sessions.

A number of self-help books are available. *AIDS: A Self-Care Manual* (Moffat *et al.,* 1987) contains information on a variety of HIV-related subjects for HIV-positive individuals and those who are close to them. *When Someone You Know Has AIDS: A Practical Guide* (Martelli *et al.,* 1987) describes how one can support and care for a person with AIDS.

Addresses and numbers of agencies that supply support and information about AIDS are available in many self-help books. The addresses of two national organizations are:

AIDS Action Council	Centers for Disease Control and
Federation of AIDS-	Prevention, AIDS Activity
Related Organizations	Building 3, Room 5B-1
1115 1/2 Independence	1600 Clifton Road
Avenue, SE	Atlanta, GA 30333
Washington, DC 20003	

PROGNOSIS

At 1 year following diagnosis of AIDS, 31% of patients have died; at 2 years, 56%; and at 3 years, 76% (Chamberland & Curran, 1990).

REFERENCES

Ayers, M. R., Abrams, D. I., Newell, T. G., & Friedrich, F. (1987). Performance of individuals with AIDS on the Luria–Nebraska Neuropsychological Battery. *International Journal of Clinical Neuropsychology, 3,* 101–105.

Bornstein, R. A., Nasrallah, H. A., Para, M. F., Whitacre, C. C., Rosenberger, P., Fass, R. J., & Rice, R. (1992). Neuropsychological performance in asymptomatic HIV infection. *Journal of Neuropsychiatry and Clinical Neurosciences, 4,* 386–394.

Bornstein, R. A., Poraza, A. M., Para, M. F., Whitacre, C. C., Fass, R. J., Rice, R. R., & Nasrallah, H. A. (1993). Effect of minor head injury on neuropsychological performance in asymptomatic HIV-1 infection. *Neuropsychology, 7,* 228–234.

Busch, K. A., & Maxwell, S. (1990). Somatic treatment of psychiatric symptoms in HIV disease. In D. G. Ostrow (Ed.), *Behavioral aspects of AIDS* (pp. 267–278). New York: Plenum Press.

Centers for Disease Control (1986). Classification system for human T-lymphotropic virus type III/lymphadenopathy–associated virus infections. *Morbidity and Mortality Weekly Report, 35,* 334–339.

Centers for Disease Control (1987). Revision of the case definition for acquired immunodeficiency syndrome. *Morbidity and Mortality Weekly Report Supplement, 36,* 1s–15s.

Chaisson, R. E., & Volberding, P. A. (1990). Clinical manifestations of HIV infection. In G. L. Mandell, R. G. Douglas, & J. E. Benett (Eds.), *Principles and practice of infectious diseases* (3rd ed.) (pp. 1059–1092). New York: Churchill-Livingston.

Chamberland, M. E., & Curran, J. W. (1990). Epidemiology and prevention of AIDS and HIV infection. In G. L. Mandell, R. G. Douglas, & J. E. Benett (Eds.), *Principles and practice of infectious diseases* (3rd ed.) (pp. 1029–1046). New York: Churchill-Livingston.

De La Paz, R., & Enzmann, D. (1988). Neuroradiology of acquired immunodeficiency syndrome. In M. L. Rosenblum, R. M. Levy, & D. E. Bredesen (1988), *AIDS and the nervous system* (pp. 121–153). New York: Raven Press.

Ewing, E. P. (1990). Etiology, epidemiology, and CDC definition. In V. V. Joshi (Ed.), *Pathology of AIDS and other manifestations of HIV infection* (pp. 7–20). New York: Igaku-Shoin.

Fernandez, F., & Levy, J. K. (1990). Diagnosis and management of HIV primary dementia. In D. G. Ostrow (Ed.), *Behavioral aspects of AIDS* (pp. 235–246). New York: Plenum Press.

Franzblau, A., Letz, R., Hershman, D., Mason, P., Wallace, J. I., & Bekesi, G. (1991). Quantitative neurologic and neurobehavioral testing of persons infected with human immunodeficiency virus type 1. *Archives of Neurology, 48,* 263–268.

Fultz, P. (1989). The biology of human immunodeficiency viruses. In R. A. Kaslow & D. P. Francis (Eds.), *The epidemiology of AIDS: Expression, occurrence, and control of human immunodeficiency virus type 1 infection* (pp. 3–17). New York: Oxford University Press.

Goedert, J. J., & Blattner, W. A. (1988). The epidemiology and natural history of human immunodeficiency virus. In V. T. DeVita, S. Hellman, & S. A. Rosenburg (Eds.), *AIDS:Etiology, treatment, and prevention* (pp. 33–60). Philadelphia: J. B. Lippincott.

Grant, I., Atkinson, J. H., Hesselink, J. R., Kennedy, C. J., Richman, D. D., Spector, S. A., & McCutchan, J. A. (1987). Evidence for early central nervous system involvement in the acquired immunodeficiency syndrome (AIDS) and other human immunodeficiency virus (HIV) infections. *Annals of Internal Medicine, 107,* 828–836.

Grant, I., Olshen, R. A., Atkinson, J. H., Heaton, R. K., Nelson, J., McCutchan, J. A., & Weinrich, J. D. (1993). Depressed mood does not explain neuropsychological deficits in HIV-infected persons. *Neuropsychology, 7,* 53–61.

Handelsman, L., Aronson, M., Maurer, G., Weiner, J., Jacobson, J., Bernstein, D., Ness, R., Herman, S., Losonczy, M., Song, I. S., Holloway, K., Horvath, T., Donnelly, N., Hirschowitz, J., & Rowan, A. J. (1992). Neuropsychological and neurological manifestations of HIV-1 dementia in drug users. *Journal of Neuropsychiatry and Clinical Neurosciences, 4,* 21–28.

Hinkin, C. H., Van Gorp, W. G., Satz, P., Weisman, J. D., Thommes, J., & Buckingham, S. (1992). Depressed mood and its relationship to neuropsychological test performance in HIV-1 seropositive individuals. *Journal of Clinical and Experimental Neuropsychology, 14,* 289–297.

Kaemingk, K. L., & Kaszniak, A. W. (1989). Neuropsychological aspects of human immunodeficiency virus infection. *Clinical Neuropsychologist, 3,* 309–326.

Kokkevi, A., Hatzakis, A., Maillis, A., Pittadaki, J., Zalonis, J., Samartis, D., Touloumi, G., Mandalaki, T., &

Stefanis, C. (1991). Neuropsychological assessment of HIV-seropositive haemophiliacs. *AIDS, 5,* 1223–1229.

Levin, B. E., Berger, J. R., Didona, T., & Duncan, R. (1992). Cognitive function in asymptomatic HIV-1 infection: The effects of age, education, ethnicity, and depression. *Neuropsychology, 6,* 303–313.

Libman, H., & Witzburg, R. A. (Eds.) (1993). *HIV infection: A Clinical Manual* (2nd ed.). Boston: Little, Brown, and Company.

Mann, J. M., & Chin, J. (1988). AIDS: A global perspective. *New England Journal of Medicine, 319,* 302–303.

Marder, K., Stern, Y., Malouf, R., Tang, M., Bell, K., Dooneief, G., El-Sadr, W., Goldstein, S., Gorman, J., Richards, M., Sano, M., Sorrell, S., Todak, G., Williams, J. B., Ehrhardt, A., & Mayeux, R. (1992). Neurologic and neuropsychological manifestations of human immunodeficiency virus infection in intravenous drug users without acquired immunodeficiency syndrome: Relationship to head injury. *Archives of Neurology, 49,* 1169–1175.

Martelli, L. J., Peltz, F. D., & Messina, W. (1987). *When someone you know has AIDS: A practical guide.* New York: Crown.

Martin, E. M., Robertson, L. C., Sorensen, D. J., Jagust, W. J., Mallon, K. F., & Chirurgi, V. A. (1993). Speed of memory scanning is not affected in early HIV-1 infection. *Journal of Clinical and Experimental Neuropsychology, 15,* 311–320.

Masur, H. (1990). Therapy for AIDS. In G. L. Mandell, R. G. Douglas, & J. E. Benett (Eds.), *Principles and practice of infectious diseases* (3rd ed.) (pp. 1102–1111). New York: Churchill-Livingston.

McDougal, J. S., Mawle, A. C., & Nicholson, J. K. A. (1989). The immune system: Pathophysiology. In R. A. Kaslow & D. P. Francis (Eds.), *The epidemiology of AIDS: Expression, occurrence, and control of human immunodeficiency virus type 1 infection* (pp. 18–41). New York: Oxford University Press.

Miller, D. (1990). Diagnosis and treatment of acute psychological problems related to HIV infection and disease. In D. G. Ostrow (Ed.), *Behavioral aspects of AIDS* (pp. 187–206). New York: Plenum Press.

Miller, E. N., Selnes, O. A., McArthur, J. C., Satz, P., Becker, J. T., Cohen, B. A., Sheridan, K., Machado, A. M., Van Gorp, W. G., & Visscher, B. (1990). Neuropsychological performance in HIV-1-infected homosexual men: The Multicenter AIDS Cohort Study (MACS). *Neurology, 40,* 197–203.

Miller, R., & Bor, R. (1988). *AIDS: A guide to clinical counselling.* London: Science Press.

Moffat, B., Spiegel, J., Parrish, S., & Helquist, M. (1987). *AIDS: A self-care manual.* Santa Monica: IBS Press.

Navia, B. A. (1990). The AIDS dementia complex. In J. L. Cummings (Ed.), *Subcortical dementia* (pp. 181–198). New York: Oxford University Press.

Navia, B. A., & Price, R. W. (1987). The acquired immunodeficiency syndrome dementia complex as the presenting or sole manifestation of human immunodeficiency virus infection. *Archives of Neurology, 44,* 65–69.

Olsen, W. L., & Cohen, W. (1988). Neuroradiaology of AIDS. In M. P. Federle, A. J. Megibow, & D. P. Naidlich (Eds.), *Radiology of AIDS* (pp. 21–46). New York: Raven Press.

Posner, M. I., & Mitchell, R. F. (1967). Chronometric analysis of classification. *Psychological Review, 74,* 392–409.

Price, R. W., Sidtis, J. J., Navia, B. A., Pumarole-Sune, T., & Ornitz, D. B. (1988). In M. L. Rosenblum, R. M. Levy, & D. E. Bredesen (Eds.), *AIDS and the nervous system* (pp. 203–219). New York: Raven Press.

Robertson, K. R., & Hall, C. D. (1992). Human immunodeficiency virus–related cognitive impairment and the acquired immunodeficiency syndrome dementia complex. *Seminars in Neurology, 12,* 18–27.

Saykin, A. J., Janssen, R. S., Sprehn, G. C., Kaplan, J. E., Spira, T. J., & Weller, P. (1987). Neuropsychological dysfunction in HIV-infection: Characterization in a lymphadenopathy cohort. *International Journal of Clinical Neuropsychology, 10,* 81–95.

Selnes, O. A., Miller, E., McArthur, J., Gordon, B., Munoz, A., Sheridan, K., Fox, R., & Saah, A. J. (1990). HIV-1 infection: No evidence of cognitive decline during the asymtomatic stages. *Neurology, 40,* 204–208.

Sidtis, J. J., & Price, R. W. (1990). Early HIV-1 infection and the AIDS dementia complex. *Neurology, 40,* 323–326.

Silberstein, C., McKegney, F., O'Dowd, M., Selwyn, P., Schoenbaum, E., Drucker, E., Feiner, C., Cox, C., & Friedland, G. (1987). A prospective longitudinal study of neuropsychological and psychosocial factors in asymptomatic individuals at risk to HTLV-III/LAV infection in a methadone program: Preliminary findings. *International Journal of Neuroscience, 32,* 669–676.

Skoraszewski, M. J., Ball, J. D., & Mikulka, P. (1991). Neuropsychological functioning of HIV-infected males. *Journal of Clinical and Experimental Neuropsychology, 13,* 278–290.

Steger, K. A. (1993). Epidemiology, natural history, and staging. In H. Libman & R. A. Witzburg (Eds.) *HIV infection: A clinical manual* (2nd ed., pp. 3–24). Boston: Little, Brown, & Co.

Van Gorp, W. G., Miller, E. N., Satz, P., & Visscher, B. (1989). Neuropsychological performance in HIV-1 immunocompromised patients: A preliminary report. *Journal of Clinical and Experimental Neuropsychology, 11,* 763–773.

Wilkie, F. L., Eisdorfer, C., Morgan, R., Loewenstein, D. A., & Szapocznik, J. (1990). Cognition in early human immunodeficiency virus infection. *Archives of Neurology, 47,* 433–440.

Working Group of the American Academy of Neurology AIDS Task Force (1991). Nomenclature and research case definitions for neurologic manifestations of human immunodeficiency virus-type 1 (HIV-1) infection. *Neurology, 41,* 778–785.

Yarchoan, R., & Pluda, J. M. (1988). Clinical aspects of infection with AIDS retrovirus: Acute HIV infection, persistent generalized lymphadenopathy, and AIDS-related complex. In V. T. DeVita, S. Hellman, & S. A. Rosenburg (Eds.), *AIDS: Etiology, treatment, and prevention* (pp. 107–120). Philadelphia: J. B. Lippincott.

Brain Tumors

DESCRIPTION

Brain Tumors

A brain tumor is a mass of tissue that grows and persists independently of its surrounding structures in the brain and has no physiological function (Kolb & Whishaw, 1985). Brain tumors are classified primary if they originate from the tissues of the brain and secondary if they result from metastases from other parts of the body. Intrinsic, intraaxial, or intracerebral tumors are contrasted with extrinsic, extraaxial, or extracerebral tumors.

Astroglial Neoplasm

An astroglial tumor is a tumor arising from astrocytes, or star-shaped neuroglia (Black, 1991). Historically, there have been a variety of classification schemata developed. Bailey and Cushing (1926) proposed 11 categories of gliomas (tumors arising from neuroglia) based on the cells from which the tumors originated. Kernohan *et al.,* (1949) developed a classification of gliomas based on the degree of cellular anaplasia or dedifferentiation. Gliomas were rated as astrocytomas of Grades I–IV. Astrocytomas of lower grade tend to progress toward higher grade. More recently, a three-stage classification scheme has been proposed and is defined below (Weir, 1973).

Astrocytoma

An astrocytoma is "a mildly hypercellular tumor with pleomorphism but no vascular proliferation or necrosis" (Black, 1991, p. 1557).

Anaplastic Astrocytoma

An anaplastic astrocytoma "has vascular proliferation, moderate pleomorphism, and moderate hypercellularity" (Black, 1991, p. 1557).

Glioblastoma Multiforme

The glioblastoma multiforme exhibits necrosis in addition to the characteristics of the anaplastic astrocytoma (Black, 1991).

Ependymoma

An ependymoma is a glial tumor in which the cells resemble the ependymal cells that line the cerebral ventricles (Harsh & Wilson, 1990).

Oligodendroglioma

An oligodendroglioma is a relatively benign tumor with cells that resemble oligodendrocytes, which are cells that myelinate CNS neurons (Harsh & Wilson, 1990).

Acoustic Neuroma

An acoustic neuroma is a benign tumor that grows from the nerve sheath of the VIIIth (auditory–vestibular) cranial nerve (Adams & Victor, 1989).

Pituitary Adenoma

A pituitary adenoma arises in the anterior pituitary (Adams & Victor, 1989).

Cerebral Metastases

These tumors result from metastases to the brain from systemic cancer (Black, 1991).

PREVALENCE, INCIDENCE, AND RISK FACTORS

Incidence

The incidence of primary brain tumors in adults is approximately 4.5/100,000 (Cohen, 1991; Schoenberg, 1991). Between 18% and 25% of patients who are autopsied as a consequence of cancer have metastases to the CNS (Cohen, 1991).

Environmental Toxins

Cranial irradiation and exposure to some chemicals may lead to an increased incidence of astrocytomas and meningiomas (Schoenburg, 1991).

Glioma

Approximately 45% of intracranial tumors are gliomas (Adams & Victor, 1989).

Glioblastoma Multiforme

Approximately 20% of intracranial tumors are glioblastoma multiforme (Adams & Victor, 1989). It is most frequent between the ages of 45 and 65 years (Jelsma & Bucy, 1969). Males are affected more than females, 55–65% to 35–45% (Reitan & Wolfson, 1985b).

Astrocytoma

Approximately 10% of intracranial tumors are astrocytomas (Adams & Victor, 1989). The age of onset is most commonly in the 3rd or 4th decade (Heffner, 1991).

Ependymoma

Approximately 6% of intracranial tumors are ependymomas (Adams & Victor, 1989). Incidence peaks occur at ages 5 and 34 (Ilgren *et al.*, 1984). Males are affected more than females in a ratio of 3:2 (Harsh & Wilson, 1990).

Oligodendroglioma

Fewer than 5% of primary brain tumors are oligodendrogliomas (Heffner, 1991). They tend to occur in the 3rd through 5th decades (Harsh & Wilson, 1990). Sixty percent of patients are male (Reitan & Wolfson, 1985b).

Meningioma

Approximately 15% of intracranial tumors are meningiomas (Adams & Victor, 1989).

Acoustic Neuroma

Approximately 7% of intracranial tumors are acoustic neuromas (Adams & Victor, 1989). Neurofibromatosis is associated with acoustic neuromas (Black, 1991).

Pituitary Adenoma

Approximately 7% of intracranial tumors are pituitary adenomas (Adams & Victor, 1989). They become increasingly likely with age. By the age of 80, small adenomas are found in more than 20% of pituitary glands (Adams & Victor, 1989).

Metastatic Carcinoma

Approximately 15–25% of intracranial tumors are metastatic carcinoma (Lohr & Cadet, 1987).

ETIOLOGY AND PATHOLOGY

A brain tumor shares its space within the skull with the brain, which already occupies 1200 cm^3 of space (Shapiro & Shapiro, 1986). A total of 100 g of tumor and edema is usually lethal. Tumor growth involving expansion of the tumor volume and cerebral edema produces increased intracranial pressure and generalized symptoms (Shapiro & Shapiro, 1986). Focal symptoms are produced by direct compression or infiltration where they are located. As the tumor enlarges, herniation may be produced. Anaplasia, or backward growth, suggests that tumor cells have gone from a more differentiated to a less differentiated state, that the cells are more primitive, and give the tumor a poorer prognosis (Heffner, 1991). Necrosis is mediated by a tumor necrosis factor that is produced by macrophages and is an indicator of more rapid growth and poorer outcome (Heffner, 1991). The relative frequencies of tumors in various locations of the brain are: posterior fossa, 30%; frontal, 22%; temporal, 22%; parietal, 12%; pituitary, 10%; and occipital, 4% (Lohr & Cadet, 1987).

The genesis of primary brain tumors has been explained in terms of the inappropriate expression of oncogenes in neoplastic cells and the loss of tumor-suppressor sequences in neoplastic cells.

Glioblastoma Multiforme

The cellular elements in glioblastomas are extremely varied. These tumors usually arise from the white matter and are rare in the posterior fossa. Glioblastomas are highly malignant and rapidly growing (Harsh & Wilson, 1990).

Astrocytoma

Astrocytomas may originate anywhere within the CNS. They commonly are slow growing and tend to infiltrate white matter (Adams & Victor, 1989).

Ependymoma

These tumors are generally slow growing and well-differentiated; however, about 10% show malignant histological changes (Ringertz & Reymond, 1949). Ependymomas account for approximately 25% of tumors located near the fourth ventricle. Two thirds of ependymomas are infratentorial (Reitan & Wolfson, 1985b).

Oligodendroglioma

More than 80% of tumors are found in the white matter of the cerebral hemisphere. In one study, 47% were frontal, 31% parietal, 19% temporal, and 3% were located in the lateral ventricles (McKeran & Thomas, 1980).

Meningioma

Meningiomas originate from the arachnoid layer of the brain (Black, 1991). They tend to occur in the cerebral convexity, parasagittal region, sphenoid wing, parasellar region, and spinal canal (Heffner, 1991). Malignant meningiomas are rare (Weiss, 1991).

Acoustic Neuroma

Acoustic neuromas are extraaxial tumors of the peripheral nervous system and are composed of Schwann cells and endoneurial fibroblasts (Heffner, 1991).

Pituitary Adenoma

Tumors usually arise as discrete nodules in the anterior pituitary gland. The tumor grows, pressing on the pituitary gland, extending out of the sella, and pressing on the optic chiasm. It may grow into the cavernous sinus, third ventricle, and posterior fossa. Some 60–70% of tumors are prolactin-secreting. Between 10% and 15% secrete growth hormone and a smaller number ACTH (Adams & Victor, 1989).

Cerebral Metastases

These tumors are most likely in melanoma, breast carcinoma, small-cell lung carcinomas, and non-Hodgkin's lymphoma (Delattre *et al.,* 1988). One third of metastases to the brain originate from the lung, a lesser number from the breast, followed by melanoma, and the gastrointestinal tract (Adams & Victor, 1989). They are spread hematogenously or are disseminated through lymphatic channels. Eighty percent are in the cerebrum, 16% in the cerebellum, and 3% in the brainstem (Heffner, 1991).

MEDICAL ASSESSMENT

Brain tumors produce progressive neurological signs and symptoms, with the rate of progression depending on the location and rate of growth of the tumor and its surrounding edema (Weiss, 1991). Although the progression of symptoms is usually steady, it may be intermittent or even acute (due to hemorrhage or suddenly increased intracranial pressure). Headache may be an initial symptom in approximately 25–35% of brain-tumor patients (Lohr & Cadet, 1987). Vomiting may occur in approximately one third of patients (Lohr & Cadet, 1987). Patients may also experience giddiness or dizziness. Seizures occur in approximately 20–50% of patients (Adams & Victor, 1989). Papilledema (due to increased intracranial pressure) may be noted, but its absence does not necessarily indicate the absence of increased intracranial pressure (Lohr & Cadet, 1987). Motor, sensory, or cranial nerve abnormalities may be noted. The clinician should be alert to the possibility of false localizing symptoms and signs due to increased intracranial pressure and resultant brain herniation (Adams & Victor, 1989; Heffner, 1991).

Changes in mentation or cognition may be noted. Rapid increases in intracranial pressure due to rapidly growing tumors or blockage may result in acute confusional states. Tumors located in the frontal or temporal lobes may result in psychiatric change. A psychiatric disorder is diagnosed initially in 18–50% of patients with brain tumors (Strub & Black, 1988). "A tumor must be suspected in any person of middle age or older in whom any slowly progressive behavioral change, whether cognitive or emotional, develops. This is particularly true when a change arises in a patient who has never had any such symptoms in the past" (Strub & Black, 1988, p. 444). In such cases, Strub and Black (1988) recommend a neurological examination and preferably a CT scan before the institution of lengthy psychotherapy.

When an intracranial tumor is suspected on clinical grounds, radiological studies are undertaken (Weiss, 1991). CT scan will reveal many larger tumors and their mass effects. It may fail to detect some tumors, especially small posterior fossa tumors, isodense infiltrating gliomas, and meningeal carcinomas. Enhancing cerebral infarcts, brain abscesses, and intracranial granulomas may be mistaken for tumors (Weiss, 1991). MRI may be used to image smaller tumors and low-grade astrocytomas. MRI angiography can be used to distinguish vascular masses from tumors (Black, 1991).

Glioblastoma Multiforme

Symptoms at the time of diagnosis may be headache, 73%; hemiparesis, 70%; cranial nerve deficits, 68%; papilledema, 60%; extremity weakness, 51%; hemisensory loss, 44%; hemianopia, 39%; vomiting, 39%; decreased level of consciousness, 33%; and speech difficulty, 32% (McKeran & Thomas, 1980). The interval between appearance of symptoms and diagnosis is usually less than 6 months (Harsh & Wilson, 1990). A stepwise deterioration is seen in 53% of patients, a gradual decline in 28%, and a sudden deterioration in 19% (Harsh & Wilson, 1990).

On CT, a glioblastoma commonly appears as a homogeneous hypodense or isodense mass. The surrounding brain is likely to appear compressed and invaded. MRI can demonstrate the variegated composition of the tumor more clearly (Harsh & Wilson, 1990).

Astrocytoma

Initial symptoms may include headache, 72%; epilepsy, 40–75%; and vomiting, 31% (Reitan & Wolfson, 1985b). The interval between initial appearance of symptoms and diagnosis may be several years (Harsh & Wilson, 1990).

On CT, low-grade astrocytomas may appear as low-density areas. MRI is more sensitive than CT to astrocytomas.

Ependymoma

Nonanaplastic ependymomas may exhibit relatively slow growth, which can result in a 1- to 2-year interval between appearance of initial symptoms and diagnosis. In about one third of patients, the presentation can be acute, often due to obstruction of CSF flow (Harsh & Wilson, 1990). On CT, the tumors are usually isodense or hyperdense and have intratumoral lucency. MRI is superior in delineating fourth-ventricle tumors (Harsh & Wilson, 1990).

Oligodendroglioma

There is usually a long interval (4 years) between appearance of symptoms and diagnosis. Seizures eventually occur in 85% of patients and are often the presenting symptom (Harsh & Wilson, 1990). Signs and symptoms at presentation may be headache, 80%; mental change, 50%; hemiparesis, 50%; papilledema, 50%; and extremity weakness, 45% (Horrax & Wu, 1951; McKeran & Thomas, 1980). On CT, part of the tumor is usually isodense or hypodense, while part is hyperdense due to calcification. On MRI, the tumor is hypointense on T1-weighted images and hyperintense on T2-weighted images (Harsh & Wilson, 1990).

Meningioma

Meningiomas may be imaged using CT. They present as well-defined lesions that are easily enhanced using a contrast medium (Black, 1991). They are likely to occur along dural planes and to have lobulated, sharply demarcated contours. They may also be detected with MRI using a gadolinium contrast medium (Black, 1991).

Acoustic Neuroma

Hearing loss is the first symptom in 70% of patients (Ojemann & Martuza, 1990). Hearing loss (generally high frequency) is found in 98% of patients at the time they seek medical attention (Ojemann & Martuza, 1990). Difficulty understanding words is often noted by the patient before hearing loss is diagnosed, especially when using the telephone (Rand, et al., 1982). Tinnitus, dizziness, unsteadiness, vertigo, retroauricular fullness, and headache may also be initial symptoms (Ojemann & Martuza, 1990). Additional symptoms may include facial palsy, diplopia, hoarseness, difficulty swallowing, facial pain or numbness, ataxia, and normal-pressure hydrocephalus syndrome (Ojemann & Martuza, 1990).

Brainstem auditory evoked response tests will indicate the presence of 98% of tumors (Ojemann & Martuza, 1990). High-resolution contrast CT scan can identify tumors 1.5 cm or more in diameter (Ojemann & Martuza, 1990). However, MRI with enhancement is the best method of imaging (Black, 1991).

Pituitary Adenoma

Patients present with hypersecretion of hormones, hypopituitarism, complete or partial bitemporal hemianopia, and headache. Tumors producing prolactin produce amenorrhea and galactorrhea in premenopausal women and loss of libido, visual loss, and headache in men. Tumors producing growth hormone cause gigantism in childhood and acromegaly in adulthood. Oversecretion of ACTH by a pituitary adenoma may result in Cushing's disease.

MRI is the imaging method of choice because it allows the evaluation of the tumor and its relation to the chiasm, hypothalamus, and cavernous sinus and can be used to distinguish the tumor from an aneurysm. Assessment for endocrine abnormalities may also be performed (Black, 1991).

Cerebral Metastases

Headache is the most common presenting symptom, followed by mental status changes (Heffner, 1991). Some 5–10% of patients experience an apoplectic onset due to seizures or raised intracranial pressure. On CT, 40% of patients will exhibit a solitary lesion. MRI is more sensitive than CT in demonstrating small lesions (Weiss, 1991).

NEUROPSYCHOLOGICAL ASSESSMENT

Due to advances in brain imaging, neuropsychological assessment rarely plays a significant role in the diagnosis of brain tumors. Nevertheless, clinical neuropsychologists should be able to recognize the signs associated with medically significant brain lesions and be able to make an appropriate referral. Clinical signs associated with brain tumors are reported in the *MEDICAL ASSESSMENT* section above.

Neuropsychological evaluation is likely to be performed after a tumor has been diagnosed to determine the degree of cerebral involvement and to provide a behavioral baseline and accounting of strengths and deficits. The baseline can be used to track recurrence or progression. The evaluation may include recommendations for postsurgical rehabilitation (Bigler, 1988).

Tumors may develop in any part of the brain. Many different speeds of development and sizes of lesion may be manifested. Since neuropsychological findings depend on these factors, there is no one type of neuropsychological profile seen with brain tumors. Tumors often have primary, more focal, lateralized effects related to the core of the tumor and secondary diffuse, nonlateralized effects related to "distance" effects (Bigler, 1988; Reitan & Wolfson, 1985b).

Although tumor patients have often been included in the "brain-damaged" groups of neuropsychological studies, there is a paucity of research concerning the neuropsychological correlates of cerebral neoplasms. The following discussion summarizes the results of some of the few studies that have been completed.

Behavior Rating Scales

The Karnofsky performance score assigns patients a score ranging from 10 to 100 according to their ability to do daily tasks (Karnofsky et al., 1951).

Cognitive Functioning

According to Reitan and Wolfson (1985a), the four most sensitive indicators of the HRNB (Halstead Impairment Index, CT, TMTB, and TPT Localization) "consistently show striking deviations from some of the better scores" (p. 105) in individuals with brain tumors. Hom and Reitan (1984) found that left cerebral hemisphere neoplasms impaired verbal abilities more than right cerebral hemisphere neoplasms. Right cerebral hemisphere neoplasms impaired abilities related to IQ more than did left cerebral hemisphere neoplasms. On the Wechsler–Bellvue, Verbal subtests, I, C, DS, A, S, and V exhibited significant differences. For Performance subtests, only BD exhibited a significant difference. Right hemisphere neoplasms resulted in more significantly impaired performance on the TPT than did left hemisphere neoplasms. The FTT was impaired contralateral to the cerebral hemisphere damaged by the neoplasm (Hom & Reitan, 1984).

Smith (1966) found patients with left hemisphere frontal tumors to be impaired on PC and all Verbal subtests.

Hochberg and Slotnick (1980) assessed patients who were at least 1-year postcraniotomy for astrocytoma and who, despite adequate self-care skills, could not return to school or occupation. Patients were tested on the CT, TPT, BVRT, A-WRAT, HVOT, SDMT, TMTA& B, and FTT. VIQ was found to be in the average range. Impaired performance was noted for all patients on the CT and TPT-Location.

Lilja et al. (1992) compared patients with tumors of high malignancy with patients with tumors of low malignancy. Differences were found on BD, verbal fluency, and the BVRT. Differences were noted in spontaneity of speech. The absence of impairment in the low-malignancy group was explained in terms of the slow and diffuse growth of Grade I and II astrocytomas.

Personality Functioning

Between 60% and 90% of patients with tumors of the frontal lobes have been reported to have personality changes, including apathy, irresponsibility, childishness, and inappropriate behavior (Frazier, 1936). Hallucinations and delusions may occur in 5–20% of patients. Anxiety and depression may be common early accompaniments of temporal lobe tumors (Mulder & Daly, 1952). Hallucinations are observed in approximately 30% of patients (Keschner et al., 1938).

MEDICAL TREATMENT

Corticosteroids are administered to reduce cerebral edema (Weiss, 1991). Osmotic agents such as mannitol may be used to treat dramatic increases in intracranial pressure.

Surgical intervention is often performed to obtain histological confirmation of a diagnosis, to restore pressure-related neurological dysfunction, and to remove as much of the tumor as is feasible. Microsurgical techniques, advanced stereotaxic and ultrasound technology, and intraoperative monitoring of evoked responses have improved the effectiveness of tumor resection (Black, 1991).

Radiation therapy is commonly used in the management of malignant tumors (Black, 1991). Focal-radiation techniques are being increasingly used. Brachytherapy involves the stereotaxic implantation of a radiation source in the tumor (Wara, 1985). The linear accelerator, multiple-source cobalt irradiator or "gamma knife," and proton beam are used as sources of focal radiation (Black, 1991).

Chemotherapy continues to be explored as a therapy for brain tumors. The results of this modality of therapy (except with young children who cannot tolerate radiation and in other special cases) remain controversial (Black, 1991).

Glioblastoma Multiforme

Treatment usually includes preoperative treatment with corticosteroids, prophylactic anticonvulsants, and reduction of elevated intracranial pressure. A maximal resection of the tumor is performed followed postoperative radiation chemotherapy.

Ependymoma

Treatment is surgical resection followed by radiation (Harsh & Wilson, 1990).

Astrocytoma

Surgical resection followed by radiation is the preferred mode of therapy (Black, 1991).

Oligodendroglioma

Total surgical resection is the preferred therapy. Postoperative radiation may increase duration of survival (Harsh & Wilson, 1990).

Meningioma

Depending on the location and other properties of the tumor, total surgical resection may be possible.

Acoustic Neuroma

Microsurgery is the preferred treatment. Over 95% of patients with small or medium tumors return to their previous activities (Ojemann & Martuza, 1990). Mortality is from 2% to 4% (Black, 1991).

Pituitary Adenoma

Microsurgical removal of the tumor results in visual improvement in about 70–80% of patients (Weiss, 1991). Proton–beam radiation may be used to destroy the tumor in some cases (Kjellberg, 1975). Radiation therapy has reduced the rate of postoperative recurrence.

Cerebral Metastases

Corticosteroids may be palliative. Depending on the patient's physical condition, surgery may be performed for accessible, solitary tumors. Radiotherapy may be appropriate for patients with multiple metastases (Weiss, 1991).

PSYCHOSOCIAL THERAPIES

Counseling may be of assistance to the patient and family. Cognitive rehabilitation may also be appropriate in some instances. Research in these areas is virtually nonexistent.

PROGNOSIS

Glioblastoma Multiforme

The 1-year survival ranges from 36% to 44% (Jaeckle, 1991).

Astrocytoma

The survival rate varies greatly depending on the extent of surgical removal. Predictors of favorable outcome include youth, normal level of consciousness, and absence of changes in personality. Approximately 50% of infiltrating astrocytomas are malignant at the time of recurrence (Harsh & Wilson, 1990).

Ependymoma

Surgical intervention combined with radiation therapy yields a 5-year survival rate of 49–83% (Harsh & Wilson, 1990).

Oligodendroglioma

The survival rate varies with histological grade. The 5-year survival rate for patients with lowest-grade tumors was 71%. The rate for patients with highest-grade tumors was 0% (Smith et al., 1983).

Meningioma

Complete tumor removal may be achieved in 60% of patients (Weiss, 1991). Even after apparently complete tumor removal, there is a recurrence rate of approximately 10% at 10 years. In one study of patients who had partial resection, 60% had recurrence (i.e., a worsening of symptoms due to persistent tumor growth) with a mean time of 66 months. When resection was followed by radiation, 32% had a recurrence with a mean time of 125 months (Barbaro et al., 1987).

Cerebral metastases

The survival rate varies depending on the histology of the underlying tumor (Weiss, 1991).

REFERENCES

Adams, R. D., & Victor, M. (1989). *Principles of neurology* (4th ed.). New York: McGraw-Hill.

Bailey, P., & Cushing, H. (1926). *A classification of tumors of the glioma group on a histogenetic basis with a correlated study of prognosis.* Philadelphia: J. B. Lippincott.

Barbaro, N. M., Gutin, P. H., Wilson, C. B., Sheline, G. E., Boldrey, E. B., & Wara, W. M. (1987). Radiation therapy in the treatment of partially resected meningiomas. *Neurosurgery, 20,* 525–528.

Bigler, E. D. (1988). *Diagnostic clinical neuropsychology* (2nd ed.). Austin: University of Texas Press.

Black, P. M. (1991). Brain tumors: Second of two parts. *New England Journal of Medicine, 324,* 1555–1564.

Cohen, M. E. (1991). Primary and secondary tumors of the nervous system. In W. G. Bradley, R. B. Daroff, G. M. Fenichel, & C. D. Marsden (Eds.), *Neurology in clinical practice,* Volume II, *The neurological disorders* (pp. 989–990). Boston: Butterworth-Heinemann.

Delattre, J. Y., Krol, G., Thaler, H. T., & Posner, J. B. (1988). Distribution of brain metastases. *Archives of Neurology, 45,* 741–744.

Frazier, C. H. (1936). Tumor involving the frontal lobe alone: A symptomatic survey of one hundred and five verified cases. *Archives of Neurology and Psychiatry, 35,* 525–571.

Harsh, G. R., & Wilson, C. B. (1990). Neuroepithelial tumors of the adult brain. In J. R. Youmans (Ed.), *Neurological surgery: A comprehensive reference guide to the diagnosis and management of neurosurgical problems* (3rd ed.) (pp. 3040–3136). Philadelphia: W. B. Saunders.

Heffner, R. R. (1991). Pathology of the nervous system. In W. G. Bradley, R. B. Daroff, G. M. Fenichel, & C. D. Marsden (Eds.), *Neurology in clinical practice,* Volume II, *The neurological disorders* (pp. 991–1007), Boston: Butterworth-Heinemann.

Hochberg, F. H., & Slotnick, B. (1980). Neuropsychologic impairment in astrocytoma survivors. *Neurology, 30,* 172–177.

Hom, J., & Reitan, R. M. (1984). Neuropsychological correlates of rapidly vs. slowly growing intrinsic cerebral neoplasms. *Journal of Clinical Neuropsychology, 6,* 309–324.

Horrax, G., & Wu, W. Q. (1951). Post-operative survival of patients with intracranial oligodendroglioma and special reference to radical tumor removal: A study of 26 patients. *Journal of Neurosurgery, 8,* 473–479.

Ilgren, E. B., Stiller, C. A., Hughes, J. T., Silberman, D., Steckel, N., & Kaye, A. (1984). Ependymomas: A clinical and pathological study. Part I. Biologic features. *Clinical Neuropathology, 3,* 113–121.

Jaeckle, K. A. (1991). Clinical presentation and therapy of nervous system tumors. In W. G. Bradley, R. B. Daroff, G. M. Fenichel, & C. D. Marsden (Eds.), *Neurology in clinical practice,* Volume II, *The neurological disorders* (pp. 1008–1030), Boston: Butterworth-Heinemann.

Jelsma, R., & Bucy, P. C. (1969). Glioblastoma multiforme: Its treatment and some factors affecting survival. *Archives of Neurology, 20,* 161–171.

Karnofsky, D. A., Burchenal, J. H., Armistead, G. C., Southham, C. M., Bernstein, J. L., Craver, L. F., & Rhoads, C. P. (1951). Triethylene melamine in the treatment of neoplastic disease. *Archives of Internal Medicine, 87,* 477–516.

Kepes, J. J. (1982). *Meningiomas: Biology, pathology, and differential diagnosis.* New York: Masson.

Kernohan, J. W., Mabon, R. F., Svien, H. J., & Adson, A. W. (1949). A simplified classification of gliomas. *Proceedings of the Staff Meetings of the Mayo Clinic, 24,* 71–75.

Keschner, M., Bender, M. B., & Strauss, I. (1938). Mental symptoms associated with brain tumor. *JAMA, 110,* 714–718.

Kjellberg, R. N. (1975). A system of therapy of pituitary tumors: Bragg peak proton hypophysectomy. In H. G. Seydel (ed.), *Tumors of the nervous system* (pp. 145–174). New York: Wiley.

Kolb, B., & Whishaw, I. Q. (1985). *Fundamentals of human neuropsychology* (2nd ed.). New York: W. H. Freeman.

Lilja, A., Salford, L. G., Smith, G. J., Hagstadius, S., Risberg, J., Brun, A., & Ohman, R. (1992). Neuropsychological indexes of a partial frontal syndrome in patients with nonfrontal gliomas. *Neuropsychology, 6,* 315–326.

Lohr, J. B., & Cadet, J. L. (1987). Neuropsychiatric aspects of brain tumors. In R. E. Hales & S. C. Yudolfsky (Eds.), *The American Psychiatric Press textbook of neuropsychiatry* (pp. 351–364). Washington, DC: American Psychiatric Press.

McKeran, R. O., & Thomas, D. G. T. (1980). The clinical study of gliomas. In D. G. T. Thomas & D. I. Graham (Eds.), *Brain tumors: Scientific basis, clinical investigation and current therapy* (pp. 194–230). Boston: Butterworth.

Mulder, D. W., & Daly, D. (1952). Psychiatric symptoms associated with lesions of the temporal lobe. *JAMA, 150,* 173–176.

Ojemann, R. G., & Martuza, R. L. (1990). Acoustic neuroma. In J. R. Youmans (Ed.), *Neurological surgery: A comprehensive reference guide to the diagnosis and management of neurosurgical problems* (3rd ed.) (pp. 3316–3350). Philadelphia: W. B. Saunders.

Rand, R. W., Dirks, D. D., Morgan, D. E., & Bentson, J. R. (1982). Acoustic neuromas. In J. R. Youmans (Ed.), *Neurological surgery* (2nd ed.) (pp. 2967–3003). Philadelphia: W. B. Saunders.

Reitan, R. M., & Wolfson, D. (1985a). *The Halstead–Reitan Neuropsychological Test Battery: Theory and clinical interpretation.* Tucson: Neuropsychology Press.

Reitan, R. M., & Wolfson, D. (1985b). *Neuroanatomy and neuropathology: A clinical guide for neuropsychologists.* Tucson: Neuropsychology Press.

Ringertz, N., & Reymond, A. (1949). Ependymomas and choroid plexus papillomas. *Journal of Neuropathology and Experimental Neurology, 8,* 355–380.

Schoenburg, B. S. (1991). Epidemiology of primary intracranial neoplasms: Disease distribution and risk factors. In M. Salcman (Ed.), *Concepts of neurosurgery,* Volume 4, *Neurobiology of brain tumors* (pp. 3–18). Baltimore: Williams & Wilkins.

Shapiro, W. R., & Shapiro, J. R. (1986). Primary brain tumors. In A. K. Asbury, G. M. McKhann, & W. I. McDonald (Eds.), *Diseases of the nervous system: Clinical neurobiology* (pp. 1137–1154). Philadelphia: W. B. Saunders.

Smith, A. (1966). Intellectual functions in patients with lateralized frontal tumors. *Journal of Neurology, Neurosurgery, and Psychiatry, 29,* 52–59.

Smith, M. T., Ludwig, C. L., Godfrey, A. D., & Armbrustmacher, V. W. (1983). Grading of oligodendrogliomas. *Cancer, 52,* 2107–2114.

Strub, R. L., & Black, F. W. (1988). *Neurobehavioral disorders: A clinical approach.* Philadelphia: F. A. Davis.

Wara, W. M. (1985). Radiation therapy for brain tumors. *Cancer, 55,* 2291–2295.

Weir, B. (1973). The relative significance of factors affecting postoperative survival in astrocytomas, grades 3 and 4. *Journal of Neurosurgery, 38,* 448–452.

Weiss, H. D. (1991). Neoplasms. In M. A. Samuels (Ed.), *Manual of neurology: Diagnosis and therapy* (pp. 213–239). Boston: Little, Brown.

Anoxia–Hypoxia

DESCRIPTION

Anoxia–Hypoxia

Anoxia refers to a lack of oxygen. *Hypoxia* refers to a deficiency in oxygen. *Hypoxemia* refers to a lesser deficiency in oxygen. Subtypes of anoxia–hypoxia include the following:

1. *Anoxic anoxia–hypoxia* is "diminished oxygen in the arterial blood despite normal ability of the blood to contain and carry oxygen" (e.g., drowning) (Reitan & Wolfson, 1985, p. 258).
2. *Anemic anoxia–hypoxia* occurs when there is a deficiency in the oxygen-carrying power of the blood (e.g., carbon monoxide poisoning).
3. *Histotoxic anoxia–hypoxia* involves dysfunction of the brain's respiratory enzymes or a metabolic blockade of cellular respiration (e.g., cyanide poisoning) (Dutka & Hallenbeck, 1991).
4. *Hypoglycemic anoxia–hypoxia* results from a deficiency in glucose.
5. *Overutilization anoxia–hypoxia* occurs when there is an increased demand for oxygen utilization relative to supply (e.g., status epilepticus) (Rowe *et al.,* 1985).
6. *Stagnant anoxia–hypoxia* or *ischemic anoxia–hypoxia* occurs when blood flow ceases (Dutka & Hallenbeck, 1991).

Cardiopulmonary Arrest

Cardiopulmonary arrest is the sudden cessation of cardiac and respiratory functioning resulting in a lack of arterial blood pressure.

Cardiopulmonary Bypass Surgery

In open heart surgery, all venous blood from the vena cavae and right atrium of the heart is rerouted by cannulae to a pump oxygenator, where oxygen is taken up and carbon dioxide removed, and then conducted via cannula to the patient's arterial system. Through this technique, the heart and lung can be bloodless during the operation (Stanton, 1988).

Chronic Obstructive Pulmonary Disease

Chronic obstructive pulmonary disease (COPD) is a condition in which there is a chronic obstruction of airflow due to chronic bronchitis or emphysema or both (Ingram, 1980). *Chronic bronchitis* involves excessive tracheobronchial mucus production sufficient to produce cough with expectoration for at least 3 months of the year for 2 consecutive years. Emphysema is distention of the air spaces distal to the terminal bronchiole and destruction of the alveolar septa (Ingram, 1980). COPD is also termed chronic airflow obstruction (CAO) or chronic obstructive lung disease (COLD).

INCIDENCE AND RISK FACTORS

Cardiopulmonary Arrest

Age

Peaks occur between birth and 6 months and between 45 and 75 years of age. The incidence of arrest increases with age in adulthood (Myerburg & Castellanos, 1988).

Gender

Arrests occur in males vs. females in a 3:1 ratio (Myerburg & Castellanos, 1988).

Additional Risk Factors

Additional factors are hypertension, obesity, previous myocardial infarction, cigarette consumption, social isolation, and a high level of life stress (Myerburg & Castellanos, 1988).

Chronic Obstructive Pulmonary Disease

Prevalence

Chronic bronchitis occurs in approximately 20% of adult males, but only a minority are clinically disabled. Adult lungs are rarely without some emphysema (Ingram, 1980).

Gender

Chronic bronchitis is more common in men than in women. Well-defined but usually limited and symptomless emphysema is found in approximately two thirds of males and one fourth of females (Ingram, 1980).

Age

Emphysema tends to increase in the 5th decade and above (Ingram, 1980).

Risk Factors

Smoking is the single most important factor in the development of COPD. Air pollution, occupational exposures to solvents, and infection are risk factors and can aggravate COPD (Ingram, 1980).

ETIOLOGY AND PATHOLOGY

Cardiopulmonary Arrest

The brain accounts for approximately 20% of the body's oxygen utilization (Norenberg & Bruce-Gregorios, 1991). Due to the brain's high metabolic activity and the lack of sufficient stores of oxygen in the brain, a decrease in oxygen tension (PaO_2) to 40–50 mm Hg leads to impaired cognitive functioning. A PaO_2 below 30 mm Hg for 10 sec will result in loss of consciousness.

A cerebral blood flow of 15 ml/100 g per min is necessary to prevent brain injury. During arrest, both cerebral blood flow and oxygen delivery rapidly cease. Total circulatory arrest for 10–15 sec will result in loss of consciousness (Norenberg & Bruce-Gregorious, 1991). There may be a brief tonic spasm and extension with opisthotonus. The EEG flattens and evoked potential responses are not obtainable (Bass, 1985). Synaptic transmission ceases. As perfusion decreases, cell injury begins to occur. Potassium leaks from cells, lactate increases to toxic levels, and calcium accumulates in cells. Changes in calcium levels are believed to be particularly important in ischemic injury (White *et al.,* 1984). Calcium uncouples oxidative phosphorylation and activates membrane phospholipases, processes that result in the enzymatic breakdown of phospholipids and the production of free radicals, thromboxanes, and leukotrienes and may result in cell death. Cell damage may not end as soon as systemic circulation is restored.

In adults, in the absence of drugs or hypothermia, 5–10 min of complete circulatory arrest without resuscitative efforts results in irreversible brain damage (Bass, 1985). Neurons are the cells in the brain most sensitive to ischemia. The CA1 and CA4 sectors of the hippocampus; the parahippocampal gyrus; cortical layers III, V, and VI; and Purkinje cells are selectively vulnerable (Dutka & Hallenbeck, 1991). Boundary zones or watershed areas, areas of the brain in the most distal reaches of two adjoining arterial trees, tend to be more vulnerable (Snyder, 1991).

Cardiopulmonary Bypass Surgery

Embolic phenomena and inadequate cerebral perfusion may result in neurological deficit (Prough & Angert, 1987).

MEDICAL ASSESSMENT

Chronic Obstructive Pulmonary Disease

The degree of obstruction, extent of disability, and reversibility are assessed. Emphysema is not reversible (Ingram, 1980).

NEUROPSYCHOLOGICAL ASSESSMENT

Cardiopulmonary Arrest

There are few group neuropsychological studies of patients who have suffered cardiopulmonary arrest. Case studies suggest that the most profound cognitive deficit resulting from cardiopulmonary arrest is an impaired ability to learn new information. Cummings *et al.*

(1984) reported the case of an individual who developed severe amnesia following cardiopulmonary arrest. Although DS, speech, language, and visuospatial functioning appeared to be
intact, he was not oriented to place and time and could not recall three words after 3 min.
LM-WMS and Paired-Associate Learning were severely impaired. At autopsy, the patient
was found to have bilateral anoxic lesions primarily limited to the hippocampus. Volpe and
Hirst (1983) assessed three patients who had suffered anoxic–ischemic injury. Impairment
was noted primarily in memory functioning. Anterograde amnesia has also been noted in
reported cases of attempted hanging (Berlyne & Strachan, 1968; Medalia et al., 1991). More
severe cases of anoxia following cardiac arrest may exhibit a wider range of symptoms.
Parkin et al. (1987) described a patient who had a severe memory deficit, perceptual problems,
and emotional disturbances of shallow quality. Some language ability and a sense of humor
were preserved.

Rowe et al. (1985) compared 17 (9 acute, 8 chronic) cardiopulmonary arrest patients
with 20 (10 acute, 10 chronic) closed head injury patients on the WAIS-R, PPT, SDMT, and
HVOT. For the acute groups, no difference was noted on any of the tests. The performance
of chronic cardiopulmonary arrest patients was significantly less than that of the chronic head
injury patients on the WAIS-R Performance subtests, simultaneous bilateral performance on
the PPT, both written and oral modalities on the SDMT, and the HVOT. The authors concluded
that the results suggested that the rate or extent of recovery of impaired visual–motor–spatial
neuropsychological functioning following cardiopulmonary arrest is less than the rate or
extent of recovery of other neuropsychological functions.

Roine et al. (1993) found the MMSE to be impaired at 1 day following arrest in patients
who had been resuscitated from out-of-hospital ventricular fibrillation. MMSE scores rose to
normal limits at 3 months postarrest. The results of neuropsychological testing at 12 months
suggested a low-normal level of cognitive functioning except for the WMS delayed recall
score, which was clearly subnormal. Speech, reading, writing, and visual perception were
relatively unchanged. Memory, visuoconstructive functions, programming of activity, voluntary hand movements, and arithmetic were more vulnerable. PIQ was more affected than
VIQ. Depressive symptoms were noted in 35% of patients at 3 months and in 31% of patients
at 12 months.

Cardiopulmonary Bypass Surgery

Studies of patients who have undergone cardiopulmonary bypass surgery find impairment
in some areas of cognitive functioning immediately after surgery. An overall improvement,
or at least a rebound in functioning to normal levels, is found for most patients. Juolasmaa
et al. (1981) administered a battery of tests 5 months pre- and 5 months postsurgery. The
tests included the WAIS, FTT, LM-WMS, Associative Learning, BVRT, BMGT, and Hand
Tapping. They reported a trend toward improvement in intellectual performance after surgery,
though much of this improvement may have been due to practice effect. Improvement was
most notable for tests of visual functioning. A significant relationship was found between
the degree of postoperative cognitive impairment and the presence of postoperative psychosis
or delirium. BD, BVMGT, and FTT appeared to be most sensitive to the residual effects of
CNS dysfunction. Patients with mitral valve disease were more prone to postoperative cognitive impairment than were patients with aortic valve disease. A high level of hypochondriasis
and anxiety appeared to increase the likelihood of cognitive impairment after surgery.

Savageau et al. (1982a) evaluated patients preoperatively and 9 days postoperatively on
VR-WMS (Forms I and II) and the TMTA&B. Of these patients, 70% remained within one
standard deviation of their preoperative performance on all test scores. Decrements of greater

than one standard deviation were observed on all test scores for 11–17% of the patients. Impairment was noted primarily on the TMTA&B. Correlates of significantly impaired test performance were age greater than 60 years, end-diastolic pressure greater than 30 mm Hg, moderate to severe enlargement of the heart, use of propranolol or chlordiazepoxide hydrocloride, duration of operation, estimate of blood loss greater than 2000 ml, hypotension, difficult intubation, insertion of an intraaortic balloon, electrolyte abnormalities, longer stay in the intensive care unit, bizarre behavior or disorientation, and depression. At 6 months, only 5% of patients showed a consistent postoperative test score deterioration (Savageau *et al.*, 1982b). Cognitive decrements at 6 months were correlated with total estimated blood loss greater than 3000 ml, administration of propranolol during the operation, fatigue, depression, and worries related to the operation. It was concluded that sustained postoperative neuropsychological dysfunction 6 months after cardiac surgery is rare.

Raymond *et al.* (1984) tested bypass and general surgical patients on the WAIS, SRT, RPM, and BVRT. In the early postoperative period, the bypass group performed more poorly on motor, visuospatial, WAIS IQ, DS, and the SRT. These differences disappeared at 6–8 weeks.

Schall *et al.* (1989) found cardiac transplantation patients to have preoperative neuropsychological deficits in memory, higher-level processing of information, and motor speed. Shaw *et al.* (1986) found that 79% of bypass patients showed impairment in some aspect of cognitive function at the 7th postoperative day. Shaw *et al.* (1987) found that 57% had impairment on at least one test. Of these patients, 71% had no significant symptoms, 27% had minor problems, and 2% were seriously disabled. Impairments were noted on the TMTB, VR-WMS, associate learning, and BD. Sotaniemi *et al.* (1986) reported that bypass patients who exhibited problems on neurological evaluation exhibited cognitive impairments at 5-year follow-up.

In contrast, Smith (1988) found cardiopulmonary-bypass and non-cardiopulmonary-bypass patients to have comparative levels of neuropsychological deficits. Hammeke and Hastings (1988) did not find impairment in their bypass patients at 6 months. Kareken *et al.* (1992) found that bypass and valve replacement patients 2–3 years after surgery did not endorse cognitive problems.

Chronic Obstructive Pulmonary Disease

Neuropsychological impairments have been found in patients suffering from COPD (Adams *et al.*, 1980; Prigatano & Levin, 1988). In major studies of COPD patients, nocturnal oxygen therapy trial and positive-pressure breathing trial patients were found to be impaired relative to controls on an extensive neuropsychological battery (Grant *et al.*, 1982; Prigatano *et al.*, 1983). Increased hypoxemia was associated with increased neuropsychological impairment (Grant *et al.*, 1987). Continuous oxygen therapy was noted to be more effective than nocturnal oxygen therapy at 12-month follow-up. Neuropsychological performance and survival were improved for continuous oxygen therapy (Heaton *et al.*, 1983). Cohen *et al.* (1986) reported that patients receiving long-term oxygen therapy did not exhibit impaired intellectual functioning during a 4-hr period of oxygen withdrawal. Patients with moderate to severe COPD exhibited impairment in most ability areas assessed on an extended HRNB (Grant *et al.*, 1982). Patients with milder COPD were found to exhibit impairments on a subset of neuropsychological subtests (Prigatano *et al.*, 1983).

Impairment Indexes

Patients with mild COPD were impaired on the Halstead Impairment Index and the Average Impairment Rating (Prigatano *et al.*, 1983).

Attention

Patients with mild COPD were impaired on DSym-WAIS (Prigatano *et al.*, 1983). DS was not impaired.

Memory

Patients with mild COPD were impaired on the LM-, VR-, and PA-WMS Immediate and Delayed (Prigatano *et al.*, 1983).

Intellectual Functioning

Patients with mild COPD were impaired on VIQ, PIQ, FSIQ, and I-WAIS (Prigatano *et al.*, 1983).

Speech/Language

Patients with mild COPD were impaired on V-WAIS and the AST (Prigatano *et al.*, 1983). No impairment was noted on C- or S-WAIS or the SSPT or SR.

Arithmetic

Patients with mild COPD were not impaired on A-WAIS (Prigatano *et al.*, 1983).

Visuospatial Functioning

Patients with mild COPD were impaired on PC-, BD-, PA-, and OA-WAIS (Prigatano *et al.*, 1983). The TMTA was unimpaired.

Sensory Functioning

Patients with mild COPD were impaired on the TPT-Time (TPT Memory and Location were unimpaired) (Prigatano *et al.*, 1983).

Motor Functioning

Patients with mild COPD were impaired on the GP and GS (Prigatano *et al.*, 1983). The FTT was unimpaired.

Executive Functioning

Patients with mild COPD were impaired on the CT and TMTB (Prigatano *et al.*, 1983).

Personality

The most common profile on the MMPI was suggestive of depression (42%), followed by unclassified (18%), normal (14.7%), hypochondriasis (8.7%), depression–hysteria (6.7%), and manipulative character disorder (6.7%) (McSweeny *et al.*, 1982). On the Profile of Mood States, patients described themselves as tense, depressed, confused, fatigued, and sapped of vigor (McSweeny et al., 1982). Relatives viewed patients as socially withdrawn and somewhat obstreperous on the Katz Adjustment Scale (Katz & Lyerly, 1963). Patients reported much greater impairment on the Sickness Impact Profile (McSweeny et al., 1982). Recreational activities, home management, sleep, and rest were impaired.

High-Altitude Hypoxemia

Mountaineers experience hypoxemia when ascending to high altitudes. At 5486 m (18,000 ft), partial oxygen pressure is approximately one half of that at sea level (Clark et al., 1983). Mountain sickness can range from mild acute mountain sickness to life-threatening high altitude pulmonary edema and cerebral edema. Symptoms may include decreased visual acuity and auditory acuity, impaired memory and concentration, judgment, clumsiness, delusions, hallucinations, and slurred speech. Berry et al. (1989) found DSym and the FTT impaired during induced isocapnic (steady-state CO_2) hypoxemia. However, performance rebounded to equal or above hypoxemia levels following hypoxemia.

Pre- and posttesting of participants in Himalayan mountain expeditions, in an effort to determine whether mountaineers experience residual cognitive impairment, has yielded mixed results. Hornbein et al. (1989) found impairment in VR-WMS and the FTT. More aphasic errors were made by mountaineers. In contrast, Clark et al. (1983) found no impairment on pre–post testing on an extensive battery of neuropsychological tests. They concluded that if healthy people do not suffer additional physical insults, acute CNS effects of low oxygen tensions are reversible. Jason et al. (1989) also found no impairment on pre–post testing of a group of mountaineers.

Nocturnal Hypoxia

Nocturnal hypoxia due to sleep-disordered breathing has been associated with impairments in verbal and nonverbal intelligence, verbal and nonverbal memory, and expressive verbal fluency (Berry et al., 1986).

Attention

DS was unimpaired (Berry et al., 1986).

Memory

VR-WMS has been found to be unimpaired but LM-WMS impaired in patients with nocturnal hypoxia (Berry et al., 1986). The ROCFT:M was impaired.

Intelligence

VIQ and PIQ have been noted to be impaired (Berry et al., 1986).

Speech/Language

Verbal fluency, using the letters ''f,'' ''a,'' and ''s,'' has been found to be impaired in patients with nocturnal hypoxia (Berry et al., 1986).

Visuospatial Functioning

Performance on the HVOT has been found to be unimpaired in patients with nocturnal hypoxia (Berry *et al.*, 1986).

Motor Functioning

The FTT was unimpaired (Berry *et al.*, 1986).

Executive Functioning

The WCST has been found to be unimpaired in patients with nocturnal hypoxia (Berry *et al.*, 1986).

MEDICAL TREATMENT

Cardiopulmonary Arrest

Treatment will involve cardiopulmonary resuscitation (CPR) (the establishment of an airway, mouth-to-mouth respiration, and chest compression) and any or all of the following measures: advanced life support, defibrillation—cardioversion, and pharmacotherapy (Myerburg & Castellanos, 1988).

A number of therapies have been developed to protect the integrity of the brain. Both barbiturates and hypothermia reduce cerebral metabolism, but have been found to be of limited benefit (Bass, 1985). Dilantin may be given if there is a possibility of seizures. Calcium-blocking agents may both offset direct cellular toxic reactions and counteract vaso-constriction during reperfusion (Bass, 1985).

Chronic Obstructive Pulmonary Disease

Treatment involves cessation of smoking, avoidance of pollutants, and immediate treatment of pulmonary infections. Exercise programs may result in improved exercise tolerance. Bronchodilators may alleviate symptoms. Bronchopulmonary drainage is maintained. If hypoxemia is severe, portable oxygen therapy may be considered (Ingram, 1980).

PSYCHOSOCIAL THERAPIES

Cardiopulmonary Arrest

To understand the patient's point of view, therapists might benefit from reading the autobiographical account by Meltzer (1983) of his recovery from cardiopulmonary arrest and resultant impairments in recent and remote memory.

Cardiopulmonary Bypass Surgery

Patients facing bypass surgery should have a presurgical psychological interview (Thompson, 1980). To minimize postoperative psychological complications, the patient should be educated about the surgical procedure. Fears of death and morbidity should be discussed. It is recommended that a loved one be present both before and after the operation. Room changes should be explained to the patient. The patient should be taken on a tour of the recovery room and intensive care unit, where basic procedures are explained and postoperative care-takers introduced. This should be done several days before surgery, before last-minute anxiety interferes with learning. Such preoperative preparation has been shown to result in an approximate 50% decrease in postoperative psychosis (Kornfeld *et al.*, 1974).

If a patient develops an altered mental status postoperatively, he or she should be evaluated for organic or psychological pathology. Postoperative psychosis may develop in as many as one third of bypass patients (Lazarus & Hagen, 1968). Onset is usually 2–4 days after surgery (Abram, 1975). Patients who have greater anxiety or depression preoperatively are at greater risk postoperatively. In addition to somatic therapy (small doses of minor tranquilizers or haloperidol in the case of severe agitation), orienting and reassuring the patient may be therapeutic (Thompson, 1980). Delirium often clears completely within a week.

Numerous books have been written for patients who face bypass surgery. Among them are *Open Heart Surgery: A Guidebook for Patients and Families* (Yalof, 1983) and *Coronary Bypass Surgery: Who Needs It?* (Kra, 1986).

Chronic Obstructive Pulmonary Disease

McSweeny *et al.* (1982) suggested that the COPD-associated features of advanced age, low social position, and neuropsychological deficit make it less likely that these patients will respond to traditional therapy. They suggest that psychological interventions should be part of a standard patient education program that might include didactic lectures and structured exercises. The content of the program might include skills for coping with the psychosocial effects of COPD for patients and families. Patients should be taught how to maximize access to reinforcing activities.

PROGNOSIS

Cardiopulmonary Arrest

A study of 210 patients who had experienced coma due to cerebral hypoxia–ischemia revealed that 13% of patients had regained independent function during the first postarrest year (Levy *et al.*, 1985). Patients with an absence of pupillary light reflexes never regained independent daily function. Patients with the best chance of regaining independence were identified as follows: (1) first-day motor response of withdrawal or better and first-day eye-opening improved at least 2 grades; (2) motor responses of withdrawal or better and normal spontaneous eye movements at day 3; (3) obeying commands at 1 week; and (4) normal oculocephalic response at week 2.

Chronic Obstructive Pulmonary Disease

Generally, there is a slow yet relentless diminution in ventilatory function in patients with COPD (Ingram, 1980). After an initial episode of respiratory failure, the 5-year survival rate averages only 15–20%.

REFERENCES

Abram, H. S. (1975). Psychiatry and surgery. In A. M. Freeman, H. I. Kaplan, & B. J. Sadock (Eds). *Comprehensive textbook of psychiatry/II,* Volume 2 (pp. 1759–1765). Baltimore: Williams and Wilkins.

Adams, K. M., Sawyer, J. D., & Kvale, P. A. (1980). Cerebral oxygenation and neuropsychological adaptation. *Journal of Clinical Neuropsychology, 2,* 189–208.

Bass, E. (1985). Cardiopulmonary arrest: Pathophysiology and neurologic complications. *Annals of Internal Medicine, 103,* 920–927.

Berlyne, N., & Strachan, M. (1968). Neuropsychiatric sequelae of attempted hanging. *British Journal of Psychiatry, 114,* 411–421.

Berry, D. T. R., Webb, W. B., Block, A. J., Bauer, R. M., & Switzer, D. A. (1986). Nocturnal hypoxia and neuropsychological variables. *Journal of Clinical and Experimental Neuropsychology, 8,* 229–238.

Berry, D. T. R., McConnell, J. W., Phillips, B. A., Carswell, C. M., Lamb, D. G., & Prine, B. C. (1989). Isocapnic hypoxemia and neuropsychological functioning. *Journal of Clinical and Experimental Neuropsychology, 11,* 241–251.

Clark, C. F., Heaton, R. K., & Wiens, A. N. (1983). Neuropsychological functioning after prolonged high altitude exposure in mountaineering. *Aviation Space and Environmental Medicine, 54,* 202–207.

Cohen, R. D., Galko, B. M., Contreras, M., Kenny, F. T., & Rebuck, A. S. (1986). Neuropsychological effects of short-term discontinuation of oxygen therapy. *Archives of Internal Medicine, 146,* 1557–1559.

Cummings, J. L., Tomiyasu, U., Read, S., & Benson, D. F. (1984). Amnesia with hippocampal lesions after cardiopulmonary arrest. *Neurology, 34,* 679–681.

Dutka, A. J., & Hallenbeck, J. M. (1991). Anoxic and ischemic encephalopathies: Pathophysiology of anoxic–ischemic brain injury. In W. G. Bradley, R. B. Daroff, G. M. Fenichel, & C. D. Marsden (Eds.), *Neurology in clinical practice: The neurological Disorders,* Volume II (pp. 1353–1358). Boston: Butterworth-Heineman.

Grant, I., Heaton, R. K., McSweeny, A. J., Adams, K. M., & Timms, R. M. (1982). Neuropsychologic findings in hypoxemic chronic obstructive pulmonary disease. *Archives of Internal Medicine, 142,* 1470–1476.

Grant, I., Prigatano, G. P., Heaton, R. K., McSweeny, A. J., Wright, E. C., & Adams, K. M. (1987). Progressive neuropsychologic impairment and hypoxemia: Relationship in chronic obstructive pulmonary disease. *Archives of General Psychiatry, 44,* 999–1006.

Hammeke, T. A., & Hastings, J. E. (1988). Neuropsychologic alterations after cardiac operation. *Journal of Thoracic and Cardiovascular Surgery, 96,* 326–331.

Heaton, R. K., Grant, I., McSweeny, A. J., Adams, K. M., & Petty, T. L. (1983). Psychologic effects of continuous and nocturnal oxygen therapy in hypoxemic chronic obstructive pulmonary disease. *Archives of Internal Medicine, 143,* 1941–1947.

Hornbein, T. F., Townes, B. D., Schoene, R. B., Sutton, J. R., & Houston, C. S. (1989). The cost to the central nervous system of climbing to extremely high altitude. *New England Journal of Medicine, 321,* 1714–1719.

Ingram, R. H. (1980). Chronic bronchitis, emphysema, and chronic airways obstruction. In K. J. Isselbacher, R. D. Adams, E. Braunwald, R. G. Petersdorf, & J. D. Wilson (Eds.), *Harrison's principles of internal medicine* (pp. 1235–1241). New York: McGraw-Hill.

Jason, G. W., Pajurkova, E. M., & Lee, R. G. (1989). High-altitude mountaineering and brain function: Neuropsychological testing of members of a Mount Everest expedition. *Aviation Space and Environmental Medicine, 60,* 170–173.

Juolasmaa, A., Outakoski, J., Hirvenoja, R., Tienari, P., Sotaniemi, K., & Takkunen, J. (1981). Effect of open heart surgery on intellectual performance. *Journal of Clinical Neuropsychology, 3,* 181–197.

Kareken, D. A., Williams, J. M., Mutchnik, M. G., Harter, G., Torres, I., & George, W. E. (1992). Self-report of cognitive function after cardiac surgery. *Neuropsychology, 6,* 197–209.

Katz, M. M., & Lyerly, S. B. (1963). Methods of measuring adjustment and behavior in the community. *Psychological Reports, 13,* 503–535.

Kornfeld, D. S., Heller, S. S., Frank, K. A., & Moskowitz, R. (1974). Personality and psychological factors in postcardiotomy delirium. *Archives of General Psychiatry, 31,* 249–253.

Kra, S. J. (1986). *Coronary bypass surgery: Who needs it?* New York: W. W. Norton.

Lazarus, H. R., & Hagen, J. H. (1968). Prevention of psychosis following open heart surgery. *American Journal of Psychiatry, 124,* 1190.

Levy, D. E., Caronna, J. J., Singer, B. H., Lapinski, R. H., Frydman, H., & Plum, F. (1985). Predicting outcome from hypoxemic–ischemic coma. *Journal of the American Medical Association, 253,* 1420–1426.

McSweeny, A. J., Grant, I., Heaton, R. K., Adams, K. M., & Timms, R. M. (1982). Life quality of patients with chronic obstructive pulmonary disease. *Archives of Internal Medicine, 142,* 473–478.

Medalia, A. A., Merriam, A. E., & Ehrenreich, J. H. (1991). The neuropsychological sequelae of attempted hanging. *Journal of Neurology, Neurosurgery, and Psychiatry, 54,* 546–548.

Meltzer, M. L. (1983). Poor memory: A case report. *Journal of Clinical Psychology, 39,* 3–10.

Myerburg, R. J., & Castellanos, A. (1988). Sudden cardiac death. In Braunwald, E. (Ed.), *Heart disease: A textbook of cardiovascular medicine,* Volume 1 (3rd. ed.) (pp. 742–777). Philadelphia: W. B. Saunders.

Norenberg, M. D., & Bruce-Gregorios, J. (1991). Nervous system manifestations of systemic disease. In R. L. Davis & D. M. Robertson (Eds.), *Textbook of neuropathology* (2nd ed) (pp. 461–534). Baltimore: Williams & Wilkins.

Parkin, A. J., Miller, J., & Vincent, R. (1987). Multiple neuropsychological deficits due to anoxic encephalopathy: A case study. *Cortex, 23,* 655–665.

Prigatano, G. P., & Levin, D. C. (1988). Pulmonary system. In R. E. Tarter, D. H. Van Thiel, and K. L. Edwards (Eds.), *Medical neuropsychology: The impact of disease on behavior* (pp. 27–73). New York: Plenum Press.

Prigatano, G. P., Parsons, O., Wright, E., Levin, D. C., & Hawryluk, G. (1983). Neuropsychological test performance in mildly hypoxemic patients with chronic obstructive pulmonary disease. *Journal of Consulting and Clinical Psychology, 51,* 108–116.

Prough, D. S., & Angert, K. C. (1987). Prolonged drowsiness. In J. G. Reves & K. D. Hall (Eds.), *Common problems in cardiac anesthesia* (pp. 494–499). Chicago: Year Book Medical Publishers.

Raymond, M., Conklin, C., Schaeffer, J., Newstadt, G., Matloff, J. M., & Gray, R. J. (1984). Coping with transient intellectual dysfunction after coronary bypass surgery. *Heart and Lung, 13,* 531–539.

Reitan, R. M., & Wolfson, D. (1985). *Neuroanatomy and neuropathology: A clinical guide for neuropsychologists.* Tucson: Neuropsychology Press.

Roine, R. O., Kajaste, S., & Kaste, M. (1993). Neuropsychological sequelae of cardiac arrest. *JAMA, 269,* 237–242.

Rowe, R. J., Sobota, W. L., & Cowan, D. M. (1985). Neuropsychological impairment and recovery patterns following cardiopulmonary arrest. Paper presented at the meeting of the International Neuropsychological Society, February 1985, San Diego, CA.

Savageau, J. A., Stanton, B. A., Jenkins, C. D., & Klein, M. D. (1982a). Neuropsychological dysfunction following elective cardiac operation. I. Early assessment. *Journal of Thoracic and Cardiovascular Surgery, 84,* 585–594.

Savageau, J. A., Stanton, B. A., Jenkins, C. D., & Frater, R. W. M. (1982b). Neuropsychological dysfunction following elective cardiac operation. II. A six-month reassessment. *Journal of Thoracic and Cardiovascular Surgery, 84,* 595–600.

Schall, R. R., Petrucci, R. J., Brozena, S. C., Cavarocchi, N. C., and Jessup, M. (1989). Cognitive function in patients with symptomatic dilated cardiomyopathy before and after cardiac transplantation. *Journal of the American College of Cardiology, 14,* 1666–1672.

Shaw, P. J., Bates, D., Cartlidge, N. E., French, J. M., Heaviside, D., Julian, D. G., & Shaw, D. A. (1986). Early intellectual dysfunction following coronary bypass surgery. *Quarterly Journal of Medicine, 225,* 59–68.

Shaw, P. J., Bates, D., Cartlidge, N. E., French, J. M., Heaviside, D., Julian, D. G., & Shaw, D. A. (1987). Long-term intellectual dysfunction following coronary artery bypass graft surgery: A six month follow-up study. *Quarterly Journal of Medicine, 239,* 259–268.

Smith, P. L. (1988). The cerebral complications of coronary artery bypass surgery. *Annals of the Royal College of Surgeons of England, 70,* 212–216.

Snyder, B. D. (1991). Anoxic and ischemic encephalopathies: Introduction and clinical aspects. In W. G. Bradley, R. B. Daroff, G. M. Fenichel, & C. D. Marsden (Eds.), *Neurology in clinical practice: The neurological disorders,* Volume II (pp. 1353–1358). Boston: Butterworth-Heineman.

Sotaniemi, K. A., Mononen, M. A., & Hokkanen, T. E. (1986). Long-term cerebral outcome after open-heart surgery: A five-year neuropsychological follow-up study. *Stroke, 17,* 410–416.

Stanton, B. A. (1988). Neurological, cognitive, and psychiatric sequelae associated with the surgical management of cardiac disease. In R. E. Tarter, D. H. Van Thiel, and K. L. Edwards (Eds.), *Medical neuropsychology: The impact of disease on behavior* (pp. 27–73). New York: Plenum Press.

Thompson, T. L. (1980). Psychiatric aspects of open heart surgery. In F. Guerra & J. A. Alderte (Eds.), *Emotional and psychological responses to anesthesia and surgery* (pp. 51–63). New York: Grune & Stratton.

Volpe, B. T., & Hirst, W. (1983). The characterization of an amnesic syndrome following hypoxic ischemic injury. *Archives of Neurology, 40,* 436–440.

White, B. C., Wiegenstein, J. G., & Winegar, C. D. (1984). Brain ischemic anoxia: mechanisms of injury. *JAMA, 251,* 1586–1590.

Yalof, I. L. (1983). *Open heart surgery: A guidebook for patients and families.* New York: Random House.

Alcohol

DESCRIPTION

Alcohol may have short-term effects on the CNS (intoxication and withdrawal) or long-term effects (alcoholism, alcoholic *Wernicke–Korsakoff syndrome,* and *alcoholic dementia*). The properties of each of these five disease states associated with alcohol use are described below.

INCIDENCE AND RISK FACTORS

Gender

The lifetime expectancy rate of alcoholism among males in the United States is 3–5%; for females, it is 0.1–1% (Fialkov, 1985).

Family

Siblings and children of alcoholics appear to be at risk. Female siblings of male alcoholics have a lifetime expectancy rate of alcoholism of 5%; the male sibling rate is 46%. Daughters of alcoholics have an expectancy of 3–8%, while sons have an expectancy of 20–50% (Fialkov, 1985).

Hyperactivity

A history of hyperactivity has been associated with alcoholism (Fialkov, 1985).

Genetic

Research has suggested the possibility of a genetic predisposition (Fialkov, 1985).

Culture

Prevalence bears a complex relationship to societal group and culture.

ETIOLOGY AND PATHOLOGY

Alcohol Intoxication

Alcohol appears to act directly on neuronal membranes, although the precise mechanism is not known (Adams & Victor, 1989).

Alcoholism

Bilateral cortical atrophy and atrophy of the vermis of the cerebellum may occur. Neuron loss and regressive changes in remaining neurons are often evident (Freund, 1985).

Alcoholic Wernicke–Korsakoff Syndrome

Malnutrition (thiamine deficiency) and prolonged ingestion of alcohol are likely etiological factors. The paraventricular gray matter structures of the diencephalon and brainstem are often affected. Lesions in the dorsomedial nucleus of the thalamus and mamillary bodies in combination with cortical atrophy are commonly observed (Greenberg & Diamond, 1985).

MEDICAL ASSESSMENT

Alcohol Intoxication

Acute intoxication is usually evidenced by facial flushing, nystagmus, dysarthria, and ataxia. Psychomotor skills, attention, and memory are impaired. Blood alcohol levels are elevated (Adams & Victor, 1989).

Alcohol Withdrawal

After prolonged drinking, abstinence from alcohol may result in tremulousness, nausea, tachycardia, hallucinosis, and withdrawal seizures. Severe withdrawal may result in delirium tremens, which is characterized by extreme confusion, delusions, hallucinations, tremor, agitation, sleeplessness, dilated pupils, fever, tachycardia, and profuse perspiration (Adams & Victor, 1989).

Alcoholism

A number of physical findings may be diagnostic of alcoholism. Physiological dependency is evidenced by (1) withdrawal syndrome, (2) tolerance—blood alcohol level of greater than 150 mg without gross evidence of intoxication or the consumption of one fifth of a gallon of whiskey or an equivalent amount of another alcoholic beverage daily for more than one day by a 180-pound individual, (3) alcoholic hepatitis, and (4) alcoholic cerebellar degeneration. Behavioral criteria may include (1) drinking despite strong medical contraindication known to the patient or (2) drinking despite strong identified social contraindication (Mendelson & Mello, 1985). CT may reveal enlargement of the CSF space, enlarged cortical sulci, and enlarged lateral and third ventricles (Wilkinson, 1987). Abnormalities may be found in evoked potential studies (Porjesz & Begleiter, 1987).

Alcoholic Wernicke–Korsakoff Syndrome

Symptoms of Wernicke's encephalopathy include ophthalmoplegia (nystagmus, lateral rectus palsies, and gaze palsies), ataxia, and an acute confusional state characterized by sleepiness, inattention, and disorientation (Victor *et al.,* 1989).

Alcoholic Dementia

Alcoholic dementia is obvious, widespread intellectual impairment in the alcoholic, persisting despite 3 or more weeks of abstinence, that interferes with social and occupational functioning. Causes other than alcohol consumption are ruled out (Goldstein, 1985).

NEUROPSYCHOLOGICAL ASSESSMENT

Alcoholism

Alcohol intoxication and withdrawal can have profound effects on cognitive and motor function depending on the degree of intoxication and the intensity of the withdrawal. During the period of withdrawal, which may take up to 3 weeks, a significant improvement in cognitive functioning may occur. Neuropsychological assessment is usually performed to determine relatively lasting effects of alcohol abuse. It is essential, therefore, to determine through interview or biomedical screening whether the patient is using alcohol or substitute drugs (Parsons & Farr, 1981). In interpreting test results, the examiner should be aware that many alcoholics (40%) have had a head injury that may contribute to cognitive impairments. Alcohol can indirectly alter cognition by affecting organ systems (circulatory, gastrointestinal, renal systems, and the liver) in addition to the CNS.

Most detoxified alcoholics will perform within normal limits on standard clinical memory assessment (C. Ryan & Butters, 1986). However, deficits may be noted on unfamiliar, nonverbal problem-solving tasks and tasks that require hypothesis-testing strategies. Impairment may be noted in visuospatial functioning.

Attention

Although DS is likely to be unimpaired, DSym may exhibit impairment (Parsons & Farr, 1981).

Memory

The WMS Memory Quotient is not likely to be depressed (Kleinknecht & Goldstein, 1972). Patients may be impaired on the Indexes of the WMS-R (J. J. Ryan & Lewis, 1988). Special tests that present verbal material and require the patient to count backward by 3s to prevent rehearsal are sensitive to memory impairment in alcoholics.

Intelligence

PA may exhibit impairment. None is likely on I or C (Parsons & Farr, 1981).

Speech/Language

Verbal abilities may be grossly intact. Performance is usually unimpaired on the Verbal subtests of the WAIS-R, with the exception of A-WAIS-R (Parsons & Farr, 1981).

Visuospatial Functioning

Performance on visuoconstructional tasks such as BD, OA, and PA may be impaired (Parsons & Farr, 1981).

Sensory Functioning

Sensory functioning may be intact except for individuals suffering from peripheral neuropathies. Performance on the tactual–spatial task TPT (time and location) is impaired (Parsons & Farr, 1981).

Motor Functioning

Motor functioning is usually grossly intact, although there may be some motor slowing.

Executive Functioning

Impairment on tests of mental flexibility, nonverbal concept formation, and reasoning is common. Impairment may be noted on the TMTB, CT (Parsons & Farr, 1981), and WCST (Klisz & Parsons, 1979).

LNNB

Scales most useful in discriminating alcoholics from controls may be: (1) Pathognomic, (2) Receptive Speech (C5), (3) Arithmetic (C9), (4) Visual (C4), and (5) Intelligence (C11) (Moses & Maruish, 1988).

Personality

Research has not been successful in defining an "alcoholic personality."

Alcoholic Wernicke–Korsakoff Syndrome

The profile of cognitive impairments is similar to that found in alcoholism, with the addition of a severe memory impairment.

Memory

Severe anterograde amnesia is definitive of Korsakoff's syndrome. The patient may have difficulty recalling everyday events and any new factual information. Memory gaps may be filled in with fictional information—confabulation. Impairment may be found in paired-associate learning and ACT (Cermak & Butters, 1972). Remote memory may exhibit a temporal gradient of impairment, with more remote events being recalled more accurately. DS is unimpaired (Butters, 1981; Brandt & Butters, 1986).

Personality

Impulsiveness, aggression, and alcohol abuse may be replaced by apathy, passivity, lack of initiative, and disinterest in alcohol (Brandt & Butters, 1986; Walsh, 1991).

Alcoholic Dementia

Alcoholic dementia shows impaired performance on all tests of cognitive functioning, with greater impairment on tests of nonverbal intelligence and visuospatial abilities. Marked impairment in language functioning (e.g., word finding), as is characteristic of Alzheimer's disease, is not found (Goldstein, 1985).

MEDICAL TREATMENT

Since alcohol use, especially long-term alcohol use, may have effects on the circulatory system, gastrointestinal system, liver, and renal system, medical treatment may involve organ systems in addition to the CNS (Adams & Victor, 1989).

Alcohol Intoxication

Alcohol is metabolized within 24 hr. Medical treatment may limit or lessen the ethanol blood level in cases of severe intoxication. Respiratory support is provided if needed (Adams & Victor, 1989).

Alcohol Withdrawal

Benzodiazepines are often prescribed to control withdrawal symptoms. Clonidine is also being used for this purpose. Withdrawal seizures may be treated with phenytoin (Adams & Victor, 1989).

Alcoholism

Disulfiram (Antabuse) is sometimes prescribed to assist the patient in remaining abstinent. If the patient drinks alcohol while taking disulfiram, he or she may develop headaches, diaphoresis, nausea, vomiting, and orthostatic hypotension. Knowledge of this consequence may act as a deterrent to drinking (Adams & Victor, 1989; Jaffe & Ciraulo, 1985).

Alcoholic Wernicke–Korsakoff Syndrome

Thiamine is administered, and an appropriate diet is prescribed (Victor et al., 1989).

PSYCHOSOCIAL THERAPIES

Alcoholism

Abstinence should be the treatment goal (with rare exceptions). Reasons include the lack of solid evidence for controlled-drinking treatment and the possibility that death may result from the decision of alcoholics to resume drinking. Treatment goals may include improvements in other areas of the patient's behavior and environment. Goldman (1990) has reported behavioral improvement and generalization of training in recovering alcoholics.

Cognitive Rehabilitation

Hannon *et al.* (1989) found memory training to result in little improvement of alcoholics' performance on standardized memory tests. Binder and Schreiber (1980) found that recovering alcoholics were able to use mnemonic strategies such as visual imagery to improve paired-associate learning.

Behavioral Therapy

Covert sensitization (aversion through verbal means), response prevention (prevention of drinking in settings that elicit drinking behavior), chemical aversion, contingency contracting, cognitive–behavioral therapies, and social skills training may be effective in treating alcoholism. Programs often include a combination of techniques (Nathan & Niaura, 1985; Hay & Nathan, 1982).

Family Therapy

Involvement of the family is often essential to successful treatment of alcoholism. The family has usually become organized around the alcoholic's behavior, and family members have defined their roles in reference to the alcoholic. Changing the alcoholic's behavior therefore entails changing the organization of the family.

Group Therapy

Group therapy may assist the patient in overcoming denial and may provide emotional support.

Alcoholics Anonymous

AA is a lay organization of individuals who have had problems with alcohol. It provides support from understanding individuals and an opportunity to regain lost self-esteem and social status and to develop a new approach to life. AA participation is a significant component of many treatment programs.

Alcoholic Wernicke–Korsakoff Syndrome

Therapy will depend on the degree of cognitive impairment. If new learning and recent memory are severely impaired, the patient may require 24-hr supervision. If there is less impairment, the therapies listed under *Alcoholism* above may be appropriate. Research has not shown remediation of the Korsakoff patient's memory impairment to be effective.

PROGNOSIS

Alcoholism

The most rapid recovery of cognitive functioning occurs in the first 3–6 weeks following the beginning of detoxification. Improvement in cognitive functioning may continue at a much slower pace for several years. The extent of recovery, assuming abstinence, is difficult to predict and may vary in individual cases. A general account of recovery of cognitive function has been authored by Goldman (1987). Social stability, less severity of psychiatric symptoms, the absence of loneliness or apathy, association with nondrinking social groups, and onset of alcohol dependence at a later age are associated with a better prognosis (Akerlind *et al.,* 1988; Vaillant, 1983).

Alcoholic Wernicke–Korsakoff Syndrome

There may be a 17% mortality rate in the acute phase of Wernicke's encephalopathy. Oculomotor abnormalities, gait ataxia, and the acute confusional state begin to respond within days to weeks. While other symptoms may appear to recover completely, in about 40% of cases, some degree of nystagmus and gait ataxia may persist. The anterograde and retrograde amnesia of the alcoholic Korsakoff's syndrome patient may be relatively permanent (Victor *et al.,* 1989).

REFERENCES

Adams, R. D., & Victor, M. (1989). *Principles of neurology.* New York: McGraw-Hill.

Akerlind, I., Hornquist, J. O., & Bjurulf, P. (1988). Prognosis in alcoholic rehabilitation: The relative significance of social, psychological, and medical factors. *International Journal of the Addictions, 23,* 1171–1195.

Binder, L. M., & Schreiber, V. (1980). Visual imagery and verbal mediation as memory aids in recovering alcoholics. *Journal of Clinical Neuropsychology, 2,* 71–74.

Brandt, J., & Butters, N. (1986). The alcoholic Wernicke–Korsakoff syndrome and its relationship to long-term alcohol abuse. In I. Grant & K. M. Adams (Eds.), *Neuropsychological assessment of neuropsychiatric disorders* (pp. 441–471). New York: Oxford University Press.

Butters, N. (1981). The Wernicke–Korsakoff syndrome: A review of psychological, neuropathological and etiological factors. In M. Galanter (Ed.), *Currents in alcoholism,* Volume VIII, *Recent advances in research and treatment* (pp. 5–27). New York: Grune & Stratton.

Cermak, L. S., & Butters, N. (1972). The role of interference and encoding in the short-term memory deficits of Korsakoff patients. *Neuropsychologia, 11,* 85–94.

Fialkov, M. J. (1985). Biologic and psychosocial determinants in the etiology of alcoholism. In R. E. Tarter & D. H. Van Thiel (Eds.), *Alcohol and the brain: Chronic effects* (pp. 245–264). New York: Plenum Press.

Freund, G. (1985). Neuropathology of alcohol abuse. In R. E. Tarter & D. H. Van Thiel (Eds.), *Alcohol and the brain: Chronic effects* (pp. 3–18). New York: Plenum Press.

Goldman, M. (1987). The role of time and practice in recovery of function in alcoholics. In O. A. Parsons, N. Butters, & P. E. Nathan (Eds.), *Neuropsychology of alcoholism: Implications for diagnosis and treatment* (pp. 291–321). New York: Guilford Press.

Goldman, M. (1990). Experience-dependent neuropsychological recovery and treatment of chronic alcoholism. *Neuropsychological Review, 1,* 75–101.

Goldstein, G. (1985). Dementia associated with alcoholism. In R. E. Tarter & D. H. Van Thiel (Eds.), *Alcohol and the brain: Chronic effects* (pp. 283–294). New York: Plenum Press.

Greenberg, D. A., & Diamond, I. (1985). Wernicke–Korsakoff syndrome. In R. E. Tarter & D. H. Van Thiel (Eds.), *Alcohol and the brain: Chronic effects* (pp. 295–314). New York: Plenum Press.

Hannon, R., de la Cruz-Schmedel, D. E., Cano, T. C., Moreira, K., & Nasuta, R. (1989). Memory retraining with adult male alcoholics. *Archives of Clinical Neuropsychology, 4,* 227–232.

Hay, W. M., & Nathan, P. E. (Eds.). (1982). *Clinical case studies in the behavioral treatment of alcoholism.* New York: Plenum Press.

Jaffe, J. H., & Ciraulo, D. (1985). Drugs used in the treatment of alcoholism. In J. H. Mendelson & N. K. Mello (Eds.), *The diagnosis and treatment of alcoholism* (pp. 355–390). New York: McGraw-Hill.

Kleinknecht, R. A., & Goldstein, S. G. (1972). Neuropsychological deficits associated with alcoholism. *Quarterly Journal of Studies on Alcohol, 33,* 999–1019.

Klisz, D., & Parsons, O. A. (1977). Hypothesis testing in younger and older alcoholics. *Journal of Studies on Alcohol, 38,* 1718–1729.

Mendelson, J. H., & Mello, N. K. (1985). Diagnostic criteria for alcoholism and alcohol abuse. In J. H. Mendelson & N. K. Mello (Eds.), *The diagnosis and treatment of alcoholism* (pp. 1–20). New York: McGraw-Hill.

Moses, J. A., & Maruish, M. E. (1988). A critical review of Luria–Nebraska Neuropsychological Battery literature. VII. Specific neurologic syndromes. *International Journal of Clinical Neuropsychology, 10,* 178–188.

Nathan, P., & Niaura, B. A. (1985). Behavioral treatment and assessment of alcoholism. In J. H. Mendelson & N. K. Mello (Eds.), *The diagnosis and treatment of alcoholism* (pp. 391–456). New York: McGraw-Hill.

Parsons, O. A., & Farr, S. P. (1981). The neuropsychology of alcohol and drug use. In S. B. Filskov & T. J. Boll (Eds.), *Handbook of clinical neuropsychology* (pp. 320–365). New York: Wiley.

Porjesz, B., & Begleiter, H. (1987). Evoked brain potentials and alcoholism. In O. A. Parsons, N. Butters, & P. E. Nathan (Eds.), *Neuropsychology of alcoholism: Implications for diagnosis and treatment* (pp. 45–63). New York: Guilford Press.

Ryan, C., & Butters, N. (1986). The neuropsychology of alcoholism. In D. Wedding, A. M. Horton, Jr., & J. Webster (Eds.), *The neuropsychology handbook: Behavioral and clinical perspectives* (pp. 376–409). New York: Springer.

Ryan, J. J., & Lewis, C. V. (1988). Comparison of normal controls and recently detoxified alcoholics on the Wechsler Memory Scale—Revised. *The Clinical Neuropsychologist, 2,* 173–180.

Vaillant, G. E. (1983). *The natural history of alcoholism.* Cambridge, MA: Harvard University Press.

Victor, M., Adams, R. D., & Collins, G. H. (1989). *The Wernicke–Korsakoff syndrome and related neurologic disorders due to alcoholism and malnutrition.* Philadelphia: F. A. Davis.

Walsh, K. W. (1991). *Understanding brain damage: A primer of neuropsychological evaluation.* Edinburgh: Churchill-Livingston.

Wilkinson, D. A. (1987). Discussion: CT scan and neuropsychological assessments of alcoholism. In O. A. Parsons, N. Butters, & P. E. Nathan (Eds.), *Neuropsychology of alcoholism: Implications for diagnosis and treatment* (pp. 76–102). New York: Guilford Press.

Drugs and Neurotoxins

This chapter summarizes very briefly some of the cognitive and behavioral effects that may be produced by drugs and neurotoxins. For more detailed information, the practitioner is referred to *Neuropsychological Toxicology* (Hartman, 1988) and *Neurotoxins in Clinical Practice* (Goetz, 1985). A list of drugs that may cause psychiatric symptoms can be found in *The Medical Letter* (1989). A description of the special batteries and techniques that have been developed for the evaluation of patients who have been exposed to toxins is beyond the scope of this book. The practitioner may consult *Foundations of Environmental and Occupational Neurotoxicology* (Valciukas, 1991) and the *Neurotoxicity Guidebook* (Singer, 1990).

ALUMINUM

Classification. Metal.

Use. Manufacturing.

Acute Physiological and Psychological Effects. Dialysis encephalopathy may manifest as dementia, speech disorder, apraxia, myoclonus, asterixis, and abnormal EEG. Deficits may be noted in attention and executive functioning in patients with lower vocabulary scores (Bolla *et al.*, 1992).

ANTIDEPRESSANTS (TRICYCLIC)

Classification. Tricyclic antidepressant medications.

Use. Medical treatment of depression.

Acute Physiological and Psychological Effects. Toxic doses may produce acute agitation, confusion, mydriasis, and convulsions (Goetz, 1985).

Chronic Physiological and Psychological Effects. Lesser doses may produce postural or intentional tremor, blurred vision, and postural hypotension (Goetz, 1985). Studies of the effects of tricyclics on cognitive functioning have yielded mixed results (Hartman, 1988).

BENZODIAZEPINES

Classification. Antianxiety medications.

Use. Prescribed for anxiolytic, hypnotic, muscle-relaxing, and anticonvulsant effects.

Acute Physiological and Psychological Effects. Memory and delayed recall may be impaired (Lucki *et al.,* 1986). Acquisition may be impaired (Barbee *et al.,* 1992).

Chronic Physiological and Psychological Effects. Critical flicker fusion, learning, memory, manual dexterity, DSym, and cancellation may exhibit impairment (Wittenborn, 1980).

CARBAMAZEPINE (TEGRETOL)

Classification. Antiepileptic.

Use. Medical treatment of epilepsy.

Physiological and Psychological Effects. Although the results of some studies have suggested that carbamazepine has less effect on cognition than other antiepileptic medications such as phenytoin (Dodrill & Troupin, 1977; Smith *et al.,* 1987), further analyses and studies have suggested that no significant differences exist (Dodrill & Troupin, 1991; Meador *et al.,* 1990). Recent reviews of the cognitive effects of antiepileptic medications include those by Dodrill (1991), Smith (1991), and Trimble (1987).

CARBON DISULFIDE

Classification. Organic solvent.

Use. Manufacture of rayon, cellophane, adhesives, rubber, lacquers, varnishes, and adhesives.

Acute Physiological and Psychological Effects. Acute intoxication may result in an agitated delirium (Hanninen, 1971).

Chronic Physiological and Psychological Effects. Cranial and peripheral neuropathies, irritability, and emotional lability may be noted (Feldman *et al.,* 1980). Reaction time, vigilance, dexterity, visual–motor abilities, and constructional abilities may be impaired (Hartman, 1988).

CARBON MONOXIDE

Classification. Gas.

Sources. Hot water heaters, space heaters, furnaces, automobile exhaust, cigarette smoke, volcanoes, forest fires.

Acute Physiological and Psychological Effects. Neurological sequelae may be numerous and varied, from focal deficits to global dysfunction. The emergence of impairments may be delayed from several days to weeks. Symptoms may include irritability, violent behavior, personality disturbances, inappropriate euphoria, confusion, and impaired judgment (Goetz, 1985). A list of acute effects at various levels of exposure may be found in Hartman (1988, p. 247).

COPPER

Classification. Metal.

Use. Manufacturing and vitamin–mineral supplements.

Chronic Physiological and Psychological Effects. Copper toxicity is a part of Wilson's disease, which is transmitted as an autosomal recessive trait with a prevalence of 1/35,000. Onset is usually in the 2nd or 3rd decade. Neurological manifestations may include tremor of the limbs or head, dysarthria, dysphagia, and hoarseness. Kayser–Fleischer rings, a rusty-brown discoloration of the cornea, are pathognomonic for the disease (Adams & Victor, 1989). Severe psychiatric symptomatology has been found in some patients (Oder *et al.,* 1991).

Impairments have been noted in a wide variety of perceptual, motor, and cognitive functioning (Bornstein *et al.,* 1985; Reitan & Wolfson, 1985). Impairment in memory functioning has been noted in neurologically impaired patients with Wilson's disease (Issacs-Glaberman *et al.,* 1989; Medalia *et al.,* 1988). Oder *et al.* (1991) found no impairment on the MMSE.

COCAINE

Classification. Stimulant.

Use. Local anesthetic; abused drug.

Acute Physiological and Psychological Effects. Initially produces euphoria, a sense of well-being, and restlessness. These effects change to irritation, restless, and depression.

Chronic Physiological and Psychological Effects. Continued use may result in paranoid ideation, depression, irritability, anxiety, and loss of motivation. Cocaine psychosis may occur with toxic levels of use. Following chronic abuse, abstinence may result in insomnia, restlessness, anorexia, and depression. Testing of abstinent cocaine abusers on the LNNB revealed impairment on the Rhythm (C2) and Expressive Speech (C6) Scales [Press, 1983 (cited in Hartman, 1988)].

ETHYLENE OXIDE

Classification. Gas.

Use. Sterilization of materials that would be damaged by heat sterilization; manufacture of fumigants, pigments, and rocket propellants.

Chronic Physiological and Psychological Effects. Impaired performance has been noted in hand–eye coordination [Estrin *et al.,* 1986 (cited in Hartman, 1988)].

LEAD

Classification. Heavy metal.

Use. Ceramic glazes, batteries, paint pigments, leaded gasoline.

Physiological and Psychological Effects. Complaints may include forgetfulness, fatigue, restlessness, apathy, sensorimotor problems, and gastrointestinal problems. Cognitive impairments may include new learning, visuospatial functioning, psychomotor speed, and manual dexterity (Hartman, 1987, 1988). BD, DSym, and the RAVLT have been reported to be impaired [Bleecker, Agnew, Keogh, & Stetson, 1982 (cited in Hartman, 1988)]. Depression and anger may be noted. Braun and Daigneault (1991) found no impairment in executive functions but impaired motor functioning in lead-smelter workers.

LITHIUM

Classification. Alkali metal.

Use. Medication for bipolar and unipolar manic disorders and for cluster headaches.

Acute Physiological and Psychological Effects. Toxic levels may result in dysarthria, as well as gait and limb ataxia, clouding of consciousness, confusion, delirium, and coma (Adams & Victor, 1989).

Chronic Physiological and Psychological Effects. Blood levels in the upper therapeutic range may result in a fast-frequency action tremor (Adams & Victor, 1989). According to Hartman (1988, p. 212), "the better-controlled studies have not found lithium to significantly affect memory." Impairments may be noted in motor or perceptual speed or both: DSym, TMTB, FTT, TPT, and BD.

MARIJUANA

Classification. Psychoactive drug [Δ-9-tetrahydrocannabinol (THC)].

Use. Abused drug; medical treatment of open angle glaucoma and asthma.

Acute Physiological and Psychological Effects. Attention, memory, speech, spatial abilities, and flexibility may be impaired (Hartman, 1988). Operation of vehicles may be affected for hours after intake.

Chronic Physiological and Psychological Effects. The results of studies of the effects of chronic marijuana use on cognition are mixed.

MERCURY

Inorganic

Classification. Metal.

Use. Manufacture of electrical apparatus, chlorine production, paint, dentistry, pesticides, and paper production.

Acute Physiological and Psychological Effects. Mental irritability and a rapid onset of weakness in the lower limbs may follow acute exposure (Goetz, 1985).

Chronic Physiological and Psychological Effects. Progressive personality change, tremor, and weakness in the limbs may be noted. Fatigue, irritability, insomnia, and depression may be interrupted by periods of excitability. Vertigo, nystagmus, blurred vision, narrowing of visual fields, optic neuritis and atrophy, and ataxia may be observed (Goetz, 1985). Impairments may be found in motor functioning, memory, visuospatial abilities, and reaction time (Hartman, 1988). Uzzell and Oler (1986) found impairments in Recurrent Figures and SCL-90-R (obsessive compulsion, anxiety, and psychoticism) and no impairment on the WAIS, RAVLT, PASAT, BGT, GP, or FTT.

Organic

Classification. Phenyl, methyl, ethyl, and diethyl mercury.

Use. Prevention of seed-borne diseases of cereals.

Acute Physiological and Psychological Effects. ''The clinical triad of organic mercury toxicity is peripheral neuropathy, ataxia, and cortical blindness'' (Goetz, 1985, p. 26). Initial symptoms may be paresthesias of the extremities, constriction of visual fields, and ataxia (Goetz, 1985).

Chronic Physiological and Psychological Effects. In chronic disease, a gradual weakness develops, and increased reflexes, jaw jerk, fasciculations, and atrophy may be observed (Goetz, 1985).

NEUROLEPTICS

Classification. Major tranquilizers; antipsychotic medications.

Use. Medical treatment of confusional states and schizophrenia.

Acute Physiological and Psychological Effects. Performance on some tasks involving sustained attention may be impaired (Cassens *et al.,* 1990), including DSym and the CPT. Acute administration of chlorpromazine (200–300 mg/day) may result in impaired performance on the FTT (Cassens *et al.,* 1990).

Chronic Physiological and Psychological Effects. Chronic administration may improve performance on the CPT (Cassens *et al.,* 1990). No impairment has been noted in performance on verbal tasks. Some improvement in Similarities performance has been noted with chlorpromazine, trifluoperazine, and carphenazine. No impairment may be noted in the ability to perform orally presented arithmetic problems and abstract proverbs. WMS performance has been generally unaffected. FTT impairment is not observed after chronic administration. Impairment has not been noted on the Bender or the TMTA&B. Findings have been inconsistent on OA, PC, and the PMT. Improved performance has been found on BD and PA (Cassens *et al.,* 1990).

ORGANOPHOSPHATES

Classification. Inhibit acetylcholinesterase and pseudocholinesterase.

Use. Insecticides.

Acute Physiological and Psychological Effects. In mild poisoning, patients complain of fatigue, headache, dizziness, nausea, and vomiting. Tremor, numbness, and tingling may be noted (Goetz, 1985). Neuropathy may be noted.

Chronic Physiological and Psychological Effects. Impairments may be found on intelligence and memory testing (Metcalf & Holmes, 1969). Impaired performance may be noted on the Bender and the TMTB (Korsak, 1977). Reidy *et al.* (1992) reported deficits in psychomotor speed, dexterity, and visual memory in workers exposed to pesticides.

PHENYTOIN (DILANTIN)

Classification. Antiepileptic medication.

Use. Medical treatment of epilepsy.

Physiological and Psychological Effects. Studies have demonstrated impaired performance on tests of memory, concentration, problem-solving, and speed of response (Trimble, 1987). Dodrill and Temkin (1989) showed that when the FTT was co-varied out, no significant differences remained between high and low serum level groups. They concluded that ''losses in cognitive abilities could not be associated with PHT [phenytoin] even though markedly elevated blood levels had been achieved'' (Dodrill & Temkin, 1989, p. 453). A 5-year follow-up of patients taking phenytoin revealed no insidious cognitive losses (Dodrill & Wilensky, 1992). Recent reviews of the cognitive effects of antiepileptic medications include those by Dodrill (1991), Smith (1991), and Trimble (1987).

SOLVENTS (MISCELLANEOUS ORGANIC)

Classification. Compounds that can dissolve non-water-soluble materials such as fats, oils, resins, and plastics.

Use. Manufacture of paints, adhesives, glues, polymers, and synthetic fabrics; painting, varnishing, and laying carpet (Hartman, 1988).

Acute Physiological and Psychological Effects. Complaints may include headache, dizziness, fatigue, paresthesias, pain, weakness, concentration, memory, and problem-solving. Impairments have been noted on the SDMT and the DSym test (Bowler *et al.*, 1992).

Chronic Physiological and Psychological Effects. Impairments have been noted in reaction time, DS, DSym, BD, and FM-WMS (Lindstrom, 1980; Lindstrom & Wickstrom, 1983).

TOLUENE

Classification. Solvent, aromatic hydrocarbon.

Use. Cleaner, degreaser, solvent, and adhesive.

Acute Physiological and Psychological Effects. Acute exposure may result in exhilaration followed by fatigue, mild confusion, ataxia, and dizziness (Goetz, 1985). Decrements in simple and choice reaction time have been demonstrated (Hartman, 1988).

Chronic Physiological and Psychological Effects. Tremulousness, unsteadiness, emotional liability, jaw jerk, snout, and primitive reflexes have been reported (Goetz, 1985). Impairment has been noted in attention, memory, and visuospatial function (Hormes *et al.*, 1986).

TRICHLOROETHYLENE

Classification. Solvent.

Use. Dry cleaning, household cleaner, lubricants, degreasers, and adhesives.

Acute Physiological and Psychological Effects. Inhalation may rapidly produce a state of euphoria (Goetz, 1985).

Chronic Physiological and Psychological Effects. Patients may report headache, dizziness, fatigue, and diplopia (Steinberg, 1981). Neurological effects may include involvement of the trigeminal nerve, retinobulbar neuropathy, optic atrophy, oculomotor disturbances, and primarily distal peripheral neuropathy (Goetz, 1985). Studies of neuropsychological sequelae have been inconsistent in the effects demonstrated.

REFERENCES

Adams, R. D., & Victor, M. (1989). *Principles of neurology* (4th ed.). New York: McGraw-Hill.

Barbee, J. G., Black, F. W., & Todorov, A. A. (1992). Differential effects of alprazolam and buspirone upon acquisition, retention, and retrieval processes in memory. *Journal of Neuropsychiatry and Clinical Neurosciences, 4,* 308–314.

Bolla, K. I., Briefel, G., Spector, D., Schwartz, B. S., Wieler, L., Herron, J., & Gimenez, L. (1992). Neurocognitive effects of aluminum. *Archives of Neurology, 49,* 1021–1026.

Bornstein, R. A., McLean, D. R., & Ho, K. (1985). Neuropsychological and electrophysiological examination of a patient with Wilson's disease. *International Journal of Neuroscience, 26,* 239–247.

Bowler, R., Sudia, S., Mergler, D., Harrison, R., & Cone, J. (1992). Comparison of Digit Symbol and Symbol Digit Modalities Tests for assessing neurotoxic exposure. *The Clinical Neuropsychologist, 6,* 103–104.

Braun, C. M. J., & Daigneault, S. (1991). Sparing of cognitive executive functions and impairment of motor functions after industrial exposure to lead: A field study with control group. *Neuropsychology, 5,* 179–193.

Cassens, G., Inglis, A. K., Appelbaum, P. S., & Gutheil, T. G. (1990). Neuroleptics: Effects on neuropsychological function in chronic schizophrenic patients. *Schizophrenia Bulletin, 16,* 477–499.

Dodrill, C. B. (1991). Behavioral effects of antiepileptic drugs. In D. Smith, D. Treiman, & M. Trimble (Eds.), *Advances in neurology,* Volume 55 (pp. 213–224). New York: Raven Press.

Dodrill, C. B., & Temkin, N. R. (1989). Motor speed is a contaminating factor in evaluating the "cognitive" effects of phenytoin. *Epilepsia, 30,* 453–457.

Dodrill, C. B., & Troupin, A. S. (1977). Psychotropic effects of carbamazepine in epilepsy: A double-blind comparison with phenytoin. *Neurology, 27,* 1023–1028.

Dodrill, C. B., & Troupin, A. S. (1991). Neuropsychological effects of carbamazepine and phenytoin: A reanalysis. *Neurology, 41,* 141–143.

Dodrill, C. B., & Wilensky, A. J. (1992). Neuropsychological abilities before and after 5 years of stable antiepileptic drug therapy. *Epilepsia, 33,* 327–334.

Feldman, R. G., Ricks, N. L., & Baker, E. L. (1980). Neuropsychological effects of industrial toxins: A review. *American Journal of Industrial Medicine, 1,* 211–227.

Goetz, C. G. (1985). *Neurotoxins in clinical practice.* New York: Spectrum.

Hanninen, H. (1971). Psychological picture of manifest and latent carbon disulfide poisoning. *British Journal of Industrial Medicine, 28,* 374–381.

Hartman, D. E. (1987). Neuropsychological toxicology: Identification and assessment of neurotoxic syndromes. *Archives of Clinical Neuropsychology, 2,* 45–65.

Hartman, D. E. (1988). *Neuropsychological toxicology: Identification and assessment of human neurotoxic syndromes.* New York: Pergamon Press.

Hormes, J. T., Filley, C. M., & Rosenberg, N. L. (1986). Neurologic sequelae of chronic solvent vapor abuse. *Neurology, 36,* 698–702.

Issacs-Glaberman, K., Medalia, A., & Scheinberg, I. H. (1989). Verbal recall and recognition abilities in patients with Wilson's disease. *Cortex, 25,* 353–361.

Korsak, R. J., & Sato, M. M. (1977). Effects of chronic organophosphate pesticide exposure on the central nervous system. *Clinical Toxicology, 11,* 83–95.

Lindstrom, K. (1980). Changes in psychological performance of solvent-poisoned and solvent-exposed workers. *American Journal of Industrial Medicine, 1,* 69–84.

Lindstrom, K., & Wickstrom, G. (1983). Psychological function changes among maintenance house painters exposed to low levels of organic solvent mixtures. *Acta Psychiatrica Scandinavica, 67,* 81–91.

Lucki, I., Rickels, K., & Geller, A. M. (1986). Chronic use of benzodiazepines and psychomotor and cognitive test performance. *Psychopharmacology, 88,* 426–433.

Meador, K. J., Loring, D. W., Huh, K., Gallagher, B. B., & King, K. W. (1990). Comparative cognitive effects of anticonvulsants. *Neurology, 40,* 391–394.

Medalia, A., Issacs-Glaberman, K., & Scheinberg, I. H. (1988). Neuropsychological impairment in Wilson's disease. *Archives of Neurology, 45,* 502–504.

The Medical Letter (1989). Drugs that cause psychiatric symptoms. *The Medical Letter, 31,* 113–118.

Metcalf, D. R., & Holmes, J. H. (1969). EEG, psychological and neurological alteration in humans with organophosphorous exposure. *Annals of the New York Academy of Science, 160,* 357.

Oder, W., Grimm, G., Kollegger, H., Ferenci, P., Schneider, B., & Deecke, L. (1991). Neurological and neuropsychiatric spectrum of Wilson's disease: A prospective study of 45 cases. *Journal of Neurology, 238,* 281–287.

Reidy, T. J., Bowler, R. M., Rauch, S. S., & Pedroza, G. I. (1992). Pesticide exposure and neuropsychological impairment in migrant farm workers. *Archives of Clinical Neuropsychology, 7,* 85–95.

Reitan, R. M., & Wolfson, D. (1985). *Neuroanatomy and neuropathology: A clinical guide for neuropsychologists.* Tucson: Neuropsychology Press.

Singer, R. (1990). *Neurotoxicity guidebook.* New York: Van Nostrand Reinhold.

Smith, D. B. (1991). Cognitive effects of antiepileptic drugs. In D. Smith, D. Treiman, & M. Trimble (Eds.), *Advances in neurology,* Volume 55 (pp. 197–211). New York: Raven Press.

Smith, D. B., Mattson, R. H., Cramer, J. A., Collins, J. F., Novelly, R. A., Craft, B., & VA Cooperative Study Group (1987). Results of a nationwide Veterans Administration cooperative study comparing the efficacy and toxicity of carbamazepine, phenobarbital, phenytoin, and primidone. *Epilepsia, 28*(Supplement 3), S50–S58.

Steinberg, W. (1981). Residual neuropsychological effects following exposure to trichloroethylene (TCE): A case study. *Clinical Neuropsychology, 2,* 1–4.

Trimble, M. R. (1987). Anticonvulsant drugs and cognitive function: A review of the literature. *Epilepsia, 28*(Supplement 3), S37–S45.

Uzzell, B. P., & Oler, J. (1986). Chronic low-level mercury exposure and neuropsychological functioning. *Journal of Clinical and Experimental Neuropsychology, 8,* 581–593.

Valciukas, J. A. (1991). *Foundations of environmental and occupational neurotoxicology.* New York: Van Nostrand Reinhold.

Wittenborn, J. R. (1980). Behavioral toxicity of psychotropic drugs. *Journal of Nervous and Mental Disease, 168,* 171–176.

50

Schizophrenia

DESCRIPTION

For a diagnosis of schizophrenia, DSM III-R requires, in the *active phase:* (1) psychotic symptoms such as delusions, hallucinations, incoherence or marked loosening of associations, catatonic behavior, flat or grossly inappropriate affect, and/or bizarre delusions; (2) areas such as work, social relations, and self-care markedly below the highest premorbid level; (3) ruling out of Schizoaffective Disorder and Mood Disorder with Psychotic Features; and (4) continuous signs of disturbance for at least 6 months. The *prodromal phase* is a clear deterioration in functioning before the active phase. The *residual phase* follows the active phase. The prodromal and residual phases are defined as manifesting at least two listed symptoms, among which are: marked social isolation, marked impairment in role functioning, markedly peculiar behavior, marked impairment in personal hygiene, blunted or inappropriate affect, circumstantial speech, odd beliefs or magical thinking, unusual perceptual experiences, and marked lack of initiative. Organic factors should be ruled out. DSM III-R should be consulted for a precise definition (American Psychiatric Association, 1987).

INCIDENCE AND RISK FACTORS

Incidence

A World Health Organization cross-cultural study revealed a range of 0.15–0.42 case/1000. There was not a great variability at geographically distinct research sites (World Health Organization, 1979). The lifetime prevalence is 1.0–1.9% (Sederer, 1991).

Age

The prevalence is greatest in the age range 15–50 years, although late onset has been described.

Gender

Schizophrenia occurs equally in males and females. Onset is earlier in males (Sederer, 1991).

Socioeconomic Status

The prevalence is greatest at lower economic levels (Kohn, 1968).

Genetics

Family studies, twin studies, and adoption studies suggest a major genetic contribution (Gelder *et al.*, 1989).

ETIOLOGY AND PATHOLOGY

The etiology of schizophrenia is unknown. A number of neurological abnormalities have been noted. CT studies have revealed cerebral atrophy, ventricular enlargement (Weinberger *et al.*, 1980), and density changes in left frontal regions. PET studies have revealed decreased cerebral blood flow and functioning in the frontal lobes (Buchsbaum, 1990). Cerebellar atrophy has been reported (Yates *et al.*, 1987).

Numerous theories of schizophrenia have been propounded. On the basis of the fact that dopamine is released during amphetamine psychosis and the fact that neuroleptic medications block dopamine, it has been proposed that abnormal dopamine neurotransmitter activity is an essential feature of schizophrenia (Gelder *et al.*, 1989). Debate over this hypothesis continues.

MEDICAL ASSESSMENT

A thorough history, mental status examination, and physical are performed. Routine laboratory testing is ordered. Although CT or MRI scans are not always ordered, they may be useful in ruling out various organic etiologies (Sederer, 1991).

NEUROPSYCHOLOGICAL ASSESSMENT

Neuropsychological studies of schizophrenia have resulted in mixed findings. This ambiguity may be due to vagueness and differences in the diagnosis of schizophrenia. The term "has been applied to a wide variety of conditions that have little in common" (Goldstein, 1986, p. 147). There is also a great deal of behavioral variation within the disorder even when it is more rigorously defined. The disorder may be influenced by variables such as long-term effects of hospitalization and the effects of somatic therapies.

Patients diagnosed as schizophrenic may be referred for neuropsychological testing to rule out competing or additional organic disorders. However, neuropsychological investigations have often failed to confirm the utility of neuropsychological tests in distinguishing brain-damaged and schizophrenic patients (Heaton & Crowley, 1981; Goldstein, 1986). Acute schizophrenics are more easily discriminated than chronic schizophrenics (Heaton *et al.*, 1978).

Watson *et al.* (1968) found that the HRNB did not distinguish between organics and schizophrenics. However, DeWolfe *et al.* (1971) found differences in deficit pattern scores between chronic schizophrenics and brain-damaged patients on the WAIS and HRNB. In contrast, Chelune *et al.* (1979) reported no significant differences in their analyses of deficit pattern scores for the WAIS. Differences were found for the SSPT, Sensory–Perceptual

Errors, and TMTB. Pattern scores based on the HRNB correctly classified 80.6% of the schizophrenic and brain-damaged patients. Goldstein and Halperin (1977) found the WAIS and HRNB to discriminate long- vs. short-term hospitalization better than paranoid vs. non-paranoid or neurologically normal vs. abnormal in a group of schizophrenics. The time to write the word "television" was the best discriminator in these latter two categories. The TPT-Time was the best discriminator for length of hospitalization. According to Goldstein (1986, p. 154),

> no one has been able to successfully derive a characteristic performance pattern on standard neuropsychological tests that is specific to schizophrenia.

Both the HRNB and the LNNB have been found to predict CT abnormality in schizophrenic patients. Boucher et al. (1986) found the Halstead Impairment Index to distinguish groups of young schizophrenics with and without ventricular or sulcal enlargement or both. Pandurangi et al. (1986) found the Halstead Impairment Index capable of discriminating schizophrenics with and without CT abnormality. The Average Impairment Rating did not discriminate these groups. No significant differences were noted in FSIQ, VIQ, or PIQ. In contrast, the Average Impairment Rating suggested impairment in patients with abnormal CT scans in a study performed by Donnelly et al. (1980). Nyman et al. (1986) found performance on the BD test to be negatively correlated with the size of the third ventricle. C. J. Golden et al. (1982) reported correct classification of the chronic schizophrenics with ventricular enlargement at a statistically significant level. It should be noted that not all studies have found the HRNB or the LNNB to predict morphological abnormalities (Carr & Wedding, 1984).

Neuropsychological evaluation can assist in the development of a treatment plan. A treatment plan for a patient diagnosed with schizophrenia will usually include treatment of positive and negative symptoms, improvement of social skills, vocational training, and improvement of adjustment to the family environment (Clarkin & Mattis, 1991). A precise understanding of the profile of the patient's cognitive and emotional functioning is essential to the appropriate formulation of such a plan.

Impairment may be found in attention (especially maintenance and ability to shift attention), verbal and nonverbal memory (chronic schizophrenics), and complex perception in the visual modality. Acute patients tend to overinclude and chronic patients underinclude when categorizing (Cutting, 1985).

Language functioning may be impaired. Andreasen (1979) examined the speech of schizophrenics for 18 disorders of thought, language, and communication. Derailment (56%) was most common, followed by loss of goal (44%), poverty of content of speech (40%), tangentiality (36%), illogicality (27%), and pressure of speech (27%). Phonemic abnormalities are not marked; syntax is generally intact; semantics may be intact; pragmatics (socially derived rules that speakers and listeners use to establish coherence across groups of sentences) (Best, 1989) may be impaired (Cutting, 1985). Impairment has been noted on verbal subtests of the WAIS and WAIS-R (Flor-Henry, 1990). In comparing schizophrenic patients to depressed patients, Dean et al. (1987) found schizophrenic patients to be more impaired on S and C. Depressed patients were more impaired on PC and OA. In a meta-analysis of research on the WAIS in schizophrenia, Aylard et al. (1984) found VIQ to be higher than PIQ.

Bigler (1988) has provided means and standard deviations for acute schizophrenics, chronic schizophrenics, and controls on the WAIS and HRNB.

Impairment Ratings

The Halstead Impairment Index suggested impairment in a group of chronic schizophrenics (Klonoff et al., 1970).

Attention

DS may be impaired (Cutting, 1980; Gruzelier *et al.*, 1988; Robertson & Taylor, 1985), but some studies have found no impairment in DS or block span (Kolb & Whishaw, 1983). CPT performance may be impaired relative to normals (Walker, 1981). WAIS-DSym may exhibit impairment (Kenny & Meltzer, 1991; Kolb & Whishaw, 1983).

Memory

LM-, PA-, and VR-WMS may be impaired for both immediate and delayed recall (Kolb & Whishaw, 1983). Impairment may be found on the ROCFT:M (Kolb & Whishaw, 1983).

General Knowledge and Social Understanding

PIQ may be impaired (Kolb & Whishaw, 1983). PA-WAIS may be impaired (Kolb & Whishaw, 1983). The SRT and ACT may exhibit impairment (Kenny & Meltzer, 1991). VIQ, PIQ, and FSIQ were impaired in patients with abnormal CT scans (Donnelly *et al.*, 1980). Comprehension was impaired in patients with abnormal CT scans (Donnelly *et al.*, 1980). PA-WAIS has been found to be impaired (Robertson & Taylor, 1985).

Speech/Language

Category word fluency has been found to be impaired (Kenny & Meltzer, 1991; Kolb & Whishaw, 1983). The SR was impaired in patients with abnormal CT scans (Donnelly *et al.*, 1980). Rhythm and SSPT were severely impaired in a group of chronic schizophrenics relative to HRNB cutoff values (Klonoff *et al.*, 1970).

Arithmetic

A-WAIS was impaired in patients with abnormal CT scans (Donnelly *et al.*, 1980).

Visuospatial Functioning

BD- and OA-WAIS may be impaired (Kolb & Whishaw, 1983). The ROCFT:C may show no impairment (Kolb & Whishaw, 1983). BD and PA were impaired in patients with abnormal CT scans (Donnelly *et al.*, 1980). The TMTA was severely impaired in a group of chronic schizophrenics relative to HRNB cutoff values (Klonoff *et al.*, 1970). PC-WAIS has been reported to be impaired (Robertson & Taylor, 1985).

Sensory Functioning

The TPT-Time and Memory were impaired in patients with abnormal CT scans (Donnelly *et al.*, 1980). The TPT-Time and Memory were severely impaired in a group of chronic schizophrenics relative to HRNB cutoff values (Klonoff *et al.*, 1970).

Motor Functioning

The FTT was severely impaired, bilaterally, in a group of chronic schizophrenics relative to HRNB cutoff values (Klonoff et al., 1970).

Executive Functioning

Perseveration has been noted on the WCST (Fey, 1951; Kenny & Meltzer, 1991; Kolb & Whishaw, 1983; Malmo, 1974). Impairment has been noted on the COWAT (Kenny & Meltzer, 1991), Chicago Word Fluency ("S", "C"), and design fluency (Kolb & Whishaw, 1983). The SCWT may be impaired (Kenny & Meltzer, 1991). The Halstead CT was impaired in patients with abnormal CT scans (Donnelly et al., 1980). The Halstead CT and TMTB performance was severely impaired in a group of chronic schizophrenics relative to HRNB cutoff values (Klonoff et al., 1970).

LNNB

Schizophrenics have been found to have deficits on the Motor (C1), Rhythm (C2), Receptive Speech (C5), Arithmetic (C9), Memory (C10), and Intelligence (C11), Scales (Lewis et al., 1979). Neither chronicity nor length of hospitalization affected scores. Purisch et al. (1978) found that schizophrenic patients differed significantly from brain-injured patients on all scales but Rhythm (C2), Receptive Speech (C5), Memory (C10) and Intellectual Processes (C11). A multivariate combination of scales achieved an 88% classification accuracy. Substantially the same results were obtained in a replication (Shelly & Goldstein, 1983). Moses (1984) found no significant differences on the LNNB between Schizophrenic Disorder and Schizoaffective Disorder patients. C. J. Golden et al. (1982) found the LNNB capable of distinguishing schizophrenics with and without ventricular enlargement. They provided a set of rules for distinguishing patients with ventricular enlargement via profile analysis.

Personality

MMPI Scale 8 is typically elevated above 70T in schizophrenia (Meyer, 1983). A 7-8/8-7 profile may be found in chronic schizophrenia. A 2-6-7 profile may be seen in early schizophrenia (R. Golden & Meehl, 1979).

The Structured Clinical Interview for the DSM III-R (Spitzer et al., 1987), Psychiatric Diagnostic Interview—Revised (Othmer et al., 1989), Schedule for Affective Disorders and Schizophrenia (Spitzer & Endicott, 1977), or Brief Psychiatric Rating Scale (Overall & Gorham, 1962) may be of diagnostic assistance. The Scale for the Assessment of Positive Symptoms and the Scale for the Assessment of Negative Symptoms may be useful for determining the balance of negative and positive symptoms of schizophrenia (Andreason, 1983, 1984).

Projective tests such as the R and TAT may be used to assess personality dynamics and abnormal thought processes.

Suicidality should be evaluated. Some schizophrenic patients are at high risk for suicide (Sederer, 1991).

MEDICAL TREATMENT

Neuroleptic medications are generally effective in treating the acute psychosis of schizophrenia (Baldessarini et al., 1990). Common neuroleptics are halperidol (Haldol), trifluoperazine (Stelazine), thioridazine (Mellaril), fluphenazine (Prolixin), and thiothixene (Navane). Adverse side effects may be acute dystonia (sudden, marked tonic contractions of the muscles of the tongue, neck, back, mouth, or eyes) and/or drug-induced parkinsonism—commonly treated with benztropine (Cogentin) or diphenhydramine (Benadryl), akathisia (motor restlessness), neuroleptic-induced catatonia, and tardive dyskinesia (persistent movements of the tongue, lips, and facial muscles) (Sederer, 1991). Neuroleptic malignant syndrome (muscular rigidity, fever, autonomic disfunction, and disturbances of mental status) may occur in approximately 1% of patients (Lazarus *et al.,* 1989).

Clozapine is a dibenzodiazepine that has been found to be helpful for as many as 30% of medication-resistant schizophrenic patients (Sederer, 1991).

PSYCHOSOCIAL THERAPIES

Some forms of individual therapy have been found to be helpful in schizophrenia. Therapy focused on adjustment in the present has been found to be more effective than therapy focused on the treatment relationship and the past.

Cognitive Rehabilitation

Cognitive rehabilitation may begin by increasing the patient's awareness of impairment. This awareness may be engendered in the process of providing feedback about the patient's neuropsychological evaluation. It is important to relate test findings to functional impairments and to provide hope by suggesting ways in which impairments may be remediated. If amotivation is a problem, the therapist may have to act temporarily as a "prosthetic ego" for the patient by "(a) abstracting the essential features of the patient's own goals, (b) finding stimuli that will cue the patients to their goals, and (c) using those stimuli to reactivate amotivated patients who seem to have difficulty maintaining goal-directed behavior" (Flesher, 1990, p. 229).

The appropriate approach to cognitive rehabilitation will depend on the information-processing deficit characteristic of the patient. Nonparanoid patients with a perceptually overinclusive style of information-processing may be supported in organizing their impoverished cognitive schemata and in maintaining sets. They may benefit from remediation of specific areas of cognitive impairment. The treatment environment should involve: (1) high information redundancy, (2) high predictability, (3) progressive elaboration and increase in complexity, and (4) cognitive mediation via coaching by the therapist in problem-solving and thinking (Flesher, 1990).

Therapy for the conceptually overinclusive, paranoid patient may involve teaching the patient to change set. Flesher (1990) has suggested first teaching the patient to learn to use his or her attentional capacity. The patient is then taught to attend to a broader range of stimuli and to revise schemata to accommodate new information.

Erickson and Burton (1986) provided a listing of a variety of techniques for rehabilitating psychiatric patients with cognitive deficits.

Perris (1989) has designed an extensive cognitive therapy for treating schizophrenic patients.

Family Therapy

Family intervention is essential in the treatment of schizophrenia. Patients whose families are accepting of the patient and provide an appropriate degree of emotional involvement are less likely to suffer relapses. Needs identified by families are: (1) reduction of anxiety about their family member, (2) understanding of the illness, (3) development of appropriate expectations, (4) acquisition of skill in managing their relative's unmotivated behavior, and (5) assistance at times of crisis. Detailed approaches to family therapy of schizophrenia have been developed (Anderson *et al.,* 1986).

Patient References

A number of references are available for patients and their families: *Understanding and Helping the Schizophrenic* (Areti, 1979), *The Caring Family* (Bernheim *et al.,* 1982), *Common Questions on Schizophrenia and Their Answers* (Hoffer, 1987), *Surviving Schizophrenia* (Torrey, 1983), and *Coping with Schizophrenia* (Wasaw, 1982). Issues of the *Schizophrenia Bulletin* commonly contain first-hand accounts of schizophrenia by patients or their relatives.

PROGNOSIS

If "good outcome" is defined as "discharge from hospital without readmission at any time" and "bad outcome" is defined as "continuous stay in hospital throughout follow-up or moderate to severe intellectual or social impairment at last follow-up," for first admissions, the good and bad outcome rates have been found to be approximately 30% each. For unspecified admissions, good outcome was 13% and bad outcome 45%. Approximately two thirds of first admissions are readmitted some time in the future (Cutting, 1985). The mortality rate is higher than that of the general population. Complete recovery is by no means rare (Cutting, 1985).

Women have a better outcome and a more remitting course than men (Angermeyer *et al.,* 1990). Outcome is affected by culture, life situation, and family support (Cutting, 1985). Positive prognostic signs are supportive family, family history of affective disorder, and premorbid history of good social relations and school performance, acute rather than insidious onset, lack of a family history of schizophrenia, and appropriate affect (McGlashan, 1986; Prudo & Blum, 1987).

REFERENCES

American Psychiatric Association (1987). *Diagnostic and statistical manual of mental disorders: Third edition—Revised.* Washington, DC: American Psychiatric Association.

Anderson, C. M., Reiss, D. J., & Hogarty, G. E. (1986). *Schizophrenia and the family: A practitioner's guide to psychoeducation and management.* New York: Guilford Press.

Andreasen, N. (1979). Thought, language and communication disorders. *Archives of General Psychiatry, 36,* 1315–1330.

Andreasen, N. (1983). *The Scale for the Assessment of Negative Symptoms (SANS).* Iowa City: University of Iowa Press.

Andreasen, N. (1984). *The Scale for the Assessment of Positive Symptoms (SAPS).* Iowa City: University of Iowa Press.

Angermeyer, M. C., Kuhn, L., & Goldstein, J. M. (1990). Gender and the course of schizophrenia: Differences in treated outcomes. *Schizophrenia Bulletin, 16,* 293–307.

Areti, S. (1979). *Understanding and helping the schizophrenic: A guide for family and friends.* New York: Basic Books.

Aylard, E., Walker, E., & Bettes, B. (1984). Intelligence in schizophrenia: Meta-analysis of the research. *Schizophrenia Bulletin, 10,* 430–460.

Baldessarini, R. J., Cohen, B. M., & Teicher, M. H. (1990). Pharmacological treatment. In S. T. Levy (Ed.), *Schizophrenia treatment of acute psychotic episodes* (pp. 61–118). Washington, DC: American Psychiatric Press.

Bernheim, K. F., Lewine, R. R. J., & Beale, C. T. (1982). *The caring family: Living with chronic mental illness.* New York: Random House.

Best, J. B. (1989). *Cognitive psychology* (2nd ed.). St. Paul: West Publishing.

Bigler, E. G. (1988). *Diagnostic clinical neuropsychology* (rev. ed.). Austin: University of Texas Press.

Boucher, M. L., Dewan, M. J., Donnelly, M. P., Pandurangi, A. K., Bartell, K., Diamond, T., & Major, L. F. (1986). Relative utility of three indices of neuropsychological impairment in a young, chronic schizophrenic population. *Journal of Nervous and Mental Disease, 174,* 44–46.

Buchsbaum, M. S. (1990). The frontal lobes, basal ganglia, and temporal lobes as sites for schizophrenia. *Schizophrenia Bulletin, 16,* 379–389.

Carr, E. G., & Wedding, D. (1984). Neuropsychological assessment of cerebral ventricular size in chronic schizophrenics. *International Journal of Clinical Neuropsychology, 6,* 106–111.

Chelune, G. J., Heaton, R. K., Lehman, R. A. W., & Robinson, A. (1979). Level versus pattern of neuropsychological performance among schizophrenic and diffusely brain-damaged patients. *Journal of Consulting and Clinical Psychology, 47,* 155–163.

Clarkin, J. F., & Mattis, S. (1991). Psychological assessment. In L. I. Sederer (Ed.), *Inpatient Psychiatry: Diagnosis and treatment* (3rd ed.) (pp. 360–378). Baltimore: Williams & Wilkins.

Cutting, J. (1980). Physical illness and psychosis. *British Journal of Psychiatry, 136,* 109–119.

Cutting, J. (1985). *The psychology of schizophrenia.* Edinburgh: Churchill.

Dean, R. S., Gray, J. W., & Seretny, M. L. (1987). Cognitive aspects of schizophrenia and primary affective depression. *International Journal of Clinical Neuropsychology, 9,* 33–36.

DeWolfe, A. S., Barrell, R. P., Becker, B. C., & Spaner, F. E. (1971). Intellectual deficit in chronic schizophrenia and brain damage. *Journal of Consulting and Clinical Psychology, 36,* 197–204.

Donnelly, E. F., Weinberger, D. R., Waldman, I. N., & Wyatt, R. J. (1980). Cognitive impairment associated with morphological brain abnormalities on computed tomography in chronic schizophrenic patients. *Journal of Nervous and Mental Disease, 168,* 305–308.

Erickson, R., & Burton, M. (1986). Working with psychiatric patients with cognitive deficits. *Cognitive Rehabilitation, 4,* 26–31.

Fey, E. T. (1951). The performance of young schizophrenics and young normals on the Wisconsin Card Sorting Test. *Journal of Consulting Psychology, 15,* 311–319.

Flesher, S. (1990). Cognitive habilitation in schizophrenia: A theoretical review and model for treatment. *Neuropsychology Review, 1,* 223–246.

Flor-Henry, P. (1990). Neuropsychology and psychopathology: A progress report. *Neuropsychology Review, 1,* 103–123.

Gelder, M., Gath, D., & Mayou, R. (1989). *Oxford textbook of psychiatry.* Oxford: Oxford University Press.

Golden, C. J., MacInnes, W. D., Ariel, R. N., Ruedrich, S. L., Chu, C., Coffman, J. A., Graber, B., & Bloch, S. (1982). Cross-validation of the ability of the Luria–Nebraska Neuropsychological Battery to differentiate chronic schizophrenics with and without ventricular enlargement. *Journal of Consulting and Clinical Psychology, 50,* 87–95.

Golden, R., & Meehl, P. (1979). Detection of the schizoid taxon with MMPI indicators. *Journal of Abnormal Psychology, 88,* 217–233.

Goldstein, G. (1986). The neuropsychology of schizophrenia. In I. Grant & K. M. Adams (Eds.), *Neuropsychological assessment of neuropsychiatric disorders* (pp. 147–171). New York: Oxford University Press.

Goldstein, G., & Halperin, K. M. (1977). Neuropsychological differences among subtypes of schizophrenia. *Journal of Abnormal Psychology, 86,* 34–40.

Gruzelier, J., Seymour, K., Wilson, L., Jolley, A., & Hirsch, S. (1988). Impairments on neuropsychologic tests of temporohippocampal and frontohippocampal functions and word fluency in remitting schizophrenia and affective disorders. *Archives of General Psychiatry, 45,* 623–629.

Gunderson, J. G., Frank, A. F., Katz, H. M., Vannicelli, M. L., Frosch, J. P., & Knapp, P. H. (1984). Effects of psychotherapy in schizophrenia. II. Comparative outcome of two forms of treatment. *Schizophrenia Bulletin, 10,* 564–598.

Heaton, R. K., & Crowley, T. J. (1981). Effects of psychiatric disorders and their somatic treatments on neuropsychological test results. In S. B. Filskov & T. J. Boll (Eds.), *Handbook of clinical neuropsychology* (pp. 481–525). New York: Wiley.

Heaton, R. K., Baade, L. E., & Johnson, K. L. (1978). Neuropsychological test results associated with psychiatric disorders in adults. *Psychological Bulletin, 85,* 141–162.

Hoffer, A. (1987). *Common questions on schizophrenia and their answers.* New Canaan, CT: Keats Publishing.

Kenny, J. T., & Meltzer, M. D. (1991). Attention and higher cortical functions in schizophrenia. *Journal of Neuropsychiatry, 3,* 269–275.

Klonoff, H., Fibiger, C. H., & Hutton, G. H. (1970). Neuropsychological patterns in chronic schizophrenia. *Journal of Nervous and Mental Disease, 150,* 291–300.

Kohn, M. L. (1968). Social class and schizophrenia: A critical review. In D. Rosenthal & S. S. Kety (Eds.), *The transmission of schizophrenia.* Oxford: Pergamon Press.

Kolb, B., & Whishaw, I. Q. (1983). Performance of schizophrenic patients on tests sensitive to left or right frontal, temporal, or parietal function in neurological patients. *Journal of Nervous and Mental Disease, 171,* 435–442.

Lazarus, A., Mann, S. C., & Caroff, S. N. (1989). *The neuroleptic malignant syndrome and related conditions.* Washington, DC: American Psychiatric Press.

Lewis, G., Golden, C. J., Purisch, A. D., & Hammeke, T. A. (1979). The effects of chronicity of disorder and length of hospitalization on the standardized version of Luria's neuropsychological battery in a schizophrenic population. *Clinical Neuropsychology, 1,* 13–18.

Malmo, H. P. (1974). On frontal lobe functions: Psychiatric patient controls. *Cortex, 10,* 231–237.

McGlashan, T. H. (1986). The prediction of outcome in chronic schizophrenia. *Archives of General Psychiatry, 43,* 167–176.

Meyer, R. G. (1983). *The clinician's handbook: The psychopathology of adulthood and late adolescence.* Boston: Allyn & Bacon.

Moses, J. A. (1984). Performance of schizophrenic and schizoaffective disorder patients on the Luria–Nebraska Neuropsychological Battery. *International Journal of Clinical Neuropsychology, 6,* 195–197.

Nyman, H., Nyback, H., Wiesel, F. A., Oxenstierna, G., & Schalling, D. (1986). Neuropsychological test performance, brain morphological measures and CSF monoamine metabolites in schizophrenic patients. *Acta Psychiatrica Scandinavica, 72,* 292–301.

Othmer, E., Penick, E. C., Powell, B. J., Read, M. R., & Othmer, S. C. (1989). *Psychiatric Diagnostic Interview, Revised (PDI-R).* Los Angeles: Western Psychological Services.

Overall, J. E., & Gorham, D. R. (1962). The brief psychiatric rating scale. *Psychological Reports, 10,* 799–812.

Pandurangi, A. K., Dewan, M. J., Boucher, M., Levy, B., Ramachandran, T., Bartell, K., Bick, P. A., Phelps, B. H., & Major, L. (1986). A comprehensive study of chronic schizophrenic patients. II. Biological, neuropsychological, and clinical correlates of CT abnormality. *Acta Psychiatrica Scandinavica, 73,* 161–171.

Perris, C. (1989). *Cognitive therapy with schizophrenic patients.* New York: Guilford Press.

Prudo, R., & Blum, H. M. (1987). Five-year outcome and prognosis in schizophrenia: A report from the London Field Research Center of the International Pilot Study of Schizophrenia. *British Journal of Psychiatry, 150,* 345–351.

Purisch, A. D., Golden, C. G., & Hammeke, T. A. (1978). Discrimination of schizophrenic and brain injured patients by a standardized version of Luria's neuropsychological tests. *Journal of Consulting and Clinical Psychology, 46,* 1266–1273.

Robertson, G., & Taylor, P. J. (1985). Some cognitive correlates of schizophrenic illness. *Psychological Medicine, 15,* 81–98.

Sederer, L. I. (1991). Schizophrenic disorders. In L. I. Sederer (Ed.), *Inpatient psychiatry: Diagnosis and treatment* (3rd ed.) (pp. 70–107). Baltimore: Williams & Wilkins.

Shelly, C., & Goldstein, G. (1983). Discrimination of chronic schizophrenia and brain damage with the Luria–Nebraska Battery: A partially successful replication. *Clinical Neuropsychology, 5,* 82–85.

Spitzer, R. L., & Endicott, J. (1977). *Schedule for affective disorders and schizophrenia.* New York: New York State Psychiatric Institute.

Spitzer, R. L., Williams, J., & Gibbon, M. (1987). *Structured clinical interview for DSM-IIIR (SCID).* New York: New York State Psychiatric Institute.

Torrey, E. F. (1983). *Surviving schizophrenia: A family manual.* New York: Harper & Row.

Walker, E. (1981). Attentional and neuromotor functions of schizophrenics, schizoaffectives and patients with other affective disorders. *Archives of General Psychiatry, 38,* 1355–1358.

Wasaw, M. (1982). *Coping with schizophrenia: A survival manual for parents, relatives and friends.* Palo Alto, CA: Science & Behavior Books.

Watson, C. G., Thomas, R. W., Andersen, D., & Felling, J. (1968). Differentiation of organics from schizophrenics at two chronicity levels by use of the Reitan–Halstead organic test battery. *Journal of Consulting and Clinical Psychology, 32,* 679–684.

Weinberger, D. R., Bigelow, L. B., Kleinman, J. E., Klein, S. T., Rosenblatt, J. E., & Wyatt, R. J. (1980). Cerebral ventricular enlargement in chronic schizophrenia. *Archives of General Psychiatry, 37,* 11–13.

World Health Organization (1979). *Schizophrenia: An initial follow up.* Chichester, England: Wiley.

Yates, W. R., Jacoby, C. G., & Andreasen, N. C. (1987). Cerebellar atrophy in schizophrenia and affective disorder. *American Journal of Psychiatry, 144,* 465–467.

Depression

DESCRIPTION

Major Depressive Episode (DSM III-R) is diagnosed if and only if at least five of the following symptoms (including depressed mood or loss of interest or pleasure) have been present nearly continually during the same 2-week period and represent a change in functioning: (1) depressed mood, (2) markedly diminished interest or pleasure in activities, (3) significant weight loss/gain or decrease/increase in appetite, (4) insomnia or hypersomnia, (5) psychomotor agitation, (6) fatigue, (7) feelings of worthlessness or excessive guilt, (8) diminished ability to think or concentrate, and (9) recurrent thoughts of death, suicidal ideation. Organic factors and uncomplicated bereavement must be ruled out. There have been no hallucinations or delusions in the absence of prominent mood symptoms, and the disturbance is not superimposed on Schizophrenia, Schizophreniform Disorder, Delusional Disorder, or Psychotic Disorder NOS (American Psychiatric Association, 1987).

Major Depression, Single Episode can be diagnosed when there is a single Major Depressive Episode and there has never been a Manic Episode or Hypomanic Episode (American Psychiatric Association, 1987).

Dysthymia is diagnosed if there is depressed mood for at least 2 years for adults (1 year for children and adolescents). In addition, while the patient is depressed, at least two of the following should be present: (1) poor appetite or overeating, (2) insomnia or hypersomnia, (3) low energy or fatigue, (4) low self-esteem, (5) poor concentration or difficulty making decisions, and (6) feelings of hopelessness. There should be no evidence of a Major Depressive Episode during the first 2 years or of a Manic or Hypomanic Episode, and the disturbance is not superimposed on a chronic psychotic disorder. Organic factors should be ruled out. More detailed definitions may be found in DSM III-R (American Psychiatric Association, 1987).

INCIDENCE, PREVALENCE, AND RISK FACTORS

Prevalence

The prevalence is 3% for bipolar depression for men and 4–9% for women. The lifetime prevalence rate for nonbipolar depression is 7–12% for men and 20–25% for women. The lifetime risk of bipolar depression is less than 1%. The prevalence of depressive symptoms ranges from 13% to 20% (Charney & Weissman, 1988).

Age

In nonbipolar depression, rates peak, for males, between 55 and 70 years and, for females, between 35 and 45 years (Charney & Weissman, 1988).

Gender

The rate for nonbipolar depression in women is approximately twice that in men (Charney & Weissman, 1988).

Marital Status

Married individuals have the lowest rate (Charney & Weissman, 1988).

Genetics

The role of genetics in unipolar depression has not been established (Mendlewicz, 1988).

Life Stress

Depression is associated with marital, occupational, parental, financial, and neighborhood stressors.

ETIOLOGY AND PATHOLOGY

Numerous theories of the biochemical etiology of depression have been advanced. Neurotransmitters such as norepinephrine, acetylcholine, and serotonin have been implicated in the theories, but a consensus has not yet formed (Janowsky *et al.*, 1988). Theories of the etiology of depression have been proposed based on learned helplessness and dysfunctional cognitive processing (Beck *et al.*, 1979), among many others. Depression can result from numerous systemic and neurological disorders.

A subset of depressed patients with enlarged ventricles has been identified. Older age, age of onset, delusions, and melancholia have been associated with ventricular enlargement (Dolan *et al.*, 1985).

MEDICAL ASSESSMENT

A physical evaluation to rule out "physical" causes of depression is an essential first step in assessment. Grady and Sederer (1991) have provided a list of over 40 physical conditions that should be ruled out. If examination identifies physical conditions that may be causing or contributing to the patient's depression, then these conditions can receive appropriate medical treatment. If necessary, the patient's depression can then be assessed and collateral medical and psychosocial treatment provided.

Medical evaluation therefore includes a thorough history and physical examination. The dextromethasone suppression test is sometimes ordered. Its sensitivity is 40–50% in patients with major depression (Grady & Sederer, 1991). An evaluation of suicide potential is essential for patients with depression. Briefly, this evaluation involves determining whether the patient has attempted suicide and whether the patient is experiencing any suicidal ideation and has any plan and intent. Numerous demographic risk factors and situational factors should be considered in evaluating suicide potential. An excellent yet brief review of these factors is available in *Suicide Risk: Assessment and Response Guidelines* (Fremouw *et al.*, 1990).

NEUROPSYCHOLOGICAL ASSESSMENT

Since depression is a common concomitant of systemic and neurological illnesses, knowledge of the effects of depression on neuropsychological testing is essential for the neuropsychologist. A referral question may ask the examiner to distinguish impairment due to depression from impairment due to neurological dysfunction. Sweet *et al.* (1992) have reviewed the role of depression in a variety of neurological disorders. Referrals of patients with suspected dementia often ask for a resolution of the diagnostic dilemma of dementia vs. depression. This problem is treated in more detail in Chapters 40–45.

As noted under *MEDICAL ASSESSMENT* above, it is imperative that the role of physical factors be thoroughly assessed when there is the possibility of depression. Physical illnesses and imbalances may masquerade as depression (Taylor, 1990). If the patient has not had a complete physical, he or she should be referred to a physician for medical evaluation.

The method used in assessing depression may be a significant factor in determining whether cognitive impairment should be expected. For example, Bornstein *et al.* (1991) found that impaired memory on the WMS was related to the Hamilton Depression Rating Scale, but not to the MMPI-D Scale.

In depression, verbal skills show less impairment than do visuospatial, motor, and memory skills, especially nonverbal memory. Some impairment has been noted in comprehension of narratives and fluency (Cassens *et al.*, 1990). Severity of depression has been found to be correlated with impaired memory and motor performance (Cohen *et al.*, 1982). Depressed patients may exhibit cognitive impairment on tasks that require complex processing, effortful processing, or independent structuring of information relative to preexisting knowledge (Sackheim & Steif, 1988).

Sweet *et al.* (1992) have suggested several guidelines for the neuropsychological evaluation of depressed patients: (1) supplement test scores with interview, behavioral observations, reports of activities of daily living (ADLs), and information from significant others; (2) when there is evidence of depression, use more stringent "cutoffs"; (3) avoid diagnosing brain dysfunction on findings such as decreased cognitive efficiency and mild memory problems; and (4) see the patient on more than one day and consider repeating tests.

Attention

DS has generally been found to be unimpaired (Glass & Russell, 1986). DSym has been found to be impaired (Hart *et al.*, 1987). Reaction time has been found to be slow relative to controls (Bruder *et al.*, 1975; Martin & Rees, 1966). The SCWT may be unimpaired (Cassens *et al.*, 1990).

Memory

Logical Memory and Visual Reproduction have been found to be impaired (Hart *et al.*, 1987). The RAVLT has been found to be impaired (Wolfe *et al.*, 1987). ACT has been reported to be impaired (Cohen *et al.*, 1982). Story recall has generally been reported impaired.

The TPT-Memory has been found impaired (Flor-Henry & Yeudall, 1979; Gray *et al.*, 1987). The results of studies have been mixed on paired-associate learning (Cassens *et al.*, 1990). King and Caine (1990) reported performance to be impaired on word-list learning and delayed recall, immediate recall of a story, multiple-choice recognition of the story, and immediate and delayed recall of geometric shapes. Delayed recognition of the word list was unimpaired.

General Knowledge and Social Understanding

PIQ may be inferior to VIQ (Sackheim *et al.*, 1992; Sackheim & Steif, 1988).

Speech/Language

Confrontation naming has generally not been found to be impaired (King & Caine, 1990). S, and I have been found to be unimpaired (Hart *et al.*, 1987; Saccuzzo & Braff, 1981).

Visuospatial Functioning

The TMTA has been found to be impaired (Shipley *et al.*, 1981). BD has been found to be impaired (Hart *et al.*, 1987). OA, PA, and PC have been found to be impaired relative to controls (Gray *et al.*, 1987).

Sensory Functioning

No impairment has been generally noted in sensory functioning.

Motor Functioning

Bilateral impairment has been noted on the FTT (Raskin *et al.*, 1982), but this finding has not been invariable (Gray *et al.*, 1987). Bilateral impairment has been noted on the GS and PPT (Flor-Henry & Yeudall, 1979). Severity of depression has been found to correlate negatively with grip strength (Cohen *et al.*, 1982).

Executive Functioning

Although WCST performance has been found to be unimpaired (Hart *et al.*, 1987), the Halstead CT has generally, though not invariably, been found to be impaired (Donnelly *et al.*, 1980; Savard *et al.*, 1980). The TMTB has been noted to be impaired (Shipley *et al.*, 1981). The COWAT and BDAE Animal Naming have been found to be impaired (Hart *et al.*, 1987). Generation of words beginning with a certain letter (e.g., "f") and in certain categories (e.g., animals) has been found to be impaired (King & Caine, 1990).

LNNB

Newman and Sweet (1986) found that patients with diagnoses of Major Depression had significantly greater elevations on all LNNB clinical scales. "Application of a two-elevation rule led to misdiagnosis of 40% of patients as brain damaged" (Newman & Sweet, 1986, p. 109).

Personality

On the MMPI, Scale 2 is elevated in depression. As scores rise on 8 and fall on 9, the depression is proportionately more severe (Meyer, 1983). A number of rating scales are used to assess depression: the Zung Self-Rating Depression Scale (Zung, 1965), Beck Depression Inventory (Beck *et al.,* 1961), and Hamilton Rating Scale for Depression (Hamilton, 1967). The Geriatric Depression Scale (Yesavage, 1986; Yesavage *et al.,* 1983) has been developed for elderly individuals.

MEDICAL TREATMENT

Tricyclic antidepressants will bring about improvement in 70–90% of patients with major depressive disorder. Side effects include cardiac toxicity, anticholinergic effects (e.g., dry mouth, urinary retention, and constipation), postural hypotension, dizziness, restlessness, insomnia, tremor, delirium, skin rashes, and allergic–obstructive jaundice (Grady & Sederer, 1991). Monoamine oxidase inhibitors may be prescribed if tricyclic antidepressants are found ineffective. Side effects include hypertensive reactions, especially when the drug interacts with tyramine. Tyramine is found in foods such as cheeses, wines, yogurt, yeast extract, and chocolate. The patient must be able to learn and follow a diet (Grady & Sederer, 1991). Fluoxetine (Prozac) is a bicyclic drug that has a clinical efficacy equal to that of tricyclic antidepressive agents without causing side effects such as anticholinergic effects or hypotensive effects (Cooper, 1988). Adverse effects include anxiety, nausea, and insomnia. Amphetamines are sometimes used in the treatment of elderly or medically ill patients.

Light therapy may benefit patients with seasonal affective disorder (SAD), which is characterized by onset in fall or winter and remission in the spring. SAD is characterized by a recurrent depressed mood associated with hypersomnia, overeating, and carbohydrate craving. Light therapy consists of exposure to bright lights for 2–6 h (Jacobsen & Rosenthal, 1988).

Electroconvulsive therapy (ECT) may be prescribed for patients who have not responded to or cannot tolerate antidepressant medications. Production of a seizure is essential for therapeutic effect (Fink, 1988). Adverse effects include headache and muscle spasms. Cognitive changes include postictal confusion. Anterograde and retrograde amnesia for events surrounding the course of ECT usually resolves within 30–60 days (Grady & Sederer, 1991).

PSYCHOSOCIAL THERAPIES

In an analysis of the research on depression-treatment outcome, Robinson *et al.* (1990) found psychotherapy to be as effective as medication. Some studies have found that psychotherapy combined with antidepressant medication is superior to either alone (Wolpert, 1988).

Behavior Therapy

From the behavioral perspective, depression results from a low rate of response-contingent positive reinforcement (Lewinsohn, 1974). Therapy focuses on encouraging the patient to participate in pleasant activities. Assertion skills are taught to assist the patient in eliciting social rewards. Several programs have been developed (Fuchs & Rehm, 1977; Lewinsohn *et al.,* 1985).

Cognitive Therapy

According to Beck (1976), a negative triad of cognitions involving a negative view of self, experience, and the future are involved in depression. These cognitions may not necessarily initially cause depression, but may maintain and augment it. Negative automatic thoughts, maladaptive assumptions, and negative self-schema may serve to elicit feelings of depression. In cognitive therapy, the patient is initially educated about the role of cognition in depression and the rationale behind the therapy. The patient is asked to schedule possibly pleasurable activities and to monitor automatic thoughts, especially those that are self-defeating, involve all-or-none thinking, or involve mind-reading. The patient is taught to examine the evidence or logic underlying his or her automatic thoughts. A variety of techniques are used to assist the patient in examining faulty, maladaptive assumptions and thinking (Beck *et al.,* 1979). Numerous therapy-outcome studies have demonstrated the efficacy of cognitive therapy of depression (Leahy & Beck, 1988).

PROGNOSIS

Treated depressions respond in weeks or months. Some 10–15% of patients have a chronic course (Charney & Weissman, 1988). Approximately 15% of patients with unipolar depression will take their own lives (Guze & Robins, 1970).

REFERENCES

American Psychiatric Association (1987). *Diagnostic and statistical manual of mental disorders: Third edition—Revised.* Washington, DC: American Psychiatric Association.

Beck, A. T. (1976). *Cognitive therapy and the emotional disorders.* New York: International Universities Press.

Beck, A. T., Ward, C., Mendelson, M., Mock, J., & Erbaugh, J. (1961). An inventory for measuring depression. *Archives of General Psychiatry, 4,* 561–571.

Beck, A. T., Rush, A. J., Shaw, B. F., & Emery, G. (1979). *Cognitive therapy of depression: A treatment manual.* New York: Guilford Press.

Bornstein, R. A., Baker, G. B., & Douglass, A. B. (1991). Depression and memory in major depressive disorder. *Journal of Neuropsychiatry and Clinical Neurosciences, 3,* 78–80.

Bruder, G., Sutton, S., Babkoff, H., Gurland, B., Yozawitz, A., & Fleiss, J. (1975). Auditory signal detectability and facilitation of simple reaction time in psychiatric patients and non-patients. *Psychological Medicine, 5,* 260–272.

Cassens, G., Wolfe, L., & Zola, M. (1990). The neuropsychology of depressions. *Journal of Neuropsychiatry and Clinical Neurosciences, 2,* 202–213.

Charney, E. A., & Weissman, M. M. (1988). Epidemiology of depressive and manic syndromes. In A. Georgotas & R. Cancro (Eds.), *Depression and mania* (pp. 26–52). New York: Elsevier.

Cohen, R., Weingartner, H., Smallberg, S., Pickar, D., & Murphy, D. (1982). Effort in cognition in depression. *Archives of General Psychiatry, 39,* 593–597.

Cooper, G. L. (1988). The safety of fluoxetine: An update. *British Journal of Psychiatry, 153*(Supplement 3), 77–86.

Dolan, R. J., Calloway, S. P., & Mann, A. H. (1985). Cerebral ventricular size in depressed subjects. *Psychological Medicine, 15,* 873–878.

Donnelly, E. F., Waldman, I. N., Murphy, D. L., Wyatt, R. J., & Goodwin, F. K. (1980). Primary affective disorder: Thought disorder in depression. *Journal of Abnormal Psychology, 89,* 315–319.

Fink, M. (1988). Convulsive therapy for affective disorders. In A. Georgotas & R. Cancro (Eds.), *Depression and mania* (pp. 452–460). New York: Elsevier.

Flor-Henry, P., & Yeudall, L. T. (1979). Neuropsychological investigation of schizophrenia and manic–depressive psychoses. In J. Gruzelier & P. Flor-Henry (Eds.), *Hemispheric asymmetries of function in psychopathology* (pp. 341–362). Amsterdam: Elsevier.

Fremouw, W. J., de Perczel, M., & Ellis, T. E. (1990). *Suicide risk: Assessment and response guidelines.* New York: Pergamon Press.

Fuchs, C. Z., & Rehm, L. P. (1977). A self-control behavior therapy program for depression. *Journal of Consulting and Clinical Psychology, 45,* 206–215.

Glass, C. S., & Russell, E. W. (1986). Differential impact of brain damage and depression on memory test performance. *Journal of Consulting and Clinical Psychology, 54,* 261–263.

Grady, T. A., & Sederer, L. I. (1991). Depression. In L. I. Sederer (Ed.), *Inpatient psychiatry: Diagnosis and treatment* (3rd ed.) (pp. 3–45). Baltimore: Williams & Wilkins.

Gray, J. W., Dean, R. S., Rattan, G., & Cramer, K. M. (1987). Neuropsychological aspects of primary affective depression. *International Journal of Neuroscience, 32,* 911–918.

Guze, S. B., & Robins, E. (1970). Suicide and primary affective disorders. *British Journal of Psychiatry, 117,* 437–438.

Hamilton, M. (1967). Development of a rating scale for primary depressive illness. *British Journal of Social and Clinical Psychology, 6,* 278–296.

Hart, R. P., Kwentus, J. A., Taylor, J. R., & Harkins, S. W. (1987). Rate of forgetting in dementia and depression. *Journal of Consulting and Clinical Psychology, 55,* 101–105.

Jacobsen, F. M., & Rosenthal, N. E. (1988). Seasonal affective disorder. In A. Georgotas & R. Cancro (Eds.), *Depression and mania* (pp. 104–116). New York: Elsevier.

Janowsky, D. S., Golden, R. N., Rapaport, M., Cain, J. J., & Gillin, J. C. (1988). Neurochemistry of depression and mania. In A. Georgotas & R. Cancro (Eds.), *Depression and mania* (pp. 244–264). New York: Elsevier.

King, D. A., & Caine, E. D. (1990). Depression. In J. L. Cummings (Ed.), *Subcortical dementia* (pp. 218–230). New York: Oxford University Press.

Leahy, R. L., & Beck, A. T. (1988). Cognitive therapy of depression and mania. In A. Georgotas & R. Cancro (Eds.), *Depression and mania* (pp. 517–537). New York: Elsevier.

Lewinsohn, P. M. (1974). Clinical and theoretical aspects of depression. In K. S. Calhoun, H. E. Adams, & K. M. Mitchell (Eds.), *Innovative treatment methods in psychopathology* (pp. 63–120). New York: Wiley.

Lewinsohn, P. M., Steinmetz, J. L., Antonuccio, D., & Teri, L. (1985). Group therapy for depression: The Coping with Depression course. *International Journal of Mental Health, 13,* 8–33.

Martin, L., & Rees, L. (1966). Reaction times and somatic reactivity in depressed patients. *Journal of Psychosomatic Medicine, 9,* 375–382.

Mendlewicz, J. (1988). Genetics of depression and mania. In A. Georgotas & R. Cancro (Eds.), *Depression and mania* (pp. 197–212). New York: Elsevier.

Meyer, R. G. (1983). *The clinician's handbook: The psychopathology of adulthood and late adolescence.* Boston: Allyn & Bacon.

Newman, P. J., & Sweet, J. J. (1986). The effects of clinical depression on the Luria–Nebraska Neuropsychological Battery. *International Journal of Clinical Neuropsychology, 8,* 109–114.

Othmer, E., Penick, E. C., Powell, B. J., Read, M. R., & Othmer, S. C. (1989). *Psychiatric Diagnostic Interview, Revised (PDI-R).* Los Angeles: Western Psychological Services.

Raskin, A., Friedman, A. S., & DeMascio, A. (1982). Cognitive and performance deficits in depression. *Psychopharmacology Bulletin, 18,* 196–202.

Robinson, L. A., Berman, J. S., & Neimeyer, R. A. (1990). Psychotherapy for the treatment of depression: A comprehensive review of controlled outcome research. *Psychological Bulletin, 108,* 30–49.

Saccuzzo, P., & Braff, D. L. (1981). Early information processing deficit in schizophrenia. *Archives of General Psychiatry, 38,* 175–179.

Sackheim, H. A., & Steif, B. L. (1988). Neuropsychology of depression and mania. In A. Georgotas & R. Cancro (Eds.), *Depression and mania* (pp. 265–289). New York: Elsevier.

Sackheim, H. A., Freeman, J., McElhiney, M., Coleman, E., Prudic, J., & Devanand, D. P. (1992). Effects of major depression on estimates of intelligence. *Journal of Clinical and Experimental Neuropsychology, 14,* 268–288.

Savard, R. J., Rey, A. C., & Post, R. M. (1980). Halstead–Reitan Category Test in bipolar and unipolar affective disorders: Relationship of age to phase of illness. *Journal of Nervous and Mental Disease, 168,* 297–304.

Shipley, J. E., Kupfer, D. J., Spiker, D. G., Shaw, D. H., Coble, P. A., Neil, J. F., & Cofsky, J. (1981).

Neuropsychological assessment and EEG sleep in affective disorders. *Biological Psychiatry, 16,* 907–918.

Sweet, J. J., Newman, P., & Bell, B. (1992). Significance of depression in clinical neuropsychological assessment. *Clinical Psychology Review, 12,* 21–45.

Taylor, R. L. (1990). *Distinguishing psychological from organic disorders: Screening for psychological masquerade.* New York: Springer.

Wolfe, J., Granholm, R., & Butters, N. (1987). Verbal memory deficits associated with major affective disorders: A comparison of unibolar and bipolar patients. *Journal of Affective Disorders, 13,* 83–92.

Wolpert, E. A. (1988). Cognitive therapies for depression and mania. In A. Georgotas & R. Cancro (Eds.), *Depression and mania* (pp. 538–548). New York: Elsevier.

Yesavage, J. A. (1986). The use of self-rating depression scales in the elderly. In L. W. Poon (Ed.), *Handbook for clinical memory assessment of older adults* (pp. 213–217). Washington, DC: American Psychological Association.

Yesavage, J., Brink, T., Rose, T., Lum, O., Huang, O., Adey, V., & Leirer, V. (1983). Development and validation of a geriatric depression screening scale: A preliminary report. *Journal of Psychiatric Research, 17,* 37–49.

Zung, W. W. K. (1965). A self-rating depression scale. *Archives of General Psychiatry, 12,* 63–70.

Appendix A

Performance Classifications and Statistics

Benton Performance Classifications[a]

Percentile	Classification
100%	Very superior
97%	Superior
90%	High average
73%	Average
23%	Low average
8%	Borderline
5%	Defective
<1%	Severely defective

[a] From Benton *et al.* (1983) and Benton and Hamsher (1989).

Wechsler Performance Classifications[a]

IQ	Classification
130+	Very superior
120–129	Superior
110–119	High average
90–109	Average
80–89	Low average
70–79	Borderline
<69	Mentally retarded

[a] From Wechsler (1981).

Heaton, Grant, and Matthews
Performance Classifications[a]

T-scores	Classification
55–100	Above average
45–54	Average
40–44	Below average
35–39	Mild
30–34	Mild to moderate
25–29	Moderate
20–24	Moderate to severe
0–19	Severe

[a] From Heaton et al. (1991).

Statistical Equivalences

Percentile ranks	Standard scores	T-scores	Scaled scores	Z-scores
>99	145	80	—	3.0
>99	137	75	—	2.5
99	133	72	17	—
98	130	70	16	2.0
97	127	69	—	—
96	126	67	—	—
95	124	66	15	—
94	123	—	—	—
93	122	65	—	1.5
92	121	64	—	—
91	120	—	14	—
90	119	63	—	—
89	118	—	—	—
88	—	62	—	—
87	117	—	—	—
86	116	61	—	—
85	—	—	—	—
84	115	60	13	1.0
83	114	—	—	—
82	—	59	—	—
81	113	—	—	—
80	—	—	—	—
79	112	58	—	—
78	—	—	—	—
77	111	—	—	—
76	—	57	—	—
75	110	—	12	—
74	—	—	—	—
73	109	56	—	—
72	—	—	—	—
71	—	—	—	—
70	108	—	—	—
69	—	55	—	0.5
68	107	—	—	—
67	—	—	—	—

Statistical Equivalences. (*Continued*)

66	106	54	—	—
65	—	—	—	—
64	—	—	—	—
63	105	—	11	—
62	—	53	—	—
61	104	—	—	—
60	—	—	—	—
59	—	—	—	—
58	103	52	—	—
57	—	—	—	—
56	—	—	—	—
55	102	—	—	—
54	—	51	—	—
53	101	—	—	—
52	—	—	—	—
51	—	—	—	—
50	100	50	10	0.0
49	—	—	—	—
48	—	—	—	—
47	99	—	—	—
46	—	49	—	—
45	98	—	—	—
44	—	—	—	—
43	—	—	—	—
42	97	48	—	—
41	—	—	—	—
40	—	—	—	—
39	96	—	—	—
38	—	47	—	—
37	95	—	9	—
36	—	—	—	—
35	—	—	—	—
34	94	46	—	—
33	—	—	—	—
32	93	—	—	—
31	—	45	—	−0.5
30	92	—	—	—
29	—	—	—	—
28	—	—	—	—
27	91	44	—	—
26	—	—	—	—
25	90	—	8	—
24	—	43	—	—
23	89	—	—	—
22	—	—	—	—
21	88	42	—	—
20	—	—	—	—
19	87	—	—	—
18	86	41	—	—
17	—	—	—	—
16	85	40	7	−1.0
15	—	—	—	—
14	84	39	—	—
13	83	—	—	—
12	82	38	—	—

Statistical Equivalences. (*Continued*)

11	—	—	—	—
10	81	37	—	—
9	80	—	6	—
8	79	36	—	—
7	78	35	—	−1.5
6	77	—	—	—
5	75	34	5	—
4	74	33	—	—
3	72	31	—	—
2	70	30	4	−2.0
1	67	28	3	—
<1	63	25	—	−2.5
<1	55	20	—	−3.0

REFERENCES

Benton, A. L., & Hamsher, K. (1989). *Multilingual aphasia examination* (2nd ed.). Iowa City: AJA Associates.

Benton, A. L., Hamsher, K., Varney, N. R., & Spreen, O. (1983). *Contributions to neuropsychological assessment: A clinical manual.* New York: Oxford University Press.

Heaton, R. K., Grant, I., & Matthews, C. G. (1991). *Comprehensive norms for an expanded Halstead–Reitan Battery: Demographic corrections, research findings, and clinical applications.* Odessa, FL: Psychological Assessment Resources.

Wechsler, D. (1981). *Wechsler Adult Intelligence Scale—Revised.* New York: Psychological Corporation.

Appendix B

Neuropsychological Interview Form

Name: _____ Record No.: _____
Age: _____ Date of Birth: ____/____/____ Social Security No.: _____-____-_____
Address: _____
Home Phone: ( ) _____-_____ Business Phone: ( ) _____-_____
Interviewer: _____ Date of Interview: ____/____/____
Referral Source: _____

Reason for Referral: _____
_____
_____
_____

MEDICAL DATA AND DATA FROM RECORDS
Date of Injury: ____/____/____ Time: _____
Circumstances of Injury: _____
_____

Medical Findings: [CT, MRI, EEG] _____
_____

Medical Diagnosis: [onset, course, prognosis, loss of consciousness, coma, length of
hospitalization] _____
_____
_____

Medications: [active side effects, allergies] _____
_____

MEDICAL HISTORY
Previous Neurological Disorders: [head injury, stroke, anoxia, meningitis, encephalitis,
seizures, toxic exposures] _____
_____

Systemic Disorders: _____
_____

PSYCHIATRIC HISTORY
Diagnoses: _____
Treatment: _____
Suicide: _____
SUBSTANCE USE
Tobacco: [amount, frequency, dates, treatment] _____
_____
Alcohol: _____
Other drugs: _____
_____

PATIENT'S REPORT OF ACCIDENT, INJURY, ILLNESS, AND SYMPTOMS
Current Complaints/Symptoms: _____
_____
_____
_____

Patient's Account of Injury or Illness: _____
_____

Patient's Account of Accident: _____
_____

Last Clear Memory Prior to Injury: _____
_____

First Continuous Memory After Injury: _____
_____

Vision: [double, blurred, loss, glasses] _____
Hearing: [tinnitus, hearing aid] _____
Touch: [tingling, numbness] _____
Smell: _____
Taste: _____
Pain: _____
Balance: [dizziness, fainting, falls] _____
Motor Abilities: [speed, clumsiness, tremor, dropping things] _____
_____

R/L Hand Preference: _____ Sinistrality in Family: _____
Walking: _____
Attention: [concentration, distractibility] _____
_____

Memory: [forgets day, appointments, becomes lost] _____
_____

Speech: [speaking, reading, writing] _____
_____

Arithmetic: _____
Problem-Solving and Decision-Making: _____
_____

Anxiety: _____
Depression: [withdrawal, suicidal ideation, attempt, history] _____
_____

Frustration and Anger: _____

Stressors: [family, marital, occupational, financial, school] _____

Energy Level: [fatigue] _____
Sleep: [duration, quality, naps] _____
Appetite: [increase, decrease, weight change] _____
Exercise: [frequency, duration] _____
Sexual Functioning: _____
PRE–POST INJURY EVERYDAY FUNCTIONING
Living situation: _____
ADLs: [eating, toileting, dressing] _____

Domestic Chores: [cooking, dishwashing, housecleaning, yard work] _____

Financial Responsibilities: [checkbook, pays bills] _____

Relations with Family Members: _____

Friendships and Social Activities: _____

Transportation: [handivan, bus, driving] _____

DEVELOPMENTAL HISTORY
Place of Birth: _____
Mother's Pregnancy: _____
Delivery: _____
Birth Weight: _____
Age Started: Walking _____ Talking _____
Childhood Diseases: [fevers] _____
Developmental Problems: [impairments in hearing, speaking, reading, writing,
    spelling, arithmetic, behavior, attention, enuresis, sleep disorders] _____

Primary Language: _____
Secondary Language: _____
EDUCATION
Highest Grade Completed: _____
Schools Attended: _____
Grades in Best Subjects: _____
Grades in Worst Subjects: _____
Special Education: _____
Grades Repeated: _____
Disciplinary Problems: _____
WORK HISTORY
Current Employment: [company, duration, duties, remuneration] _____

Prior Employment: [chronology, longest period of employment] _____
_____
_____
_____

MILITARY HISTORY
Branch: _____ Dates: _____
Highest Rank: _____ Duties: _____
Disciplinary Actions: _____ Discharge Status: _____
LEISURE/RECREATION
Hobbies: _____ Sports: _____
LEGAL PROBLEMS
_____

FAMILY HISTORY
Mother: [age, occupation] _____
_____
_____

Father: [age, occupation] _____
_____
_____

Siblings: [ages, occupations] _____
_____
_____
_____
_____

MARITAL HISTORY:
Spouse: [name, age, occupation] _____
_____
Years Married: _____
Children: [names, ages, schools] _____
_____
_____
_____

Appendix C

Test Abbreviations

3MS	Modified Mini-Mental State Examination
16PF	Sixteen Personality Factor Questionnaire
AC-BDAE	Auditory Comprehension
ACT	Auditory Consonant Trigrams
ACWP-MAE	Aural Comprehension of Words and Phrases
AIR	Average Impairment Rating
AST	Aphasia Screening Test (HRNB)
AT-BDAE	Apraxia Test (Supplementary)
A-WAIS-R	Arithmetic
A-WRAT-R	Arithmetic
BDAE	Boston Diagnostic Aphasia Examination
BD-WAIS-R	Block Design
BNT	Boston Naming Test
BVMGT	Bender Visual Motor Gestalt Test
BVRT: A, B, D, E	Benton Visual Retention Test
BVRT: C	Benton Visual Retention Test: Copy
BVRT: G	Benton Visual Retention Test: Multiple Choice-Memory
C1-LNNB	Motor Functions
C2-LNNB	Rhythm
C3-LNNB	Tactile Functions
C4-LNNB	Visual Functions
C5-LNNB	Receptive Speech
C6-LNNB	Expressive Speech
C7-LNNB	Writing
C8-LNNB	Reading
C9-LNNB	Arithmetic
C10-LNNB	Memory
C11-LNNB	Intellectual Processes
C12-LNNB	Intermediate Memory—Form II
CCSE	Cognitive Capacity Screening Examination
COWAT-MAE	Controlled Oral Word Association Test

CPT	Continuous Performance Test
CT	Halstead Category Test (HRNB)
CVLT	California Verbal Learning Test
C-WAIS-R	Comprehension
DCT	Dot Counting Test
DNMS	Denman Neuropsychology Memory Scale
DRS	Dementia Rating Scale
DS-WAIS-R	Digit Span
DS-WMS-R	Digit Span
DSym-WAIS-R	Digit Symbol
EDSS	Expanded Disability Status Scale
F-BDAE	Fluency
FL	Finger Localization
FM-WMS-R	Figural Memory
FR	Facial Recognition
FTT	Finger Tapping Test (HRNB)
GCS	Glasgow Coma Scale
GDS	Gordon Diagnostic Systems
GNGT	Go–NoGo Tasks
GOAT	Galveston Orientation and Amnesia Test
GP	Grooved Pegboard Test
GS	Grip Strength (HRNB)
HII	Halstead Impairment Index
HRNB	Halstead–Reitan Neuropsychological Battery
HT	Hand Test
HVOT	Hooper Visual Organization Test
ICDT	Incompatible Conditional Discrimination Tasks
I-WAIS-R	Information
I-WMS-R	Information
JLO	Judgment of Line Orientation
LBT	Line Bisection Test
LCT	Letter Cancellation Test
LDE	Lateral Dominance Examination (HRNB)
LM-WMS-R	Logical Memory
LNNB	Luria–Nebraska Neuropsychological Battery
MAE	Multilingual Aphasia Examination
MAS	Memory Assessment Scales
MC-WMS-R	Mental Control

MF	Memory for Faces
MFI	Memorization of Fifteen Items
MI	Motor Impersistence
MMPI	Minnesota Multiphasic Personality Inventory
MMPI-2	Minnesota Multiphasic Personality Inventory—2
MMSE	Mini-Mental State Examination
MST	Motor Sequencing Tasks
MTDDA	Minnesota Test for Differential Diagnosis of Aphasia
NAART	North American Adult Reading Test
NART	National Adult Reading Test (British)
N-BDAE	Naming
NCCEA	Neurosensory Center Comprehensive Examination for Aphasia
NCSE	Neurobehavioral Cognitive Status Examination
OA-WAIS-R	Object Assembly
OBD-168	Organic Brain Disorder—168
OFT	Overlapping Figures Test
OR-BDAE	Oral Reading
O-WMS-R	Orientation
PASAT	Paced Auditory Serial Addition Test
PA-WAIS-R	Picture Arrangement
PC-WAIS-R	Picture Completion
PD	Phoneme Discrimination
PMT	Porteus Maze Test
POT	Personal Orientation Test
PPT	Purdue Pegboard Test
PPVT-R	Peabody Picture Vocabulary Test—Revised
PR	Pantomime Recognition
R	Rorschach
RA-MAE	Rating of Articulation
RAVLT	Rey Auditory–Verbal Learning Test
R-BDAE	Repetition
RC-BDAE	Reading Comprehension
RCWP-MAE	Reading Comprehension of Words and Phrases
RFFT	Ruff Figural Fluency Test
RKSPE	Reitan–Klove Sensory-Perceptual Examination (HRNB)
RLASCL	Rancho Los Amigos Scale of Cognitive Levels
RLO	Right–Left Orientation
RMT	Randt Memory Test
ROCFT: C	Rey–Osterrieth Complex Figure Test: Copy
ROCFT: M	Rey–Osterrieth Complex Figure Test: Memory
RPFW-MAE	Rating of Praxic Features of Writing
RPM	Raven's Progressive Matrices
R-WRAT-R	Reading

SBIS: FE   Stanford Binet Intelligence Scale: Fourth Edition
SCWT   Stroop Color Word Test
SDL   Serial Digit Learning
SDMT   Symbol Digit Modalities Test
S-LNNB   Spelling
SNST   Stroop Neuropsychological Screening Test
SPMSQ   Short Portable Mental Status Questionnaire
SR   Seashore Rhythm Test (HRNB)
SR-MAE   Sentence Repetition
SRT   Selective Reminding Test
SSPT   Speech Sounds Perception Test (HRNB)
SSS   Subtracting Serial 7's
STAI   State–Trait Anxiety Inventory
STB-MAE   Spelling Test Battery
SVT   Symptom Validity Test
S-WAIS-R   Similarities
S-WRAT-R   Spelling

TAT   Thematic Apperception Test
TDBC   Three–Dimensional Block Construction
TFR   Tactile Form Recognition (HRNB)
TMTA   Trail Making Test A (HRNB)
TMTB   Trail Making Test B (HRNB)
TOT   Temporal Orientation Test
TPT   Tactual Performance Test (HRNB)
TT-MAE   Token Test
TTT   Tinkertoy Test
TVN   Test of Visual Neglect
TWFT   Thurstone Word Fluency Test

VFDT   Visual Form Discrimination Test
VMS-WMS-R   Visual Memory Span
VN-MAE   Visual Naming
VPA-WMS-R   Visual Paired Associates
VP-WMS-R   Verbal Paired Associates
VR-WMS-R   Visual Reproduction
VSAT   Visual Search and Attention Test
V-WAIS-R   Vocabulary

WAB   Western Aphasia Battery
WAIS-R   Wechsler Adult Intelligence Scale—Revised
W-BDAE   Writing
WCST   Wisconsin Card Sorting Test
WISC-R   Wechsler Intelligence Scale for Children—Revised
WMS   Wechsler Memory Scale
WMS-R   Wechsler Memory Scale—Revised
WPSI   Washington Psychosocial Seizure Inventory
WRAT-R   Wide Range Achievement Test—Revised

Appendix D

Test Sources

American Guidance Service
4201 Woodland Road
PO Box 99
Circle Pines, MN 55014-1796

Jastak Associates
PO Box 3410
Wilmington, DE 19804-0250

Lafayette Instrument
PO Box 5729
3700 Sagamore Parkway North
Lafayette, IN 47903

Lea & Febiger
600 South Washington Square
Philadelphia, PA 19106-4198

National Computer Systems
Professional Assessment Services
PO Box 1416
Minneapolis, MN 55440

University of Victoria Neuropsychology
   Laboratory
P.O. Box 1700
Victoria, British Columbia V8W 3P4
Canada

Oxford University Press
200 Madison Avenue
New York, NY 10016

Psychological Assessment Resources
PO Box 998
Odessa, FL 33556

The Psychological Corporation
PO Box 839954
San Antonio, TX 78283-3954

Reitan Neuropsychology Laboratory
2920 South 4th Avenue
South Tucson, AZ 85713

Western Psychological Services
12031 Wilshire Boulevard
Los Angeles, CA 90025

Index

About the Author

Robert M. Anderson, Jr., holds a Ph.D. in clinical psychology from the University of Hawaii, and a Ph.D. in the philosophy of science from the University of Minnesota. He has completed a postdoctoral fellowships in experimental neuropsychology in Karl Pribram's laboratory at Stanford University and in clinical neuropsychology at the University of Rochester Medical Center, and has been a summer fellow at the Center for Advanced Study in the Behavioral Sciences. He has worked as a neuropsychologist at Forsyth Memorial Hospital in Winston–Salem and the Rehabilitation Hospital of the Pacific in Honolulu. He is currently in private practice in Honolulu and on the Core Faculty of Forest Institute of Professional Psychology, Hawaii Campus, where he is Coordinator of the Neuropsychology Track.